Cooperation, Complicity and Conscience

Problems in healthcare, science, law
and public policy

Cooperation, Complicity and Conscience

Problems in healthcare, science, law and public policy

Edited by

Helen Watt

London – The Linacre Centre

Published by The Linacre Centre
60 Grove End Road, London NW8 9NH
www.linacre.org

British Library Cataloguing in Publication Data

A catalogue record for this book is available from
the British Library

ISBN 0 906561 10 8

Typeset by Academic + Technical, Bristol
Printed and bound by Bath Press

Foreword

Cooperation in evil or wrongdoing is one of the most perplexing areas in bioethics – and, indeed, in ethics generally. For the "working ethicist", it is the area most likely to cause anxiety, as unduly rigorist advice may lead to someone unnecessarily forfeiting his or her job, career or peace of mind. And for those facing cooperation problems in their own lives in a more immediate way, the area may be both perplexing and personally demanding.

Institutions, too, find this a difficult area practically, whether or not the intellectual problems raised are particularly abstruse. As I write this, the Hospital where the Linacre Centre is based is facing the question whether they may accommodate an NHS primary care practice, with all this means in terms of advice, prescriptions and referrals. Many other hospitals throughout the world are (or have been) faced with cooperation problems of a similarly pressing kind.

This book is offered as an interdisciplinary contribution to the subject of cooperation in evil: a rich and important but somewhat under-researched field. The book includes both general treatments of the subject (by Bishop Donal Murray, Bishop Anthony Fisher, Cathleen Kaveny and Luke Gormally) and more specific treatments of topics such as use of fetal cells in treatment and research (explored by Alexander Pruss, as a concrete example to illustrate more general points, and by Neil Scolding, coming from the viewpoint of a medical researcher). Charlie O'Donnell and Mike Delany provide "hands on" advice, based on their experience as doctors and medical students, on dealing with cooperation problems in medical training and practice. My own paper looks at the issue of cooperation in suicide on the part of doctors and nurses, while Jane Adolphe addresses problems arising for the Holy See in regard to negotiation and implementation of the UN Convention on the Rights of the Child. A debate follows between Colin Harte and John Finnis on moral problems in the context of voting, and Richard Myers ends with a general overview of conscientious objection in US law.

The papers in this collection are written by professional ethicists (philosophers, theologians, lawyers), and/or by those who have faced these issues in their own work in medical practice and research, law, and political campaigning. Most of the papers were presented at the 2003 Linacre Centre Conference at Queens' College, Cambridge, though we are also pleased to be able to include Alexander Pruss's paper, first published in the *Linacre Quarterly*. Some papers have not been included, simply because the presenters' other commitments prevented them from providing a written text in time for publication. Thanks are owing to all who contributed to an enjoyable and stimulating conference, whether or not their papers appear in this volume. I am grateful to those individuals and institutions who sponsored the Conference, particularly Ave Maria School of Law, which provided not only two speakers but generous financial support. Finally, I wish to thank my Linacre Centre colleagues – particularly Bob Bell – for their tireless and enthusiastic work in organising the Conference, and my new colleagues Patrick Carr and Lauren Dykes for their kind help in producing the proceedings.

Contents

Contents

1

Cooperation, complicity and conscience: the background to the debate

Bishop Donal Murray

I am pleased and honoured to have been asked to contribute to this book. The Linacre Centre is to be congratulated for putting before us once again a stimulating opportunity to reflect on issues with which we have to struggle in the field of bioethics.

I am particularly glad to be contributing the first chapter. This enables me to make some points about the topic before the other contributors reveal how complex it really is! Chambers Dictionary defines "complicity" as "the state or condition of being an accomplice", but goes on to offer a secondary definition in a single word: "complexity". This book will, I suspect, reveal the appropriateness of that definition.

I do not intend to try to anticipate that complexity or to address all its ramifications. Rather than attempting to look in any detail at the vast range of circumstances that may confront us, I thought it might be useful to reflect a little on the fundamental reason why these issues arise. In doing so, I will draw heavily on *Veritatis Splendor*, Pope John Paul II's crucially important encyclical on fundamental moral questions.

1. Freedom

Our everyday experience constantly brings our conscience face to face with situations of cooperation and complicity. We find ourselves saying things like, "Damned if you do, damned if you don't"; "I'm not happy with this but I don't see what choice I have got"; "you can't make an omelette without breaking eggs"; "I'll go along with you, but on your own heads be it"; or even "stop the world, I want to get off!"

The questions arise because we are free. Without freedom there would be no conscience, no decisions to be made, no responsibility to be borne. But the questions arise more specifically because of the kind of freedom we human beings possess.

In Genesis the temptation put by the serpent was that Adam and Eve should refuse to recognise human freedom as created, and therefore limited, and should attempt to act as though they possessed the kind of freedom that God alone has: "God knows that when you eat of [the fruit] your eyes will be opened and you will be like God, knowing good and evil" (Gen 3:5). When the eyes of Adam and Eve are opened they do not see the world they wanted to see but a world which has become hostile; when they try to decide their own good and evil for themselves they find that they are out of harmony with a good that is greater than they can grasp.

In *Veritatis Splendor*, John Paul II identified the question of how we understand human freedom as the underlying question in modern moral debate:

> The moral issues most frequently debated and differently resolved
> in contemporary moral reflection are all closely related, albeit in
> various ways, to a crucial issue: *human freedom.*[1]

Our freedom is not the creative freedom of God: we do not create our own universe out of nothing, hence the problem of cooperation and complicity. We share a universe, which we do not simply control, with others, who are also free; our scope for acting is limited in all sorts of ways. All of our free choices have to take account of realities which impinge on our actions but which are not products of our decisions. Some of these are simply unalterable physical facts like the law of gravity; some are the products of free decisions made by other people, like the lack of resources to carry out some procedure I might have wished to undertake.

2. Responding to evil

In this world many things happen which I believe to be wrong. In some instances I have no right to interfere or no way of intervening, except perhaps by persuasion. Some situations are such that I feel I ought not to remain silent but should express my disapproval of what is being done or my support of someone who is being unfairly treated. Some of the things that are done, I could, and perhaps should, prevent. Others seem to involve and implicate me, or to seek my cooperation, in ways that I find morally

---

[1] John Paul II, *Veritatis Splendor* (1993), 31. The official translation wrongly renders the opening phrase '*Morales quaestiones…*' as 'The human issues…'.

troubling. There is a virtually unlimited range of events and actions, some of which I might have prevented, some of which seem beyond my control. I know, however, that there is no way in which I could get around to questioning or influencing, still less preventing everything of which I disapprove. Nevertheless, there are many ways in which I may feel responsible for or tainted by things that are done by others.

In a world as full of injustice and inequality as ours, there is always an underlying question about our complicity. John Paul II spoke of "the background of the gigantic remorse caused by the fact that, side by side with wealthy and surfeited people and societies, living in plenty and ruled by consumerism and pleasure, the same human family contains individuals and groups that are suffering from hunger. There are babies dying of hunger under their mothers' eyes."[2]

Faced with such evils, we feel contaminated by them, yet utterly helpless to do anything about them. We cannot change the world by an act of will. In order to do anything significant it is often necessary to work with others, who have their own ideas and priorities quite different from mine. It may be, for instance, that the only effective way of counteracting a particular large scale evil is to persuade the government, or the European Union, to take action. But that is a sphere in which one voice may have little impact. We operate in a world that often seems highly resistant to our wishes.

In speaking about cooperation and complicity, we must beware of seeking after a kind of illusory purity which would fail to recognise that we can only live and act in this messy relationship with others and in this often murky world which cannot simply be transformed by our speaking a creative word – saying "Let there be light!" Our freedom is human, not divine.

But it is more complicated than that because it is not enough to sit back and say, "It's not my fault; I cannot solve every problem; I am not my brother's keeper; I can't change the way things are." The fact that our power is limited can become an excuse for doing less than our best. Chesterton expressed it as pointedly as only he could: "Compromise used to mean that half a loaf was better than no bread. Among modern statesmen it really seems to mean that half a loaf is better than a whole loaf."[3]

3. Embodied freedom

Veritatis Splendor stresses the fact that our freedom is embodied. Without an understanding of embodied freedom, neither the question of complicity nor our efforts to respond to the question can be coherent.

---

[2] John Paul II, *Dives in Misericordia* (1980), 11.
[3] G.K. Chesterton, *What's Wrong with the World*. San Francisco: Ignatius 1910, p. 23.

To say that our freedom is embodied is first of all to say that it is situated in the physical world and therefore in time and place. It is limited by its situation. Since we are dealing with a world we did not create, our range of choices is limited. Our imagination allows us to picture Harry Potter sitting astride a broomstick and flying through the air playing quidditch. We, however, cannot fly through the air by mounting a broomstick, even if we had a Nimbus 2000. We are limited by what is physically possible. So, for instance, in health care, much as we would wish it otherwise, we may have to conclude in a particular case that there is no possible treatment which would offer hope of a cure to a seriously ill patient.

To say that our freedom is embodied is also to say that, even in relation to the physically possible, we may be limited by our own abilities. It is entirely physically possible for human beings to speak Chinese – hundreds of millions of them, even tiny children, do so with astonishing ease. For all I know, there may be people reading this book who can speak it fluently. But, as far as I am concerned, it is not within the range of my possibilities. A decision by me to communicate with somebody in Chinese can produce no result, even though for someone else such a decision might be straightforward. So, in health care, it may be that at a particular time or in a particular place, the knowledge, or the skill, or the equipment that might have helped a patient is not available.

To say that our freedom is embodied is to say that we are limited by the possible reasons for acting that we find in the real world around us. Like the chicken, we usually cross the road in order to get to the other side. There is no use in crossing the road in order to make the sky turn green or in order to join Peter Pan in Never Never Land. If the reason for acting is unreal then the exercise of freedom is itself absurd. We can only choose to reach goals that really exist; otherwise we trap ourselves in an illusion. In health care, we are sometimes tempted to persist with a treatment which we know is simply incapable of helping the patient – to do something, even if we know it is pointless. On a wider scale, the desire to be able to cure an ailment might spur somebody to enter the field of medical research, but until such research bears fruit the desire is only a dream. We can only seek realistic goals by realistic means.

4. Arena for freedom

But there is a paradox here, and I believe it is important to keep it in mind as we discuss cooperation issues. These limitations, if we look at them from another angle, are actually the scope, the arena, the potential for our freedom.[4] Our physical situation is limited but it is precisely that situation

---

[4] Cf. John Paul II, *Veritatis Splendor*, 86.

which provides us with the very possibility of acting – and which very often prompts us to act. I cannot fly on a broomstick, but it is only because I am in one place that I can decide to move to another. As they say, "You have to start from somewhere."

Our abilities are limited but they are, first of all, abilities. I cannot speak *Chinese*, but I can *speak* and huge possibilities of self-expression, communication and relationship to others spring from that, admittedly limited, ability. Our reasons have to be real reasons if our freedom is not to be caught up in absurdity, but that reality of the world is what offers us reasons for acting and makes sense of our actions. Only because there is something at the other side of the road does it makes sense to cross it.

There is, for human beings, no act of freedom which is, so to speak, untouched by our own embodied selves, by the world around us and by the actions of other people. That is because our embodiment, the world around us, our involvement with other people make up the sphere in which we exercise our freedom. To act without paying attention to the context in which we act would not make us more free but less free. Freedom is our ability to deal with reality; it is not a means of escaping from reality.

In fact, it is this imperfect reality which, so to speak, calls our freedom into action. We are not spiritual souls, either loosely attached to, or imprisoned within, a physical body in a physical universe. We are beings who are fully part of this physical world with its limitations, but who are also, at the same time, filled with unlimited longings and hopes which can only be incompletely expressed in what one might call the limited language of physical existence. The Creator places in the human heart "a yearning for absolute truth and a thirst to attain full knowledge of it" which is seen in the human "search for *the meaning of life*."[5] That search for meaning finds its full answer only in the Incarnate Word, who fully reveals the mystery of human existence.[6] We have no way of moving towards the satisfying of that yearning except as what we are, embodied beings travelling along the often frustrating paths of this physical world.

We are responsible for what we, by our free choices, make out of the situation in which we find ourselves. That means that we need to understand the situation if we are to act with genuine freedom.

There are several ways in which that situation can affect our decisions and our responsibility. It may mean that we can, at least for the moment, see no way of achieving all of what we would wish to do, even what we may feel a strong moral demand to do. That may be because the problem is so complex

---

[5] *Ibid.*, 1.
[6] Cf. Vatican II, *Gaudium et Spes*, 22.

or difficult and there is no way of responding to it, or because my own skill is not adequate to deal with it, or because the line of action I feel obliged to follow is opposed by other people – perhaps the patient him or herself – who have a right to a say in the situation, or it may be that contrary decisions are being taken by others and I find myself in a dilemma as to whether to go along with them, to indicate disagreement with them or to try to prevent them.

We need to resist the temptation to view this simply as a struggle between some perfect disembodied freedom and all of this physical reality that gets in my way! When I face this complex situation I become morally complicit in it *only by my choice.* I am morally responsible not for the physical facts that confront me but for the choices I make. John Paul II clearly indicates that we are responsible for what we choose to do (or to fail to do):

> The object of an act of willing is in fact a freely chosen kind of behaviour. To the extent that it is in conformity with the order of reason, it is the cause of the goodness of the will; it perfects us morally, and disposes us to recognise our ultimate end in the perfect good, primordial love. By the object of a given moral act, then, one cannot mean a process or an event of the merely physical order, to be assessed on the basis of its ability to bring about a given state of affairs in the outside world.[7]

But this paragraph indicates a further complication. It points to the various dimensions of a moral action. It is the choice of a particular line of action, but also "within that choice, a decision about oneself and a setting of one's own life for or against God."[8] The physical facts that surround me, whether these are facts of nature or the result of the actions of others, cannot be morally attributed to me. On the other hand, I may be responsible for the fact that I have chosen not to try to alter those realities, for my attitude to them and for what that attitude says about me.

The physical reality around me, the physical reality of my embodied self, are not simply roadblocks around which I have to work. These are the field in which my liberty works; furthermore, my freedom can alter them. Human beings can fly, not on broomsticks but in aeroplanes. The range of the possible can be extended by human creativity and by technology. I cannot speak Chinese but it would be possible for me to set out to acquire that ability – how successfully might remain to be seen. I cannot sensibly choose to act for reasons which do not correspond to the real world, but I

---

[7] John Paul II, *Veritatis Splendor*, 78.
[8] *Ibid.*, 65.

can choose from among the many different reasons for acting that present themselves; I can purify the reasons for which I choose to act; I can seek to ensure that I act for worthy motives; I can seek realistic means of achieving the goals to which I aspire. I am not helpless before reality; I am free to work within it and in many ways I am free to modify it and to expand the potential it offers me.

Nor can I simply look at the actions of people around me and say to myself, "they do their thing and I do mine." Particularly in the area of health care, individuals rarely act entirely alone. The action of one person often needs the cooperation of other members of the health care team. One person's action involves the hospital or other institution in which he or she is working and in some sense involves all who are part of that team.

5. Preventable dilemmas

The challenge of complicity arises, for instance, when something that might be done for a particular patient in the most advanced country or the most high-tech hospital cannot be done for him or her in a less advanced location. Probably in such a case one may sadly have to conclude that there is only some inferior and less adequate treatment that can be offered to this patient in this place at this time. This is obviously a question about the allocation of scarce resources.[9]

A person who is faced with such a case can hardly avoid asking whether this situation itself may not be immoral and whether one has a responsibility to do something about it. It may be, of course, that it cannot be changed; it may even be that it should not. Resources are limited. It is simply not possible that every person should receive what would, in the abstract, be the optimum possible treatment. Health care resources have to be distributed where they will do most good, not merely in terms of the numbers treated but in order to ensure the optimal quality of care that in some cases can only be provided in centres of excellence. Such centres, in the nature of the case, may be at some distance from the person who needs a particular high-tech treatment.

Having given due weight to these issues, however, one may be convinced that in a particular instance such considerations do not justify the lack of resources; one may believe that it was unfair and unjust that this patient should have been unable to receive the treatment which would have given him or her the best chance of a cure. In that case, merely to offer the patient

---

[9] Cf. A. Fisher and L. Gormally (eds), *Healthcare Allocation: an ethical framework for public policy.* London: The Linacre Centre 2001.

an inferior treatment and to remain silent about the injustice involves becoming complicit in the unfairness. People in health care, and perhaps particularly their professional bodies, see the wider picture of the practical consequences of decisions about allocation of resources in a way that the general public can never see it. So the challenge may arise as to what a health care professional, perhaps along with professional colleagues, is going to do about this injustice.

In other words, the question of complicity may not be exhausted by satisfying oneself that one has made the best possible decision in this particular case. It may be necessary to ask whether one should have had to face this decision in the first place and, if not, how to ensure that such a situation does not arise again.

6. Working in a team

The challenge in relation to cooperation arises in a whole variety of ways. The immediate environment in which most health care personnel operate is that of hospital care or group practice. One is part of a team. What the other members of the team choose to do is primarily their own responsibility. Nevertheless, being part of a team means working together with others, or to use another word, cooperating. Being part of a team means to some degree going along with the team's actions and standards and values.

It is of course possible to work with people whose views and values are different from our own. The difficulty is to know at what point one's membership of the team amounts to endorsing an activity to which one cannot give moral approval.

This will depend in the first place on the seriousness of the issue involved. If people in the ward or the department or the team, for instance, are deliberately violating the fundamental right to life by direct abortion or euthanasia, then membership of the team becomes difficult if not impossible to justify even if an individual seeks to remain apart from these activities. If such is the officially stated policy of the hospital or practice, then the cooperation is even more explicit and difficult to justify.

In the second place it will depend on how involved one is in the activity one judges to be immoral, whether one can do anything about it, and what the consequences of trying to do something may be. It depends on the extent to which one is "a member of the team." One may have no real connection with the immoral activity. It may be, for instance, that one is unhappy about the family planning advice being given by a colleague, while one's own position against contraception is clear and well known. It may be that in a large hospital, one has no real involvement with what goes on in some other department.

On the other hand, it may be that one has a particular position of responsibility or influence which gives rise to a duty to take a stand. These and other similar considerations will, no doubt, lead to useful discussions about the practical implications of the issues we are discussing. And it may not be out of place to recall at the beginning of these discussions the warning of Aristotle:

> It is the mark of the educated person to look for precision in each class of things just so far as the nature of the subject admits.[10]

Seeking mathematical certainty where it is not to be found can be the source of a great distortion in ethical thinking. It might be argued, for instance, that utilitarianism is the fruit of a hopeless quest for mathematical exactitude.

7. Basis of morality

No doubt in the course of this book we will venture deeply into the complexity of some of these dilemmas and challenges. The context in which we need to see all of this, however, is the recognition that our freedom is not absolute. It is about the choices we make in dealing with a reality that we do not create, even though we may shape and modify it. Much as we might prefer to be able to act as God does, by a creative word which does not need to work with any raw material, and which cannot be affected or distorted by the actions of others who are shaping and modifying the same environment, this is not the reality of human freedom.

Equally important is to recognise what morality ultimately means. A choice cannot be judged to be good simply because it is a means to attain a good goal, or because the person has a good intention. Nor is it simply a matter of looking at the consequences of an action, good and bad, and weighing them up in some kind of utilitarian balance sheet.

Of course, if the action is not aimed at a good goal, if the intention is evil, if harmful consequences, which were foreseen or should have been foreseen, are brought about for no good reason, the action cannot be moral. But there is a more fundamental requirement.

An action is good when it expresses the free self-directing of the person towards his or her ultimate purpose or destiny and is in conformity with the truth about human good recognised by reason.[11] When we look at this in terms of the Gospel, we can say that the morally good action

---

[10] Aristotle, *Nicomachean Ethics*, I, 3.
[11] Cf. John Paul II, *Veritatis Splendor*, 72.

shows consistency "with that dignity and vocation bestowed on [us] by grace" and shows our likeness to the image of the Son, the first-born.[12]

The title of this book rightly suggests that issues of cooperation and complicity need to be considered in the light of conscience. It is in our conscience that we recognise the truth about human good and about the dignity and vocation to which we are called. The fundamental moral issues of our time concern the relationship of human freedom to God's will, or, to put it another way, the relationship of human freedom to the truth.[13]

Conscience is a kind of dialogue between the person and his or her deepest self, what the Bible calls, the heart:

> The heart is the dwelling-place where I am, where I live; according to the biblical expression, the heart is the place "to which I withdraw". The heart is our hidden centre, beyond the grasp of our reason and of others; only the Spirit of God can fathom the human heart and know it fully. The heart is the place of decision, deeper than our psychic drives. It is the place of truth, where we choose life or death. It is the place of encounter, because as image of God we live in relation; it is the place of covenant.[14]

Conscience is a dialogue between the individual and God, "the primordial image and the final end" of the human person.[15]

In the end, morality is about how we relate to one another and to God. It is not, first of all, about the whole range of physical consequences of our actions, some good, some evil, – which could never be fully measured – but rather about how we use our freedom. A good deal of the anguish caused by issues of complicity and cooperation springs from the realisation that everything we do has mixed consequences. Many of those consequences are things that we could never have foreseen and for which we have no moral responsibility.

The issue is precisely about what we *choose* to do. That is the significance of the word "direct" which occurs in statements about morally absolute prohibitions as formulated, for instance, in *Evangelium Vitae*: "*I confirm that the direct and voluntary killing of an innocent human being is always gravely immoral*". "*I declare that direct abortion, that is, abortion willed as an end or as a means, always constitutes a grave moral disorder*".[16] Of course some of what we choose is chosen by omission; we *freely allow*

[12] *Ibid.*, 73.
[13] Cf. *Veritatis Splendor*, 84.
[14] *Catechism of the Catholic Church*, 2563.
[15] John Paul II, *Veritatis Splendor*, 58.
[16] John Paul II, *Evangelium Vitae*, 57, 62.

something to happen through apathy or negligence or a false sense of helplessness. In speaking of sinful situations in his Apostolic Exhortation on Reconciliation and Penance, John Paul II stresses that this phrase should not disguise the personal responsibility which lies at the root of all sin. He refers to "the very personal sins of those... who take refuge in the supposed impossibility of changing the world..."[17]

That rather disturbing and challenging thought is, I think, a good indication of the complexity underlying issues of complicity and cooperation and of the honesty that is called for as we address them conscientiously. We must live in a world that we did not create, but we must not take refuge in the supposed impossibility of changing that world.

---

[17] John Paul II, *Reconciliatio et Paenitentia*, 16.

2

Why not dirty your hands?

Or: on the supposed rightness of (sometimes) intentionally cooperating in wrongdoing

Luke Gormally

1. Introduction

"Why not dirty your hands?" is a somewhat misleading title, since the thesis I want to consider is that it is sometimes right intentionally to cooperate in wrongdoing. And if it really were right one would not be dirtying one's hands thereby. Hence the clarificatory subtitle.

The purpose of considering the thesis is not to convince anyone of it, nor, on the other hand, to argue against it. The purpose of considering an argument for the thesis is to display some of the key elements of a mindset or moral outlook in which preoccupation with whether one is engaged in formal cooperation in wrongdoing is to a large extent unintelligible.

Since the mindset in question is a powerful influence in our society and culture it would be foolish to think that Catholics and other Christians might be untouched by it. And in so far as they are, they will be prone to confusion in their practical thinking about problems of cooperation.

Having brought out the principal elements of this mindset – utilitarian or consequentialist is the appropriate adjective to describe it – I would like to spend the rest of the paper calling to mind the key contrasting elements in the moral outlook of the orthodox Christian, which alone make sense of the way we discuss problems of cooperation.

2. Cooperation at the coalface

It is important to have a sense of the multifarious ways in which choices to cooperate in wrongdoing can present themselves, as well as of the ways in which what is at issue can fail to be grasped. Something of this complexity and of the ways in which what is at issue can be obfuscated were brought home to me in the winter months of 1979–1980 when I spent many hours interviewing more than thirty Catholic healthcare professionals, in different parts of England, about the ethical problems they encountered in their work, with a special focus on problems of cooperation. These professionals ranged in position from Dean of a Medical School to student nurse and all professed to be practising Catholics. The most frequently cited reason a number of them had for thinking that practices such as giving contraceptive advice or assisting in sterilization procedures were not morally problematic (i.e. presented no choice about possibly wrongful cooperation) was that both practices were in many cases entirely justifiable. Here what I was encountering was the ripple-effect among the Catholic laity of the very public rejection by many moral theologians and by a number of bishops of the teaching of *Humanae Vitae*. Some of my interviewees had, indeed, arrived at the conclusion that the Church possessed no distinctive authority to teach moral truth. None of them, however, professed to think that abortion or starving handicapped babies to death was ever justifiable. Nonetheless, some of them had participated in the acknowledged wrongdoing of abortion and the killing of handicapped babies.

In conducting interviews I used as a heuristic device some of the categories of contributory responsibility for another's wrongdoing which St Thomas identifies in his discussion of duties of restitution.[1] In particular the following ways of bearing some responsibility for what the principal perpetrator of wrongdoing gets up to seemed relevant. It is arguable that not all of these categories of contributory responsibility should be called forms of cooperation; but they are certainly forms of complicity.

- first, one can be an accomplice in the actual doing of the wrong, as someone providing assistance;
- secondly, one can give one's agreement to the wrongdoing, where prior agreement is required;
- thirdly, one can advise the principal agent to carry out the wrong;
- fourthly, one can *fail* to advise the principal agent against the wrongdoing when one *could* and *should* do so;
- fifthly, one can *fail* to order the principal agent not to act as he intends when one *could* and *should* do so;

---

[1] St Thomas Aquinas, *Summa theologiae* 1a 2ae, q.62, a.7.

- sixthly, one can provide support or concealment of a kind without which the principal agent could not carry out the wrong he proposes; and
- seventhly, one can *fail* to provide support of a kind which would have prevented the wrongdoing when one *could* and *should* provide such support.

An example of that last category was brought to my attention by a student nurse in her final year of training and who was working in what was regarded as the worst ward of a long-stay psychiatric hospital. The other staff on the ward had told her that she would be "blacked" if she attempted ordinary care of patients. Patients who soiled their beds were to be left in that condition; physical violence and mental torture were commonplace. The pressures on her to become a party to these practices were very strong. But what made her position particularly difficult was the futility of whistleblowing. Her superiors within the hospital, who could and should have prevented what was happening, were adept at burying complaints and were interested rather in taking measures designed to prevent a public enquiry into what had been going on for years. They were complicit in the wrongdoing taking place on Ward X by their failure to support a whistleblower when they could and should have provided support.

The desire to save one's own skin is a motivation which leads people into a variety of forms of cooperation in the wrongdoing of others. Not a few doctors, when juniors, have encountered the consultant who does not hesitate to intimate sabotage of their career prospects if they do not comply with his wishes. Sometimes it can require considerable courage to stand firm in face of such threats. It is likely to be the person who recognises how he ought to act who realises that courage is needed. But not all are clear-sighted. Here I want to reflect on a line of reasoning people can invoke, or be encouraged to invoke, as justification for cooperating in wrongdoing. Reflection on this reasoning can lead us to see the radical contrast between an outlook which is characteristic of the secularist mind-set so influential in our society and the outlook which should characterise a Christian.

3. The "no difference" argument

A nurse is asked to "scrub up" to assist in an abortion in theatre; a house officer is told to write up a dose of sedation for a handicapped child which she knows to be part of a regime established by the consultant in order to suppress demand-feeding by the child to ensure his early death by starvation. The nurse and the house officer might be persuaded to comply by the thought: my refusing to do so will make no difference to the outcome because if I don't do it someone else will. So what harm is avoided by my refusing to do it? If they haven't got this line of reasoning already up their sleeve there are philosophers around – bioethicists – who would like to sell it to them. And it is worth looking at what they have to say to get the measure of the underlying mindset.

So, let us turn to consider the thought: there is no good reason against my assisting in wrongdoing because my refusal to do so will make no difference.

A number of philosophers have argued for something like this claim. Here I shall consider Michael Bayles's defence of the claim which he offers precisely in commending it to doctors, nurses and lawyers.[2]

Bayles's starting point is the claim that the basis for a reasonable refusal to assist is that thereby you prevent a state of affairs in which some wrongdoing occurs. But if the wrongdoing is going to occur in any case, because someone else will provide the assistance if you don't, there is "no moral gain" from refusing to provide the assistance. "...the world is not morally worse", as he puts it, if you rather than someone else provides the assistance. In short, it makes no difference whether or not you do it, because if you don't someone else will. The conclusion is not that you have an obligation to provide the assistance, only that it is not morally wrong to do so:

> All that need be assumed is that if an act makes no difference to the occurrence of moral wrong, it is not morally wrong. To deny this premise would be irrational, for it would be to claim that doing A is wrong but refraining from doing A is not wrong, although there is no difference in the moral wrong that results.[3]

In face of the suggestion that Jack's assisting in wrongdoing might make Jack a morally worse person, Bayles's response is to say that providing such assistance cannot make Jack a morally worse person unless it is wrong *for Jack* to provide the assistance. But the conclusion of the "no difference" argument is that it would not be wrong for him to provide the assistance. While it would be better that the principal agent not do what he proposes to do, the issue, Bayles insists, is whether it is any worse if Jack aids him than if Jill does. The objection that Jack's assistance makes Jack a morally worse person either assumes that it is worse if Jack assists than if Jill does or ignores the issue.

[2] Michael Bayles, "A Problem of Clean Hands: Refusal to Provide Professional Services". 5 (1979) *Social Theory and Practice*: 165–181. Bayles's interest is in what a principal agent could reasonably think, but his argument applies, *mutatis mutandis*, to what an ancillary agent might reasonably think.
[3] *Op. cit.*, 169.

Bayles's argument assumes or implies four propositions any one of which is sufficient to render unintelligible Catholic teaching about the morality of cooperation in wrongdoing. These propositions are:

1. First: that a person is as responsible for what he foresees will be the outcome of his refusal to assist in wrongdoing as he would be for the outcome of assisting. It is to be noted that Bayles thinks a person as responsible for what someone else foreseeably does in consequence of his refusal to do it as he is for doing it himself.
2. Second: that a choice is wrong depends on a calculation of the overall utility or disutility of the foreseeable consequences of the choice.
3. Third (following from the second proposition): there are no intrinsically evil choices. There can be circumstances, for example, in which murder is the right thing to do. Readers may recall the famous case devised by the late Bernard Williams in his critique of utilitarianism in which Jim, a botanist researching plants, wanders into a small South American town to find himself, as a distinguished overseas visitor, given the choice by the local militia captain, Pedro, of killing one of the twenty Indian hostages Pedro had intended to execute. If he is willing to do the killing Pedro will spare the other nineteen hostages. If Jim refuses to kill one of them, then all twenty will be killed by Pedro. As Williams remarks, a consistent utilitarian will regard it as *obviously* right that Jim should kill one of the hostages. In truth we don't need exotic examples like this to get the point. Consider the reasoning that has from time to time been offered to justify the killing of handicapped babies: that the overall forseeable consequences for a family of life without a handicapped baby are better than the forseeable consequences of life with a handicapped baby.
4. Fourth: that it is *not* the case that the effect on the agent of his or her choices is an independent ground for determining the wrongness of choice which cannot be subsumed into some overall calculation of consequences.

Jonathan Glover in a paper on the "no difference" argument[4] took issue some years ago with Solzhenitsyn's absolutism about lying. In his Nobel laureate lecture Solzhenitsyn said:

> And the simple step of a simple courageous man is not to take part in the lie, not to support deceit. Let the lie come into the world, even dominate the world, but not through me.

---

[4] Jonathan Glover, "It makes no difference whether or not I do it". *Aristotelian Society, Supplementary Volume* 49 (1975): 171–190.

Glover's comment on this is to say that there will be cases in which

> ... to obey the principle [never be party to lying] is to do so at the cost of the total outcome being worse. The strict consequentialist will say that the principle tells us to keep our hands clean, at a cost which will probably be paid by other people. It is excessively self-regarding, placing considerations of my own feelings or purity of character far too high on the scale of factors to be considered.[5]

The formulation of this criticism reveals the assumption that what I make of myself in and through my choices is to be counted as simply one factor in the calculation of overall consequences of choice which should determine what I choose to do. And it is clear for Glover that even if I make a murderer of myself in choosing to kill someone, that consideration will not necessarily override other considerations which favour the killing. Speaking of the man who is resistant to killing the innocent, he comments that one can admire such a character-trait while thinking that it leads to the wrong decision, as would be the case if, in Bernard Williams's scenario, Jim were to refuse to shoot an Indian.

Bayles and Glover are utilitarians. A utilitarian believes that our choices should be determined by calculating which of our possible courses of action will in their consequences maximise utility, where utility for a modern utilitarian is most commonly taken to consist in the satisfaction of preferences and the satisfaction of preferences consists in states of affairs. States of affairs will be innumerably various, but the consequentialist has to assume that the calculations required in order to compare options allow us to use some common measure for purposes of comparison.

A Catholic who has reflectively assimilated the Church's moral teaching will not have any reason to think utilitarianism represents a defensible picture of what it is to be reasonable in the choices we make. But utilitarianism is such a strong presence in our society and culture that it would be foolish, as I have already remarked, to assume that all Catholics or all Christians are free of its influence.

Utilitarianism has been a decisive influence in the formulation of public policy and legislation, particularly as they govern the practice of medicine. The 1990 *Human Fertilisation and Embryology Act*, for example, rests on the ethical foundations supplied by the 1984 Warnock Report.[6] Those foundations are straightforwardly utilitarian: the law regulating the reproductive technologies and embryo research was to be based on calculating

---

[5] *Op. cit.*, 185.

[6] *Report of the Committee of Enquiry into Human Fertilisation and Embryology*. London: HMSO 1984.

the benefits of various provisions, and in the calculus of benefits it was decided, pretty arbitrarily, that the human embryo should count for relatively little compared with the value attached to the satisfaction of adult desires, whether they be the desires of the infertile, the desires of research scientists, or the desires of the biotech entrepreneurs. What we have in this country now in permissive legislation in this field is entirely in line with Warnock's thinking.

4. Human agency and responsibility in the Catholic moral tradition

I want to use Bayles's utilitarian argument for commending some intentional cooperating in wrongdoing as a foil to bring out the picture of human agency, and the picture, therefore, of human dignity, which underlies Catholic casuistry about cooperation in wrongdoing.

Necessarily as human beings we want fulfilment, we seek our flourishing. Our practical reasoning, that is, our reasoning about what to do (as distinct from our theoretical reasoning – our reasoning about what is the case) is given intelligible direction in the search for fulfilment by certain basic principles, starting points without which the exercise of practical reasoning to that end would be impossible. The fundamental principle is that good is to be done and sought and evil is to be avoided. And we have a built-in capacity for recognising what count as those fundamental features of our flourishing which are the "goods" we should seek: life enjoyed in a measure of health, truth, friendship, justice, solidarity, integrity, a right relationship to God, and others. As Germain Grisez puts it: "These basic truths about what is good for us are like a law written in our hearts to shape our deliberations and guide our free choices and actions."[7] And that law has been written in our hearts by our Creator. It is a fundamental feature of our connatural dignity as human beings – by which I mean the basic dignity which comes with coming into existence as a human being – that God has provided us with this built-in directedness to the fundamental ingredients of human flourishing.

We cannot, however, maintain, in our practical deliberation and choosing, a right relationship to the goods which make for our flourishing as human persons if we do not observe a number of moral absolutes, that is, norms which exclude in all circumstances the choice of certain types of act. Because all the basic goods as they present themselves to us in deliberation and choice are concretely aspects of one or another person's fulfilment, and because the connatural dignity of human beings is such that we should respect what is

---

[7] Germain Grisez, "Human Free Choice and Divine Causality", unpublished lecture; Ms p. 10.

integral to their fulfilment, we should never treat the goods of human persons as mere means to our own purposes. The moral absolutes set minimal conditions of respect for that dignity of human persons which is implicit in our God-given orientation to those goods. So there should be no murder, that is, no intentional killing of the innocent, because it is contrary to the dignity which belongs to us just in virtue of the fact that we are living human beings. No adultery, which is contrary to recognition of the fact that the proper expression of our sexual capacities belongs within marriage in which spouses treat each other as irreplaceable. Only in that relationship is the choice of sexual intercourse consistent with respect for the dignity of the other person. No choice of contraceptive intercourse, which is contrary to the disposition to live marriage as a relationship essentially ordered to the good of children. No lying, that is, knowingly conveying falsehood in statements which purport to convey the truth, because lying corrupts in us respect for truth. No bearing of false witness, which is contrary to the good of justice; and so on.

All these types of choice are identifiable in non-evaluative terms, so that it makes sense to ask, for example (as the utilitarian clearly does ask): Why should I never intentionally kill an innocent person? Why should I not have intercourse with someone else's spouse? Why should I not deliberately render intercourse sterile in circumstances in which it might otherwise be fertile? What are under consideration here are *types of act* identified by reference to the practical reasoning people engage in, reasoning which issues in proposals for choice. A proposal specifies what they have in mind to aim for, either as a means to their goal or as their goal. If a person chooses to act on a particular proposal, that proposal is the reason for which a person is acting, in the sense that it explains what they are up to. In scholastic terminology this is standardly referred to as the *object* of a person's act. (This fact about terminology is mentioned here to help make intelligible a text of Pope John Paul II referred to below.)

Ancient pagan philosophers recognised the importance of at least some moral absolutes if we are to be truly reasonable in the choices we make. Aristotle, for example, thought you "must always be wrong" if you committed adultery, theft or murder.[8]

Much more important than the witness of pagan thinkers is the constant testimony of Christian tradition to the indispensable role of moral absolutes in governing human choice. From Jesus's reaffirmation of the Ten

---

[8] *Nichomachean Ethics* 2.6: 1107a9–17. On Aristotle and ancient and medieval commentators on him on the topic of moral absolutes see John Finnis, *Moral Absolutes*. Washington, D.C.: Catholic University of America Press 1991, pp. 31–36.

Commandments[9] and the witness of the Apostolic tradition to their central importance in Christian life, right through to the authoritative teaching of John Paul II, the Church has been clear about the importance of moral absolutes.

In his encyclical *Veritatis Splendor* Pope John Paul, confronting the teaching of dissenting moral theologians who have denied that there can be moral absolutes, wrote:

> Reason attests that there are objects of the human act which are by their nature "incapable of being ordered to God", because they radically contradict the good of the person made in his image. These are the acts which in the Church's moral tradition have been termed "intrinsically evil" (*intrinsice malum*): they are such *always and per se*, in other words, on account of their very object, and quite apart from the ulterior intentions [by which the Pope means the further aims] of the one acting and the circumstances.[10]

And a few paragraphs later the Pope adds:

> ... in the question of the morality of human acts, and in particular the question of whether there exist intrinsically evil acts, we find ourselves faced with the *question of man himself*, of his *truth* and of the moral consequences flowing from that truth. By acknowledging and teaching the existence of intrinsic evil in given human acts, the Church remains faithful to the integral truth about man; she thus respects and promotes man in his dignity and vocation. Consequently, she must reject the theories... which contradict this truth.[11]

The theories in question developed in the minds of at least some of the dissenting moral theologians under the influence of utilitarianism.

It is a central feature of man's connatural dignity that he is able to give shape to his life in virtue of the orientations his practical intelligence gives to his will and in virtue of his ability freely to choose in ways consistent with those fundamental orientations to the basic goods. In the exercise of intelligence and choice man exhibits the truth that he is made in the image of God. If the exercise of practical intelligence recognises the normative conditions of human flourishing and our choices are consistent with moral truth then we have some share in the providential wisdom of God –

---

[9] *Matthew* 19: 16–19.
[10] Pope John Paul II, *Encyclical Letter "Veritatis Splendor"*, section 80.
[11] *Op. cit.*, section 83.

the wisdom of God for our lives manifested in the directiveness given to practical intelligence by the basic goods and by the moral absolutes.

Of course this is an inadequate statement of the extent of our potential sharing in divine wisdom in the conduct of our lives. For, because of the Fall we lost a secure orientation in our lives to what truly fulfils us and we became prone to think that it is down to us to determine what *counts* as making for our fulfilment. Hence the distorted understandings of human autonomy which have featured in human history, so that we have sought to provide for what we have taken to be our needs by inventing gods – the fundamental sin of idolatry – and by killing God in the person of Jesus. But precisely the death and resurrection of Jesus have made possible a profound sharing in the wisdom of God through the Holy Spirit, present in the Church and in her ministry of teaching and poured abroad in our hearts to give us hearts of flesh responsive to the will of God for our flourishing. The grace of conversion restores our orientation to what is good, enables us freely to choose it, and makes possible our living in what Pope John Paul calls "the order of love": that is, sharing in the inner Trinitarian life exhibited in self-giving love in our own lives.[12]

The nature of our salvation in Christ makes clear that the restoration of our dignity consists precisely in our living on God's terms. Our fulfilment as human beings lies in the Kingdom of Heaven. Heaven, however, is not an extrinsic reward for a way of life in which human choice bears no intrinsic relationship to the reality of heavenly life. On the contrary, those human goods which give point and purpose to our choices will find their transformed realisation in heaven.[13] Respect for those goods in this life and an upright dedication to sharing in their realisation serve to build up the Kingdom, most of all by shaping in us dispositions of openness to the fulfilment for which we were made. So what most of all matters in this regard is the character we acquire.

To live well we need to become the kind of persons God wants us to be. God makes available to us all that is necessary to that end.

Our ability to choose what to do with our lives and in our lives cannot have as its purpose bringing about what we may think of as "best states of affairs". For a number of reasons, of which I shall mention two. First, the significant consequences of our choices stretch way beyond our capacity to know or anticipate. Secondly, the whole ambition to compare the overall

---

[12] See Luke Gormally, "Pope John Paul II's teaching on human dignity and its implications for bioethics", in Christopher Tollefsen (ed) *John Paul II's Contribution to Catholic Bioethics*. Dordrecht: Kluwer 2004.

[13] Vatican Council II, *Pastoral Constitution on the Church in the Modern World*, "*Gaudium et Spes*", section 39.

consequences of various options assumes that there is some common measure to make the attempted comparison meaningful. But what could the common measure be that would enable us to compare the overall benefits of the consequences of either choosing to help starve a senile patient to death or choosing to help sustain her life? The choice to help starve her would certainly have as its consequence that she was killed; and might have as its further consequences that a hospital bed was released for another patient; that various doctors and nurses were relieved of the burdens of her care; that perhaps some hitherto wavering colleague was confirmed in collusion in such behaviour; and perhaps many foreseeable consequences of various kinds for the patient's relatives.

The choice to help sustain the old woman's life, on the other hand, could have as its consequences: that she was allowed to die a natural death; that some patient did not get a bed she needed; that one's medical and nursing colleagues were helped by one's willingness to care for that old woman to remain true to their professional responsibilities; that others, including relatives, were not left with uneasy consciences about the old woman's death.

There is no way the choice of what to do about feeding the patient could be rationally based on comparing the overall utility or benefit of the consequences of each option, because those consequences are incommensurable goods or evils; that is, there is no common measure which would allow us to assign comparable positive and negative values to those consequences.

While we are given a share in God's wisdom, through natural law and revelation, sufficient for us to choose rightly and shape our lives to play the roles God has for us in his providential designs, we do not have God's own knowledge of those designs. So a Christian will not let his moral outlook be infected by the secularist assumption that it is down to us to try to calculate how to bring about the best states of affairs in the world. Human responsibility cannot be of that kind. It is only in God's power to bring good out of the many evils that are truly outside our control; but we know that it is in the nature of divine wisdom to bring good out of evil. In our present condition, however, we have no comprehensive insight into God's doing of this, though many of us surely have the experience of God's gracious providence in delivering us from evil. We need to trust in that providence if we are ever tempted to start thinking like a utilitarian.

It is because the character we shape by our choices matters greatly for our living well, and because the moral absolutes are so important for shaping our choices, that the traditional casuistry about cooperation in wrongdoing is important. That casuistry is first of all concerned with whether we share the intention of the principal agent in wrongdoing, that is, with whether our actions are chosen precisely to achieve his objective. This concern reflects the moral significance of the distinction between intended and foreseen consequences of our choices, a significance which is tied to the central importance of moral absolutes and their significance for the formation of character.

Absolute prohibitions necessarily bear not on physical causation as such but on chosen courses of conduct, i.e. courses of conduct specified by the reasons for which they were chosen. Thus the prohibition of murder is not a prohibition on *any* causing of the death of innocent human beings (for you might do that as an unforeseeable consequence of something else you do) but is in its main part a prohibition on *intentionally* killing innocent human beings. A course of conduct is identifiable as intentional precisely by reference to the practical reasoning of the agent. Thus a course of conduct is a case of intentional killing if what results in the killing was brought about, or allowed to happen (when it might have been prevented) because a person chose that course of conduct in order to bring about the death of another. The purpose of securing the other person's death was the *reason* for the chosen conduct.

An absolute prohibition bears on what is intentional for two main reasons. First, because persons are most fully answerable for those courses of conduct they decide on in the light of their reasoning about their goals and the means to achieving them. At the other extreme to such fully deliberative choices are those states of affairs one brings about without intention or foresight of doing so and for which, absent culpable negligence, one is not held responsible. In between, so to speak, are states of affairs one *foresees* one will bring about but which one's reasons for acting make no part of what one seeks to achieve. The standard textbook illustration for the distinction being made here is the hastening of death which may result from the use of opiates or analgesia which are solely to control symptoms.[14] Death in this kind of case is no part of what one seeks to achieve. Of course, if what one is seeking to achieve is a relatively unimportant good and the foreseen side-effects of one's choice involve significant harm to someone, then one may for that reason be under an obligation to refrain from that choice. But sometimes unintended harm to another is a foreseeable outcome of the pursuit of objectives one has entirely good reasons to pursue, as when a surgeon undertakes high risk surgery to save someone's life, and the surgery itself kills the person.

Casuistry about material cooperation is clearly concerned with those of one's actions which, though not intended to assist wrongdoing, foreseeably do so.

---

[14] It should be noted that the standard textbook illustration fails to reflect the best of contemporary practice, since correctly administered use of opiates tends to prolong rather than shorten life.

23

The absolute prohibitions of traditional morality concern intentional actions (more broadly, intentional courses of conduct) because of the fundamental importance to human flourishing of having people *never* act for *reasons* which are directly contrary to the human good, identifiable in terms of the basic goods.

The second reason why absolute prohibitions bear on intentional actions is directly related to the first. When we act, our choices do not merely bring about states of affairs in the world. If, for example, as a doctor I embark on a regime of terminal sedation of one of my patients who is not as yet in the terminal phase of dying precisely in order to hasten that patient's death, my practical reasoning is not confined to specifying that a particular state of affairs should obtain, namely that my patient should become comatose and die. My practical reasoning importantly specifies *what I am committed to doing or to being* in order to bring about the desired state of affairs: for example, that *I* will prescribe sedation, that *I* will ensure that food and fluids are in no way delivered to the patient, that *I* will overcome the resistance, say, of nursing staff to this regime; and so on.[15] My chosen commitment to these means to my ends shapes my character. In general, reasons which specify bad objectives (whether ultimate objectives, or intermediate objectives towards achieving ultimate ones), to the realisation of which I commit myself, shape a bad character, with all the implications that has for human well-being. Thus, for example, a commitment to assist someone to kill for a particular type of reason (the mother doesn't want the unborn child, or the adult children no longer want to care for their senile mother) contributes to shaping a disposition to kill for that kind of reason. And that kind of disposition can become second nature; that's what character is – second nature. I once sat on a commission considering the physical and psychological sequelae of abortion for women. We interviewed an abortionist who claimed to have carried out about 100,000 abortions; he had been doing 100 a week for the past 20 years. He was a millionaire. He talked as if it was an utterly unproblematic way of giving women what they wanted and of earning money by doing so. I recall hearing of another abortionist who was interviewed by a pro-lifer who had gone along to tell him that he intended to picket his abortion clinic. In the course of their conversation the pro-lifer asked the abortionist, a man who had carried out a few thousand abortions but nothing like 100,000, whether he could remember having an uneasy conscience about any of the abortions

---

[15] See Luke Gormally, "Terminal Sedation and the Doctrine of the Sanctity of Life", in Torbjörn Tännsjö (ed) *Terminal Sedation: Euthanasia in Disguise?* Dordrecht: Kluwer 2004: 81–91.

he had carried out. After some thought the abortionist replied: Yes, I had an uneasy conscience about the first abortion I did and I can still remember the woman, but since then it's really been fairly routine.

In contrast to intentional courses of conduct, what I do not seek to achieve, such as the side-effects of what I do, does not involve commitments which *necessarily* serve to shape character in this kind of way. The psychology of character formation is an important part of the background to understanding the rationale of absolute prohibitions.

In saying this I do not mean to suggest that material cooperation cannot affect one's character. Professor Grisez has discussed ways in which it can,[16] and Professor Kaveny has discussed the way in which what begins as material "intimacy" with evildoing can, by a process of "contamination", transform one's original intentions.[17]

All I wish to emphasise here is that the framework of traditional morality makes clear that formal cooperation with wrongdoing will *necessarily* corrupt character. Anyone with a traditional understanding of what it means to live well will have decisive reasons against any formal cooperation in wrongdoing. But whether or not one should materially cooperate will depend on considerations other than the precise character of what one chooses to do. Those considerations, in all their complexity, are the topic of other contributions to this volume.

5. Conclusion

In this paper I have used a utilitarian line of argument, purporting to show that it can sometimes be right intentionally to cooperate in wrongdoing, in order to bring out the main features of a traditional and orthodox Christian understanding of moral responsibility. We are not responsible for producing "best states of affairs" in the world. There is no rational way of identifying such states of affairs as objects of choice. We obviously do have positive duties of justice and charity towards others in our pursuit of the human good. But more fundamental to the practical wisdom we have received for the conduct of our lives are the absolute negative duties we have to refrain from certain types of act. Failure in practice to recognise these exceptionless norms corrupts character. What we make of ourselves through our choices is what we most of all have control over and what, therefore, we are most of all

---

[16] See Germain Grisez, *The Way of the Lord Jesus*, Volume 3: *Difficult Moral Questions*. Appendix 2: "Formal and material cooperation in others' wrongdoing". Quincy, Illinois: Franciscan Press 1997: 871–897, esp. 879–880.

[17] See M. Cathleen Kaveny, "Appropriation of Evil: Cooperation's Mirror Image". 61 (2000) *Theological Studies*: 280–313, at 305ff.

answerable for. If you are a Christian you know you possess the dignity of a person whose character matters in the eyes of God; if you are a utilitarian your character can be traded in for what is often the illusory project of maximising benefit. God looks to us to cooperate in the realisation of our fulfilment. So above all we should be concerned to grow in those dispositions of mind and heart – the knowledge and love of what is truly good – which will make us fit citizens of the Kingdom of Heaven. That fundamentally is what is at issue in the casuistry about cooperation in wrongdoing.

3

Cooperation in evil: understanding the issues[1]

Bishop Anthony Fisher OP

1. Introduction

1.1. The complicity of intellectuals

In a recent book, *Complicities: The Intellectual and Apartheid,* Mark Sanders examines the complicated role of South African thinkers during the apartheid era.[2] He begins with the five-volume report of the South African Truth and Reconciliation Commission which attributed culpability not only to specific agents, but to various groups (including the churches and "the health sector") and to the wider community. It challenged South Africans to recognize "the little perpetrator" in each of them and to accept their responsibility both for what had happened and for ensuring that such evil is never repeated.[3] But, Sanders says, "until recently, there has been no full-scale philosophical exposition of complicity on which to draw".[4] He turns therefore to Émile Zola,[5]

---

[1] My thanks to Ms Georgina Meyer and Br Vincent Magat OP for their research assistance and to Prof Cathleen Kaveny for her patience.

[2] Mark Sanders, *Complicities: The Intellectual and Apartheid.* London: Duke University Press 2002.

[3] *Ibid.* p. 3.

[4] *Loc. cit.*

[5] Who in *J'accuse* (1898), an open letter to the President of France in defence of Alfred Dreyfus (the Jewish artillery officer wrongly convicted of treason), wrote: "La vérité, je la dirai... Mon devoir est de parler, je ne veux pas être complice" ("Truly, it is my duty to speak up: I will not be an accomplice to this crime.") Sanders, *op. cit.* pp. 4–5.

Karl Jaspers[6] and Jacques Derrida[7] for an explanation of how even those who do not formally support a particular evil can live symbiotically with it and have some responsibility for it. Sanders' book might have been enriched by some acquaintance with moral-theological reflection upon sin (original, social-structural and personal) and cooperation in evil. But his work still challenges us to consider the role that intellectuals – pastors, moral theologians, textbook writers, media commentators, bioethicists, ethics committee members, hospital chaplains, healthcare movers and shakers – play in complicity with evils, including those that the Church, at least, very publicly opposes.

In a world ablaze with headlines about cloning, over-the-counter abortifacients, resource shortages in hospitals, withdrawal of feeding from the unconscious, and umpteen other problems, the subject of cooperation might appear rather obscure or self-indulgent. Yet those of us who work in moral theology and especially in advising people or organizations with real dilemmas know how often cooperation issues arise. The third volume of Grisez's tour de force, *The Way of the Lord Jesus*, excellently demonstrates just how common this is.[8] But as Henry Davis remarked half a century ago, there is no more difficult question in the whole range of moral theology than that of cooperation in evil.[9] Perhaps this explains why so little has been written on it compared with the headline issues. The present book might help to fill the gap.

1.2. Traditional distinctions

We must all confront the issue of cooperation in evil because, especially for those who live "in the world", it is inevitable that they will engage in such

---

[6] Jaspers proposes a kind of "metaphysical guilt" or co-responsibility for horrendous evil in *The Question of German Guilt* (1946). He writes that "there exists a solidarity among men as human beings that makes each co-responsible for every wrong and every injustice in the world, especially for crimes committed in his presence or with his knowledge." Sanders, *op. cit.* pp. 6–7.

[7] Sanders, *op. cit.* p. 9, notes that "complicity – the foldedness or 'contamination' of oppositional pairs – has been a key concern of deconstruction from the beginning". For Derrida complicity cannot be avoided: one chooses in order to avoid the worst.

[8] Germain Grisez, *The Way of the Lord Jesus, Vol. 3: Difficult Moral Questions* (Quincy, IL: Franciscan Press 1997), including his extended essay on cooperation at pp. 871–898.

[9] Cited in James F. Keenan SJ, "Prophylactics, toleration and cooperation: contemporary problems and traditional principles". 29(2) (June 1989) *International Philosophical Quarterly*: 209, and "Collaboration and cooperation in Catholic health care". 77 (April 2000) *Australasian Catholic Record*: 163.

cooperation from time to time – indeed sometimes it is their duty to do so. Even Christ's little band paid taxes some of which were no doubt used for wicked purposes; despite his entreaties, when Jesus cured the sick some of them went on to sin some more; after repeatedly evading his persecutors, Christ eventually allowed himself to be arrested, thereby occasioning his false trial and terrible execution. All sorts of wickedness goes on in our society, and we finance it through our taxes, elect leaders who allow it and fail to do much to change things. More immediately, almost anything we do can be an occasion, opportunity or means for someone else to do something wrong. To avoid all cooperation in evil would require that we abandon almost all arenas of human activity – such as family, workplace, government, health system, Church – and could well constitute a sin of omission.[10]

Reflection upon cooperation in evil begins, therefore, with some commonplace human experiences:

- we are all involved in webs of relationships which enable people (including ourselves and others) to achieve both their good ends and bad ends whether by good means or bad means; in this context our actions inevitably affect others;
- which ends and means those other people choose are often beyond our control or influence;
- sometimes we choose to involve ourselves in other people's bad ends or means, by seduction or conspiracy or deliberate cooperation in that evil, making at least part of their bad willing our own;
- at other times we make no such choice, but the otherwise good things that we do foreseeably assist others to achieve their bad purposes;
- this is an example of an act with a double effect – one good and intended; the other bad, not intended but foreseen – and so the principles of cooperation are really expressions of the principle of double effect;
- accepting the bad "side-effects" of cooperation has implications for those who perform the act of cooperation, those who are assisted by it in performing their evil act, and other parties who may be affected; it is sometimes reasonable and sometimes unreasonable to engage in an act foreseeing and permitting such side-effects; and so
- people in this situation must decide whether to go ahead with their contemplated action despite its connection with the morally objectionable

---

[10] *Cf.* 1 Cor 5:9–10. Grisez *op. cit.* p. 871: "some unreflective and/or unsophisticated people imagine problems regarding co-operation can (and perhaps should) be avoided by altogether avoiding co-operation. That, however, is virtually impossible and sometimes inconsistent with doing one's duty."

action of another, or alter their plans, thereby possibly foregoing achieving whatever good they had proposed.[11]

I need not rehearse the history, similarities and differences between different expositions of the principles of cooperation in the Catholic moral-theological tradition.[12] Suffice it to say that by cooperation in evil traditional authors meant performing an act which in some way assists the evil activity of another agent. This could be either *positive* or *negative*, depending upon whether the cooperator does something which helps the principal agent or fails to impede the principal agent when the cooperator could have done so. It could also be either *effective* or *occasional*, depending upon how much the cooperator's act actually contributed to the principal agent's act. It could be *necessitated* or *free*, depending upon how pressured or free the cooperator was. It could be *necessary* or *contingent*, depending upon how indispensable it was to the principal agent's wrongful action. And it could be *unjust* or merely *unlawful*, depending upon whether an innocent third party was injured and a duty of restitution or reparation thereby occasioned.

The most important distinction made by these writers, however, was that between *formal* cooperation, where the cooperator's act shares in the wrongfulness of the principal agent's act – his/her wrongful end or intention or will – and *material* cooperation, where the cooperator's action, though good or neutral in itself, has the foreseen effect of facilitating the principal agent's wrongdoing.[13] Formal cooperation was subdivided by some authors into

---

[11] See M. Cathleen Kaveny, "Appropriation of Evil: cooperation's mirror image". 61 (June 2000) *Theological Studies*: 280–83. She makes a persuasive case for the category of "appropriation of evil" as a mirror image of cooperation in evil.

[12] Hereafter the "traditional authors" I refer to are those cited in Gary M. Atkinson and Albert Moraczewski OP, *A Moral Evaluation of Contraception and Sterilization.* Braintree, Mass.: Pope John Center 1979; Anthony Fisher OP, "Co-operation in evil". XLIV (3) (Feb. 1994) *Catholic Medical Quarterly*: 15–22; Kaveny *op. cit.*; Keenan *op. cit.*; Russell E. Smith, "The principles of cooperation in Catholic thought", in Peter Cataldo & Albert Moraczewski OP (eds) *The Fetal Tissue Issue: Medical and Ethical Aspects.* Braintree, Mass.: Pope John Center 1994: 81–92; such as Davis, (early) Häring, Healy, Jone, McHugh and Callan, Merkelbach, Noldin, Peschke and Prümmer, who themselves drew upon Augustine, Aquinas, Ligouri and others.

[13] St Alphonsus Liguori said that "Cooperation is formal and always sinful when it concurs in the bad will of the other; cooperation is material when it concurs only in the bad action of the other, not his intentions. The latter is licit when the action is good or indifferent in itself; and when one has a reason for doing it that is both just and proportioned to the gravity of the other's sin and to the closeness of the assistance which is thereby given to the carrying out of that sin." In his exegesis of Alphonsus and the Catholic moral tradition, Grisez (*op. cit.* p. 873) explains that "contributing to another's wrongdoing is *formal* cooperation if, and only if, the act by which one contributes agrees in bad intending with the wrongful act with which one cooperates".

"explicit" and "implicit". *Explicit* formal cooperation occurs where the cooperator clearly approves of the principal agent's evil action. *Implicit* formal cooperation, on the other hand, was said to occur when, though the cooperator denies intending the principal agent's object, no other explanation will suffice to distinguish the cooperator's object from the principal's; the cooperator's action by its very nature or by the form it takes in the concrete situation can have no other meaning. Some used this same terminology to separate the cooperator who shares in the evil ends of the principal agent from the cooperator whose ends are different but who intentionally assists the principal agent's act as a means to the cooperator's own ends.[14]

According to some of these authors, the presumption should always be *against* cooperating, even materially, in evil unless there is a sufficiently grave reason to warrant proceeding. Others thought that the presumption should be *in favour of* the cooperator's chosen good or neutral act, unless the foreseen effects of unintentionally assisting someone else's evil acts are so grave that one should abstain from so acting. Either way, while formal cooperation was generally regarded as prohibited, material cooperation was seen as permissible, even required, if certain conditions were met.

In specifying those conditions some authors distinguished *immediate* from *mediate* material cooperation on the basis of the degree to which the cooperator's act forms part of or physically overlaps with or is essential to the act of the principal agent, as opposed to being merely an occasion of or assistance to it. Mediate material cooperation was then subdivided into

---

Material cooperation, on the other hand, refers to involvement in some wrongdoer's act while "sharing no bad intending in common. Whatever is badly willed by the wrongdoer is at most only an accepted side-effect, foreseen but not intended, of the material cooperator's act." Thus the very same behaviour, viewed externally, may be either formal or material cooperation in evil, or both, or neither.

[14] Catholic Health Australia, *Code of Ethical Standards for Catholic Health and Aged Care Services in Australia*. Canberra 2001: 8.8: "Cooperation is *formal* if the intended 'object' or 'end' (including the chosen means) of one's action is precisely to contribute to the other's wrongful conduct, or if one otherwise shares in the other party's 'bad will'. For example, if a Catholic facility refers patients to another facility *intending* that they undergo abortions there rather than on its own premises, such a referral would involve formal cooperation in abortion. Likewise, if a Catholic institution entered into a contractual arrangement with another party, with the intention of providing some services prohibited by Catholic teaching, such a contract would involve formal cooperation in those prohibited services. Formal cooperation in wrongdoing is never morally permissible.

"8.9: Care must be taken to ensure that arrangements which are claimed to distance a Catholic provider from the provision of prohibited services do not implicitly involve *formal* cooperation. Sometimes there is no reasonable explanation for one's cooperation other than that one endorses the other's wrongdoing."

proximate and *remote* on the basis of how closely the cooperator's action "joined" or "touched" upon the principal's action, geographically, temporally or causally.

1.3. Traditional examples

Enough distinctions: now for some examples. In an earlier article I listed the sorts of examples that classical writers offered and which they thought were instances of formal cooperation or permissible and impermissible material cooperation in evil.[15] I will not rehearse them all here. A few chosen from the healthcare world must suffice.

Examples of *formal* and therefore forbidden cooperation included:

- a doctor or nurse assists in an illicit procedure such as an abortion or sterilisation, physically supporting every step of the principal surgeon, performing an essential part of the procedure and/or being ready to take over in case of necessity;
- a person volunteers his/her services to an abortion clinic, helping people fill out forms in order to help women seeking abortions to get them;
- a hospital administrator decides that the obstetrics department will offer sterilization and sees to it that all patients about to be sterilized fulfil the usual consent requirements;
- a physician or counsellor refers someone for abortion;
- an agency (e.g. the army, a prison) distributes or disseminates contraceptives;
- a counsellor encourages a person to engage in non-marital sexual activity or to take illicit drugs in the hope that this will lead to the client's psychological growth, or to engage in contraception, sterilization or abortion because this is "the lesser evil".

Amongst the examples of what some traditional authors regarded as *permitted* material cooperation were:

- a physician gives merely passive assistance at the preliminary instruction and preparation for an illicit operation, remaining aloof from every appearance of approval of the procedure;

---

[15] Fisher *op. cit.*; see also note 11 above. More recent examples and distinctions are offered by Benedict Ashley OP and Kevin O'Rourke OP, *Ethics of Health Care: An Introductory Textbook*. Washington DC: Georgetown University Press 1994; David Bohr, *In Christ, A New Creation: Catholic Moral Tradition*. Revised ed., Huntington: Our Sunday Visitor 1999; Orville Griese, "The principle of cooperation", in Orville Griese, *Catholic Identity in Health Care: Principles and Practice*. Braintree: Pope John Center 1987; Grisez, *op. cit.*; and C. Henry Peschke, *Christian Ethics: Moral Theology in the Light of Vatican II*. 2 Vols. Alcester: Goodliffe Neale 1977.

- an intern or nurse in an operating room performs the usual duties, such as the preparation of instruments, drugs and patients, but sometimes finds him/herself caught up in immoral procedures;
- an assistant likewise administers anaesthesia or hands over instruments during an immoral operation, if this is an accidental and quite exceptional part of the cooperator's routine work and there is a risk to the patient or to the assistant's employment if the assistant refuses;
- an engineer keeps utilities working in a hospital where abortions are done, only to make a living and further the other good activities carried out there;
- a doctor or agency distributes medicine for healing a sexually transmitted disease, taking care that this is no inducement or invitation to engage in a sinful practice;
- a company manufactures a drug or device which has good uses but which the company knows some people will abuse;
- a legislator who, having tried and failed to exclude abortion funding from a general appropriation bill, then votes for the bill only to bring about the good things it will fund.

Examples of what traditional authors regarded as *wrongful material cooperation* include:

- an intern or nurse who is frequently asked to assist in immoral procedures does so rather than protesting or looking for an alternative position where she/he will not be asked to do this;
- a pharmacist sells a substance such as a poison or a drug of addiction to someone he/she has reason to suspect will abuse it;
- a religious takes part in an abortion;
- a Catholic hospital permits abortions or sterilisations to be performed on its premises.

Rather than multiply or analyse the textbook examples – some of which could certainly be questioned – I will look in the first half of my paper at some more recent examples which have received comment from the *magisterium* of the Catholic Church, the response of some prominent theologians, and the issues both raise.

2. Five modern examples

2.1. Sterilisation in American Catholic hospitals

It was not until the 1970s that uniform *Ethical and Religious Directives for Catholic Hospitals* were adopted throughout the United States as a regulatory, educational and legal-defensive measure.[16] In the face of continuing dispute about the appropriateness of various kinds of involvement by Catholic institutions in sterilization, the bishops submitted the matter to the Sacred Congregation for the Doctrine of the Faith (hereafter "CDF"). The Congregation's 1975 response[17] indicated that direct sterilizations,[18] even those performed to avoid pathological medical conditions, were contraceptive in intent and so "intrinsically evil". The official approval and, *a fortiori,* the regulation, management and execution of direct sterilizations by and in Catholic hospitals was "absolutely forbidden" – apparently as constituting formal cooperation in evil. The document went on to explain that, with respect to other involvements

> The traditional teaching on material cooperation, with its
> appropriate distinctions between necessitated and freely-given
> cooperation, proximate and remote cooperation, remains valid,
> to be applied very prudently when the case demands it . . .
> Scandal and the danger of creating misunderstanding must be
> carefully avoided with the help of suitable explanation.

Thus even if permitting sterilizations was thought to be merely material and not formal cooperation by a Catholic agency, such cooperation was said to "accord badly with the mission confided to such an institution and [to] be contrary to the essential proclamation and defence of the moral order".

The US bishops issued a commentary on this document in 1977 and a fuller set of *Directives* in 1994.[19] While the main body of those *Directives* had been reviewed by the CDF before the bishops' vote, the Appendix on cooperation had not. It was soon subject to criticism for too readily allowing

---

[16] On the history and prehistory of these directives, see Griese *op. cit.* pp. 374–84 and Kevin O'Rourke OP, Thomas Kopfensteiner and Ron Hamel, "A Summary of the Development of the Ethical and Religious Directives for Catholic Health Care Services". 83(6) (Nov.–Dec. 2001) *Health Progress.*

[17] Congregation for the Doctrine of the Faith (CDF), *Quaecumque sterilizatio* (also known as *Haec sacra congregatio): Response to the American Bishops on the Question of Sterilization in Catholic Hospitals,* 13 March 1975 *AAS* 68: 1976, echoed in CDF, *Responses to questions regarding 'Uterine isolation' and related matters,* 31 July 1993.

[18] Defined as "actions which of themselves (*i.e.* of their own nature and condition) have a contraceptive purpose, the impeding of the natural effects of the deliberate sexual acts of the person sterilized".

[19] National Conference of Catholic Bishops (US) (NCCB), "Commentary on the Reply of the CDF on Sterilizations in Catholic Hospitals". 11 (15 Sept. 1977) *Origins:* 399–400; see also NCCB, "Statement on Tubal Ligation". (20 August 1980) *Origins* and Catholic Health Association, *Ethical and Religious Directives for Catholic Health Care Facilities,* 4th ed. (St. Louis: CHA 1994), co-published in 24 (15 December 1994) *Origins:* 449–462.

material cooperation in procedures such as abortion and sterilization on the grounds of pressure from government, finance, patients or professionals (called "duress").[20] The "duress" exception, it seems to me, was just muddled thinking. Its authors, James Keenan and Thomas Kopfensteiner, cited Henry Davis and others as arguing that a man may, under threat of death, destroy another man's property.[21] They thought this shows that even immediate material cooperation in evil, though generally prohibited, is sometimes permissible and that the tradition is "flexible" enough to accommodate this. Yet it is far from clear that the man who did this would be engaging in objective evil at all, since property rights are not absolute. And while persons and groups under great pressure can and do sometimes choose wrongly, those who under great pressure panic or erupt or are paralyzed or behave irrationally may have limited or no moral responsibility for what they do. Of course, they may be responsible for being in the situation or for being unprepared for it.[22] But there is no special "duress" exception to the principles of cooperation.

In a recent article on cooperation in evil Australian theologian Brian Lewis notes that "although the Roman Catholic Church officially condemns all contraceptive sterilisation, many Catholic moral theologians" – he cites Häring[23] – "consider that in some cases it may be morally defended. It would seem therefore that some discretion should be given to doctors regarding sterilisation in select cases".[24] On this basis, of course, hardly any

---

[20] The text reads: "Immediate material cooperation is wrong, except in some instances of duress. The matter of duress distinguishes immediate material cooperation from implicit formal cooperation. But immediate material cooperation – without duress – is equivalent to implicit formal cooperation and, therefore, is morally wrong."

[21] Keenan, "Prophylactics..." 216; Thomas Kopfensteiner, "The meaning and role of duress in the cooperation in wrongdoing". 70(2) (May 2003) *Linacre Quarterly*: 150–158.

[22] Grisez, *op. cit.* p. 896. In any case, most of the authors who used the immediate–mediate distinction did so, not so as to be "flexible" in the way Keenan admires, but precisely so as to *exclude* cases of immediate material cooperation as being as bad as formal cooperation. None thought that financial pressure would excuse such wrongdoing.

[23] The earlier Häring (Bernard Häring, *The Law of Christ* Vol. 2. Cork: Mercier Press 1963, p. 503) took a very different view: "Any pharmacist, druggist, or clerk in a drugstore who... is quite aware of the immoral objects [contraceptives] he is selling... is, in my opinion, guilty of formal cooperation in every instance of sale. He cannot be excused from guilt merely on the score of having no choice. The excuse that he does merely what he is told is vapid. Excuses of this kind have been alleged in defence of the most unheard of crimes. A conscience attuned to the divine law steers clear of such an evasion and of the evil deed. This is not to deny that the manager or owner of the store in question obviously must be charged with far greater guilt than a mere clerk."

[24] Brian Lewis, "Cooperation revisited". 77(2) (April 2000) *Australasian Catholic Record*: 158–162, at p. 162.

practice would be excluded: for it is hard to think of any mainstream secular activity without its theologian advocates today. This "pluralism" exception to the principles of cooperation is a version of what I've called the "tax-lawyer" approach to morality, according to which the role of the moral adviser is to help people find a way *around* the moral tax-law, avoiding as much tax as possible without getting caught in serious breach of the law. This particular variety relies upon shopping around for a legal opinion that supports your tax-avoidance scheme. Whatever the Church says, if you can find an opinion by a prominent theologian or two that permits the contrary, you can call that a probable or more probable or equally probable opinion – which sounds very classical – and then go for it: after all, the magisterium is just one amongst many theological voices.

Not all theologians took the duress or pluralism tracks. Orville Griese and Germain Grisez, for instance, in their thorough treatments of cooperation, both showed how hospital administrators, who commit themselves to ensuring that the sterilizations that are performed in their hospital are performed properly, are *formally* cooperating in evil – however much they claim to disapprove of it and however much they claim to be under financial or other pressure to provide it.[25] Grisez also criticised the slender list of indicia of unacceptable material cooperation in the 1994 Appendix and

---

[25] Griese *op. cit.* p. 388: "The American bishops clarified this issue in their *Commentary on the Roman Reply of 1975* by saying that if a hospital cooperates because of the *medical reasons* advanced in support of allowing the procedure (that is, the 'reasons for the sterilization'), 'the hospital can hardly maintain under these circumstances that it does not approve sterilizations done for medical reasons, and this would make cooperation formal.' Other examples of sharing the intent of the principal agent (hence, *formal* cooperation) would be the following: any service or accommodation on the part of the Catholic hospital whereby requests for immoral procedures are referred to other health facilities, agencies or individuals where such procedures are provided; any deliberate efforts on the part of individuals to induce another person to submit to an immoral procedure by means of threats, persuasion, etc.; any express approval of the plans of an individual who is determined to submit to an immoral procedure."

Grisez *op. cit.* p. 892: "Hospital administrators who, among other things, must see to it that sterilization procedures are carried out 'properly' – that is, with competent techniques to ensure that patients who undergo them will not get pregnant again – ... might prefer that no sterilization be done in their hospitals, but they cannot commit themselves to ensuring that a sterilization be done properly without intending that sterility be achieved, and they cannot intend, without choosing contrary to conscience, that any sterilization be done while believing no sterilization ought to be done." See also pp. 391–402 and Germain Grisez, *The Way of the Lord Jesus* Vol. 2: *Living a Christian Life*. Quincy IL: Franciscan Press 1993, p. 441; Matt McDonald, "The limits of cooperation". 10(11) (Dec. 2000) *Catholic World Report*.

the minimal sense of the "prophetic" responsibility of Catholic institutions to bear witness to moral truths.[26]

The CDF likewise criticized the way the 1994 Appendix was being used by some to justify various activities such as sterilization in Catholic hospitals, and pointed to the principles clearly enunciated in *Veritatis Splendor* §§71–83 and *Evangelium Vitae* §74. The bishops responded by ordering an appendectomy of the *Directives*. Two new directives forbade Catholic providers from engaging in "immediate material cooperation" in "intrinsically immoral" actions such as direct sterilization, abortion and euthanasia, and cautioned against entering into arrangements with non-Catholic organizations who engage in such practices; at worst only "mediate material cooperation" with such wrongdoing would ever be permissible.[27] The bishops also drew attention to the risk of scandal, counselled the use of [more] reliable theological advisers, directed Catholic agencies periodically to reassess whether their agreements with other parties are being implemented in a way that is consistent with Catholic teaching[28] and insisted that the bishop

---

[26] Grisez, *op. cit.* (Vol. 3), pp. 895–896. In his 1998 address to the US bishops, Pope John Paul II reminded them that when the Church teaches that abortion, sterilization or euthanasia are always morally inadmissible, she is giving expression to the universal moral law inscribed on the human heart, binding everyone's conscience, not merely that of Catholics. The Church's prohibition on such procedures in Catholic healthcare facilities is therefore not the imposition of external rules in violation of personal freedom but simply fidelity to moral reason and God's law. John Paul II charged the bishops with reminding hospital administrators and medical personnel that any failure to comply with this prohibition is both a grievous sin and a source of scandal.

[27] Catholic Health Association, *Ethical and Religious Directives for Catholic Health Care Facilities* 5th ed. St. Louis: Catholic Health Association 2001, co-published in 31 (19 July 2001) *Origins*, §§69 and 70. Hamel (Ronald P. Hamel, "Part Six of the Directives". 83(6) (Nov.–Dec. 2002) *Health Progress*) noted that "Some theologians maintain that such cooperation for reasons of duress is reflected in parts of the tradition. Although this directive may not resolve the larger theological debate, it does resolve the practice of Catholic health care institutions – they may not enter into any arrangement that involves immediate material cooperation in the wrongdoing of others when that wrongdoing consists in intrinsically evil actions." Hamel suggested that "immediate material cooperation would likely include such things as ownership, governance, or management of the entity that offers prohibited procedures; financial benefit derived from the provision of the procedures; supplying elements essential to the provision of the services such as medical or support staff or supplies; or performing or having an essential role in the procedure." Directive 70 is now followed by a footnote (n. 44) which appeals to John Paul II's reiteration of the "absolute prohibition" against abortion, direct sterilization, and euthanasia in Catholic health care facilities and to the CDF's 1975 statement on sterilization in Catholic facilities. It specifically supersedes the US Bishops' 1977 commentary.

[28] *Ibid.* §72.

has the final responsibility for addressing such issues.[29] No longer can a Catholic institution claim that financial, political or other pressure justifies cooperation in sterilisation. What impact this will have on the 48% of Catholic managed care plans and the large number of Catholic healthcare providers in the US and elsewhere who offer or contract out for sterilizations is yet to be seen. Happily the more recently promulgated Australian Catholic health directives avoid many of the pitfalls of their predecessors.[30]

2.2. *Condoms against HIV*

In 1987 the Administrative Board of the US Catholic bishops published *The Many Faces of AIDS: A Gospel Response*.[31] Amongst other things the document proposed that "if grounded in the broader moral vision" Church-sponsored educational programmes "could include accurate information about prophylactic devices" and that "if it is obvious that a person [with HIV] will not act without bringing harm to others" a health professional could reasonably advise, on a personal level, that the person use condoms to minimize the harm. Theologians such as Josef Fuchs sj, Richard McCormick sj, James Keenan sj, Jon Fuller sj and Kevin Kelly were very supportive.[32] Some suggested that this was merely an application of the

---

[29] *Ibid.* §71: "The possibility of scandal must be considered when applying the principles governing cooperation. Cooperation, which in all other respects is morally licit, may need to be refused because of the scandal that might be caused. Scandal can sometimes be avoided by an appropriate explanation of what is in fact being done at the Catholic health care facility in question. The diocesan bishop has final responsibility for assessing and addressing issues of scandal, considering not only the circumstances in his local diocese but also the regional and national implications of his decision." A footnote to §71 cites the *Catechism of the Catholic Church* §§2284 and 2287: "Scandal is an attitude or behaviour which leads another to do evil... Anyone who uses the power at his disposal in such a way that it leads others to do wrong becomes guilty of scandal and responsible for the evil that he has directly or indirectly encouraged."

[30] See Catholic Health Australia, *Code of Ethical Standards for Catholic Health and Aged Care Services in Australia*. Canberra: Catholic Health Australia 2001, especially chapter 8 on cooperation.

[31] NCCB (Administrative Board), "The Many Faces of AIDS". 17(28) (24 Dec. 1987) *Origins*: 481–489.

[32] See Jon D. Fuller sj, "Needle exchange: saving lives". 179 (18–25 July 1998) *America*: 8–11; James F. Keenan sj, "Prophylactics, toleration and cooperation: contemporary problems and traditional principles". 29(2) (June 1989) *International Philosophical Quarterly*: 205–220; Keenan, "Living with HIV/AIDS". 249 (3 June 1995) *The Tablet*: 701; Keenan, "Applying the seventeenth-century casuistry of accommodation to HIV prevention". 60 (1999) *Theological Studies*: 492–512; Richard McCormick sj, "Needle exchange saves lives". 179 (July 18–25 1998) *America*: 3; Kevin Kelly, *New Directions in Sexual Ethics: Moral Theology and the Challenge of AIDS*. London: Chapman 2000.

"principle of toleration of the lesser evil" whereby Christian leaders back at least to Augustine have done little or nothing to combat evils such as brothels because they have thought such efforts likely to be ineffectual or counter-productive. What these writers failed to explain, however, is how actively handing out information about condoms and even counselling in favour of their use could be compared with prudential silence.

Several American bishops and theologians, and eventually Cardinal Ratzinger, expressed concerns that suggesting use of condoms might be construed as approving or promoting non-marital sexual activity, cause scandal and compromise witness; some also doubted the effectiveness of the condom strategy.[33] In 1989 the Bishops' Conference issued a new letter, *Called to Compassion and Responsibility: A Response to the HIV/AIDS Crisis*, which no longer included the condom information and counselling propo-sals. While urging compassion for AIDS sufferers, the bishops said chastity was the only "morally correct and medically sure way" to prevent the disease and that young people should not be fooled by "the 'safe-sex' myth".[34]

Some were undaunted. James Keenan, a casuist with an abiding interest in AIDS issues, asserted that:

> The dissemination of this [condom] information whether read or heard by grandmothers, fathers, pastors, eucharistic ministers, high school students, prison inmates, or anyone else in no way constitutes "promoting the use of prophylactics," but rather provides "information that is part of the factual picture"... Traditionalists prefer to see a clearer description of the object of toleration or cooperation. Actually, the [1987] letter is really saying that the use of the prophylactic, not the sexual activity with the prophylactic, is being considered. They are not cooperating with the illicit sexual union, but rather with methods that protect the common good.[35]

Fuller and Keenan cite many sources in support in "At the end of the first generation of HIV prevention", in James F. Keenan (ed) *Catholic Ethicists on HIV/AIDS Prevention*. New York: Continuum 2000. See also Bohr *op. cit.* p. 229 and Lewis, *op. cit.*

[33] *E.g.* "Reaction to AIDS statement". 17 (24 Dec. 1987) *Origins*: 489–93; "Continued reaction to AIDS statement". 17 (7 Jan. 1988) *Origins*: 516–22; Germain Grisez, Letter, 158 (13 Feb 1988) *America*: 173–174; Janet Smith, "The Many Faces of AIDS and the toleration of the lesser evil". 12 (1988) *International Review of Natural Family Planning*: 82–89; Joseph Cardinal Ratzinger, "Cardinal Ratzinger's Letter on AIDS Document". 18 (7 July 1988) *Origins*: 117–8.

[34] Fuller and Keenan, *op. cit.* p. 7. Note that, following a similar intervention by the CDF in 1995, a resource pack on HIV education with advice similar to that given in the 1987 American letter was withdrawn from St Andrews-Edinburgh.

[35] Keenan, "Prophylactics..." 212.

Does anyone believe the target audience for such information is grand-mothers and Eucharistic ministers? Would any so-called "traditionalist" who liked clear act-descriptions characterise providing information about condoms as "promoting prophylaxis without sex" or, even more vaguely, "protecting the common good"? How can the condom act prophylactically except by being worn during non-marital intercourse?[36] Isn't this the sort of acrobatic act-description that brought casuistry into disrepute?[37]

But, insists Keenan, if a person "is going to have sex anyway" then such "proposals of cooperation *in no way assist the person to commit the act*".[38] Yet if they "in no way assist" why call them "cooperation"? Why call them "the lesser of two evils" unless some, supposedly lesser but real, evil will predictably be facilitated? And what are we to make of the notion of a person who is "going to have sex no matter what", who is completely beyond reasoning with or influencing and whose self-harm and harm of others must therefore be contained as far as possible?[39] There is a ring of determinism and despair in this talk, common enough amongst some secular public health officials and psychologists, but surely alien to the Catholic confidence in the power of persuasion and conversion, grace and virtue. We must never admit of the idea that some people are beyond chastity or other virtues: if we do, even implicitly, then they will surely fulfil our low expectations.

Keenan suggests that the critics of condom promotion are "fundamentally conservative" rather than "fundamentally human"; that they lack the clear distinctions and nuances of those who support condom promotion; that they radically misunderstand the Catholic moral tradition which has always been flexible and accommodationist; that they give the Catholic moral tradition a bad name by suggesting it is "a highly intolerant system which prefers to refrain from diminishing the cycle of evil"; and that they make that tradition seem "inhuman, restrictive and useless".[40] One of the

---

[36] Here I use the term "non-marital" in the sense developed by John Paul II that would even include some sexual acts between spouses.

[37] Similarly Lewis, *op. cit.* p. 160 describes the object of the act of condom information as preventing HIV, not encouraging the wearing of condoms while engaging in sexual activity so as to prevent HIV.

[38] Keenan, "Prophylactics..." 217 [author's italics].

[39] *Ibid.* 217: "the person is going to commit the act despite AIDS... We are not talking here of someone who is deciding whether or not to abstain, who is undecided. We are talking of someone, much like the wife's husband, intent on acting. We can no longer influence him by one of our values, to live chastely..."

[40] *Ibid.* 219; James F. Keenan sj, "Institutional cooperation and the Ethical and Religious Directives". 64 (Aug. 1997) *Linacre Quarterly*: 501; Keenan, "Collaboration and cooperation in Catholic health care". 77 (April 2000) *Australasian Catholic Record*: 164.

side-effects of cooperation in evil not identified in the traditional manuals is the academic controversy it can occasion, including a great deal of uncharitable *ad hominem*.

More recently, Fuller and Keenan returned to their themes by claiming that Monsignor Jacques Suaudeau of the Pontifical Council for the Family was pro-condoms for HIV reduction as "the lesser of two evils" and that this represented a "tolerant signal" from the Roman curia in line with pro-condom bishops from Brazil and elsewhere.[41] This caused considerable controversy as the Brazilian bishops denied taking a pro-condom or lesser-evil line and Suaudeau declared that he had been mischievously misinterpreted,[42] characterising the articles in *America* magazine as "a flat lie".[43] Since then several bishops' conferences and individual bishops have publicly supported the Vatican position that condom promotion is neither safe nor moral, and cooperation in it is impermissible;[44] but others have intimated support for the "lesser evil" line.[45]

2.3. *Drug injecting rooms in Australia*

In *Called to Compassion* the US bishops used the same arguments against "needle exchange" (really needle distribution) as they had used against condom promotion: that it might be construed as approving or promoting wrongful conduct (in this case drug abuse), cause scandal and compromise

---

[41] Fuller and Keenan, *op. cit.*; *cf.* Jacques Suaudeau, "Prophylactics or family values? Stopping the spread of HIV/AIDS". (19 April 2000) *L'Osservatore Romano*.

[42] Jacques Suaudeau, "Response to an erroneous interpretation of 'Prophylactics or Family Values?'". (27 Sept. 2000) *L'Osservatore Romano*: 2.

[43] "Condom claim 'a flat lie,' says Brazilian bishop". *Zenit*, 22 October 2000.

[44] *E.g.* "Bishops reject condoms in battle against AIDS". 10 Aug 2001 *National Catholic Reporter*; "Kenyan bishops oppose condom distribution programs". 3 Dec 2002 *Catholic World News*; "South African Bishops reject condoms again". Jan–Feb 2003 *Catholic Insight*. In 2003 Keenan's continuing passion for "gay" causes brought him into direct opposition to the Catholic bishops of Massachusetts (Massachusetts Catholic Bishops, *Joint Statement on the Definition of Marriage to be read in all parishes May 31–June 1 2003*, www.macathconf.org/03bishops_define_marriage_stat.htm) and to the Vatican (CDF, *Considerations regarding Proposals to Give Legal Recognition to Unions between Homosexual Persons*, 3 June 2003) in his opposition to campaigns by the Church and others to define, protect and privilege the heterosexual union of marriage: James F. Keenan SJ, *Testimony in opposition to H. 3190 to the Honorable Chairpersons and Members of the Joint Committee on the Judiciary of the Legislature of the Commonwealth of Massachusetts*, April 28, 2003 (www.massequality.org/keen.html).

[45] Mike Francis and Ellen Teague ("Vatican Cardinal breaks ranks over condoms". 5 Feb. 2005 *The Tablet*: 33) list Cardinals Godfried Danneels and George Cottier amongst those who have recently favoured condom use in certain circumstances.

witness; and that it is not an effective strategy.[46] Yet again McCormick, Keenan and Fuller came out against the bishops.[47] Keenan accused them of hesitating to engage constructively with a major public health problem, of causing scandal, of being motivated by a base desire "to keep the infection out of our ranks", the opposite of that mercy we admire in the Good Samaritan. He predicted that in time not only Catholic hospitals and theologians but increasing numbers of bishops will simply ignore Church rulings on these matters. In due course even the magisterium will have to come to terms with "the more chaotic questions" and the wisdom of the world on how to accommodate the chaos.[48]

An apparent example of such a prudent and compassionate "accommodation" was the announcement in June 1999 that the Sisters of Charity Health Service (SCHS) in Sydney would conduct the first legal trial in Australia of a "medically supervised" or "safe" injecting room for intravenous drug users. The author of the scheme, Dr Alex Wodak, explained that the proposal was "a harm-reduction approach to illicit drugs" which would help reduce mortality and morbidity for drug users and the social nuisance of public injecting.[49] For those (few) who sought to change their life-style, there would also be appropriate referral.[50]

No one doubted the sincerity of the Sisters of Charity and their employees, whose record in the care of the poor and marginalised has been outstanding. Nonetheless, the proposal had its critics. Some pointed out that drug abuse should never be reduced merely to a "health" issue or a "social" problem requiring public health "containment" measures: it is a psychological, moral and spiritual problem – as well as a medical and social one. Some recalled that drug abuse is both intrinsically evil and extrinsically very harmful[51] and

---

[46] See also New Jersey Catholic Conference, *Statement on the Establishment of a Demonstration Needle and Syringe Exchange Program in the New Jersey Department of Health*, Nov. 1993.

[47] Jon D. Fuller sj, "Needle exchange: saving lives". 179 (18–25 July 1998) *America*; James F. Keenan sj, "Applying the seventeenth-century casuistry of accommodation to HIV prevention". 60(3) (Sept. 1999) *Theological Studies*: 506; Richard McCormick sj, "Needle exchange saves lives". 179 (July 18–25 1998) *America*. Likewise Lewis, *op. cit.* p. 160.

[48] Keenan, "Applying..." 507–512.

[49] He was referring here to syringes on the streets, public injecting, opportunities for police corruption and calls upon the ambulance service.

[50] Alex Wodak, "Why trial a supervised injecting room?". 10(3) (Sept. 1999) *Bioethics Outlook*: 4–6.

[51] The Church teaches that "the use of drugs inflicts very grave damage on human health and life. Their use, except on strictly therapeutic grounds, is a grave offence" (*Catechism*, §2291). Illicit drug-taking impedes the ability of the human person to think, will and act responsibly. It destroys bodies, minds, lives. It kills. Sometimes slowly, sometimes quickly. It destroys families and harms communities.

that supporting abstinence must therefore be the focus of any genuinely Catholic drug abuse strategy.[52] All sorts of misgivings were expressed about whether a drug injecting room would work, how one would know, and whether the means to that end were morally permissible or reasonable in the circumstances. Some even claimed that since drugs are immoral, that's the end of the matter: you can't be involved with drugs, especially if you are nuns.

That last argument, of course, was too simple. We must first ask: did SCHS (owners, management, health professionals...) share in the bad will of the drug pushers and abusers? Was drug abuse the "proximate end" of their project? As Grisez pointed out, regarding hospital CEOs who say they deplore sterilisation but then allow and manage it in their institutions, people *can* formally cooperate in things they do not like. Someone who deplored drug abuse and who engaged in various projects to prevent or cure it, but who nonetheless provided some people with the wherewithal for drug abuse *so that* they could/would continue engaging in that wrongful activity, would be formally cooperating in evil – even if this action were motivated by the hope of some other good effect, such as building a relationship of trust with drug-abusers, eventual rehabilitation of some, and so on.

Nonetheless, the vast majority of those involved in the SCHS proposal might well have said that it was no part of their goal that anyone take drugs; that their scheme was aimed at discouraging drug abuse or at least at keeping people alive and (relatively) healthy despite their bad choices; that they did not want to encourage even a single additional case of injecting; that if those who entered the injecting room chose not to inject themselves with drugs, the scheme would not be thwarted but would rather be a success; and so on.

But that SCHS were not formal cooperators in drug abuse was not the end of the matter. Since establishing and running an injecting room foreseeably facilitates drug abuse and has various predictable good and bad effects, we must still consider whether it is reasonable material cooperation. Amidst both public praise and public disquiet about the proposal the local ordinary, Cardinal Clancy, referred the matter to the CDF. With the referral came a submission from the Sisters of Charity in favour of the proposal. The Congregation, however, found against. Cardinal Ratzinger's letter was

---

[52] *Cf.* John Paul II, "Address to participants in the Eighth World Congress of Therapeutic Communities, Castel Gandolfo, 7 September 1984". 24 Sept. 1984 *L'Osservatore Romano*, Eng. ed., and "Address to the participants at the International Conference on Drugs and Alcohol, 23 November 1991". XIV/2 (1991) *Insegnamenti*: 1249; Pontifical Council for Pastoral Assistance to Health Care Workers, *Charter for Health Care Workers*. Vatican City 1995: §§93–96.

never published in full.[53] But the CDF apparently gave the Sisters of Charity Health Service the benefit of the doubt in assuming that none of those involved would cooperate formally in drug taking. It nonetheless opposed the plan because of:

- insufficient focus on the goal of and appropriate means for freeing people from drug addiction;
- the danger that a supervised injecting room would actually encourage drug trafficking and abuse;
- the risk of scandal in the everyday sense of deeply disturbing people and in the theological sense of leading people into sin;
- serious doubts about the efficacy of such programmes[54] and fear that they represent the first step towards decriminalization and "normalisation" of drugs;
- the risk of compromising that clear Gospel witness which Catholic agencies should always give; and
- the danger that this will undermine respect for law and further degrade social mores.

In a recent monograph Keenan uses this as his central case *of a failure on the part of the Church to practice what she preaches.*[55] Amidst sinister talk of secret

---

[53] Only excerpts of the document were published by the Archbishop of Sydney: see CDF, *Letter to Cardinal Clancy regarding a proposed Medically Supervised Injecting Service*, part published as "The debate on medically supervised injecting rooms: Cardinal explains Holy See's decision". 7 Nov. 1999 *The Catholic Weekly* (Sydney): 1.

[54] There is considerable dispute over whether injecting rooms work. Experience around the world varies and is interpreted very differently by different commentators. Some argue that since some people are going to take drugs no matter what we do, it is better that they do so in a medically supervised environment where conditions are sterile, needles (and therefore diseases) are not shared, and health professionals are on hand to assist overdose victims. Lives will be saved; some will join rehabilitation programmes; other approaches are not working. Others argue that injecting rooms have failed where they have been tried: users will not travel inconvenient distances to use them; they often want to take their "fix" as soon as possible after buying it; of those who do use the service, little will be done to get them off drugs. In order to attract clients the clinic will avoid any strong message about the evil of drug abuse or the value of rehabilitation; it may also convey implicitly despair about the possibility of users ever getting off drugs, or public approval of drug abuse. Critics of injecting room proposals have also suggested that such programmes serve to mask inactivity and niggardliness on the part of governments, and are commonly motivated more by a desire to "clean up the streets" than a concern for the addicts. See Anthony Fisher OP, "Why some people are uneasy about injecting rooms". 10(3) (Sept. 1999) *Bioethics Outlook*: 11–16.

[55] James F. Keenan SJ, *Practice What You Preach: The Need for Ethics in Church Leadership*. Milwaukee: Marquette University Press 2000.

denunciations, pre-emptive censorship, careerist bishops, old-boy networks, homophobia and misogyny, and deliberate falsification by Church leaders, he offers his own version of the facts. A well-meaning and thoroughly thought-through proposal met knee-jerk opposition from Rome, he retrospected. At the time, however, even the SCHS's own ethical advisers had expressed surprise at how *little* consultation there had been with Church leaders, moral theologians and the wider Church.[56]

One of the central issues in cooperation in evil, to which I shall return, is the characterisation of acts and the gravaman of *formal* as opposed to *material* cooperation. Keenan claims that the *real* object of this proposal was the good one of rehabilitating drug addicts. "The Sisters," Keenan explains, had found "a way of accompanying otherwise marginalized people precisely to bring them into rehabilitation and into a drug free life-style ... to see if their presence and counsel might successfully wean addicts off their addictions."[57] Yet the published case for the injecting room put weaning addicts rather low on the list of goals. Wodak's public support for a staged process – of reclassifying drug abuse as a "public health problem" and proposing, first, injecting rooms, then decriminalisation of drugs, then prescription provision of heroin – provided little comfort for those advocating a rehabilitation and abstinence focus.[58] Nor did the proposed means seem well-suited to such a goal. Nor had the "harm reductionist" government partners in this project demonstrated much commitment to encouraging abstinence – given the long queues for "detox" in that state and inadequate follow-up support for those who were trying to get off drugs. To call this a rehabilitation programme seems to me a kind of "creative" act-description designed more to sell the project than to characterize it accurately.

Keenan next claims that the CDF "did not forbid the practice because of moral issues" at all, "but rather practical ones".[59] This distinction between moral and practical issues would mystify the great writers of the Western

---

[56] As Gleeson (Gerald Gleeson, "St. Vincent's withdraws from supervising injecting room". 10(4) (Dec. 1999) *Bioethics Outlook*: 6) put it rather diplomatically: "the SCHS would have been wise to seek more extensive ethical advice". Gleeson, perhaps influenced by Keenan's action theory, favoured injecting rooms himself: see also Gerald Gleeson, "An ethical reflection on a medically supervised injecting room". 10(3) (Sept. 1999) *Bioethics Outlook*: 7–10.

[57] Keenan, *Practice*... p. 6.

[58] *Cf.* Joe Santamaria, "Heroin injecting rooms and Catholic health care services". 11(3) (Sept. 1999) *Bioethics Research Notes*: 25–26.

[59] Keenan, *Practice*... p. 7. He also said that "the CDF's objections were not on moral grounds" (p. 16), that "the program was not viewed as immoral" by the CDF (p. 16) and that "to date, there is nothing [from the Church] to suggest that the proposal was faulty on moral grounds" (p. 19).

ethical tradition, almost all of whom have insisted that moral reasoning is *precisely* practical reasoning. That tradition never reduced morality to compliance with a few negative moral absolutes and avoidance of formal cooperation – thereby relegating most of decisionmaking, including all issues regarding material cooperation in evil and scandal, to the realm of the "non-moral". If the CDF's conclusion was that this proposal involved such grave downsides and such dubious upsides as to amount, at the very least, to illicit material cooperation in wrongdoing, this was a *moral* judgment, based upon *moral* arguments. So, too, those who supported the injecting room proposal did so because they believed the good(s) in prospect very great and the downsides relatively small and this grounded their *moral* judgment that it was permissible material cooperation. Whichever side one agrees with (if either), one is agreeing with the conclusion of a *moral* argument.

Keenan suggests that when moral theologians disagree with one another, "the care of our argumentation is often noticeably inferior to our normally good work".[60] He goes on to ask: "Why can't we agree to disagree without smearing one another's arguments?" The two instances he then cites of bad argument and smear tactics in the debate over injecting rooms in Australia are the commentaries by John Fleming (whom he also calls "Fletcher") and myself (whom he calls "the usually fair Tony Fisher" and "Fischer"). He proceeds to select – rather misleadingly – from a magazine article on the subject, ignoring completely our academic writing on the topic.[61] He suggests that our statements involved "misrepresentation" and "innuendo", were "obscurantist", "unfair" and "insidious", and were calculated to "undermine the Sisters' credibility" and "smear" their arguments. So much for agreeing politely to disagree![62] Once again an undesired but increasingly foreseeable side-effect of material cooperation in evil seems to be a theological debate that generates more heat than light....

2.4. *Counselling pregnant women in Germany*

In June 1995 the German Bundestag legalised abortion in the first twelve weeks of pregnancy provided that the woman had a certificate that she had

---

[60] Keenan, *Practice*... p. 14.

[61] See *e.g.* Fisher, "Why some people..."; John Fleming, "Drugs and Ethics", Australian Drug Summit 2000, Parliament House, Sydney, 13–15 June 2000, http://www/wesley mission.org.au/drugsummit/day1.htm.

[62] Keenan concludes his paper with a section entitled "humility" in which he confesses that "before I read Cardinal Bernadin on the *Common Ground* Project, I did not fully believe that I had an obligation to fairly represent a theologian's opinion with which I disagreed. Now, I believe I have an added obligation to represent an opponent's opinion." (p. 20).

attended a *Schwangerschaftsberatungsstellen* – an approved counselling centre. In September of that year the German Bishops' Conference criticized the law but agreed to take part in Church-state abortion counselling boards. The bishops clearly believed that Church involvement would be at most material cooperation in the evil of abortion and that many women would be dissuaded from having an abortion by Church-sponsored counselling agencies.

Four years of discussions between the German bishops and the Vatican followed. The Pope cautioned against any cooperation in the legalization or practice of abortion. The bishops and several lay organisations declared their continuing support for Church involvement in the counselling services. The Pope responded by asking them to testify more clearly to the right to life and to ensure that no Church agency issued a certificate which could be used to procure an abortion.[63] The bishops countered by asking the Pope to support their existing programme.

In June 1999 John Paul II wrote again to the German bishops, and in September Cardinals Ratzinger and Sodano reiterated, that Church agencies should only issue certificates which could not be used to facilitate the death of an unborn child. It was becoming increasingly clear, however, that such certificates, despite a declaration stamped upon them that they could not be used to secure an abortion, were being used for just that by three out of four women seeking counselling from Catholic agencies.[64] The bishops were increasingly divided. Bishop Johannes Dyba of Fulda, who had argued all along that counselling certificates amounted to "licenses to kill", had a growing number of allies.

On the other hand there were bishops who thought that if the Church withdrew from providing the counselling services it would be complicit in abortion. In October 1999 some wrote to the Pope asking if he would bear on his conscience that "German children will be murdered because the Church can no longer counsel future mothers in conflict." Cardinal Sodano responded by reaffirming the Pope's instructions. Even then some of the bishops hoped to change the Pope's mind during their *ad limina* visit to Rome. In November the Pope directed and the majority of the bishops voted to cease participation on the abortion boards. Only three said they would continue cooperating with the government programme in their dioceses.[65]

---

[63] John Paul II, "Letter to the German Bishops of 11 January 1998". 90 (1998) *AAS*: 601–607.

[64] According to figures provided by Caritas in early 1999, only 5,000 of the 20,000 who had by then sought counselling from a Catholic agency had gone forward with their pregnancy. By late 2000 the figures would have been much higher.

[65] Crista Kramer von Reisswitz, and *Inside the Vatican* Staff, "German bishops accept Pope's appeal". (Jan. 2000) *Inside the Vatican*: 25–27.

Throughout this interchange there was no suggestion that the German bishops or those conducting or staffing the pregnancy counselling agencies were engaging in formal cooperation in abortion – though it would be naïve to assume that *all* those involved in such agencies shared the bishops' abhorrence of abortion. What seemed to have been decisive here was (a) the gravity of what was at stake, i.e. innocent unborn human lives, (b) the witness which the German bishops were called to give to the sanctity of life, and (c) concern about the corrupting effects on churchworkers, pregnant women and the culture of even this much material cooperation in abortion.

2.5. Support for improving abortion laws

In a previous paper I explored John Paul II's teaching in *Evangelium Vitae*,[66] recently reiterated by the CDF in its *Doctrinal Note on Some Questions regarding the Participation of Catholics in Political Life*.[67] I agreed with the exegesis of Archbishop Bertone and Professor Finnis. I suggested that a legislator who, with a view to achieving or maintaining a permissive abortion regime, actively supports someone else's permissive law or bill or actively blocks someone else's restrictions to such a law or bill, engages in formal cooperation in the evil of the sponsor of the legislation.[68] So too does one uninterested in the abortion issue who nonetheless supports such a bill or blocks such restrictions, hoping thereby to gain some other advantage,

---

[66] John Paul II, *Evangelium Vitae*: Encyclical on the Value and Inviolability of Human Life, 25 March 1995: §73: "A particular problem of conscience can arise in cases where a legislative vote would be decisive for the passage of a more restrictive law, aimed at limiting the number of authorized abortions, in place of a more permissive law already passed or ready to be voted on. Such cases are not infrequent. It is a fact that while in some parts of the world there continue to be campaigns to introduce laws favouring abortion, often supported by powerful international organizations, in other nations – particularly those which have already experienced the bitter fruits of such permissive legislation – there are growing signs of a rethinking in this matter. In a case like the one just mentioned, when it is not possible to overturn or completely abrogate a pro-abortion law, an elected official, whose absolute personal opposition to procured abortion was well known, could licitly support proposals aimed at 'limiting the harm' done by such a law and at lessening its negative consequences at the level of general opinion and public morality. This does not in fact represent an illicit cooperation with an unjust law, but rather a legitimate and proper attempt to limit its evil aspects."

[67] CDF, *Doctrinal Note on some questions regarding the Participation of Catholics in Political Life*, 24 Nov. 2002 §4 citing *Evangelium Vitae* §73.

[68] Anthony Fisher OP, "Some problems of conscience in bio-lawmaking", in Luke Gormally (ed) *Culture of Life – Culture of Death*. London: Linacre Centre 2002: 195–226.

such as appeasing certain opponents, keeping his/her seat, or horse-trading support for some other (possibly noble) legislative objective. In such cases politicians can be guilty of formal cooperation in the evils of bad lawmaking and of abortion itself, even if they disapprove of abortion and say so publicly.

Evangelium Vitæ says as much. So too it says that when it is not possible to defeat a pro-abortion law or bill, a politician could in certain circumstances licitly support a proposal aimed at "limiting the harm done" by that bad law or bill.[69] (There are big magisterial italics or "scare quotes" around the phrase "limiting the harm done".) That politician would not thereby be responsible for the far-from-perfect state of the law, despite the undesired support that such material cooperation might lend to offences against life.

The recent CDF document suggests that Christians ought not to remove themselves from political life but should rather play their full role as citizens.[70] The document emphasizes the importance of being guided by a genuinely Christian conscience, seeking always the common good, and being willing, like St Thomas More, to give witness to the faith in public life. It warns against cultural and moral relativism and disingenuous appeals to tolerance or to the autonomy of lay involvement in political life which sanction "the decadence of reason" and the disintegration of those "non-negotiable ethical principles, which are the underpinning of life in society". Thus Catholics have grave obligations to defend the right to life, marriage and the family, a drug-free society etc., and never to vote for a programme or law which contradicts the fundamental contents of faith and morals.

The Congregation also recognizes "the legitimate plurality of temporal options" that arise from "the contingent nature of certain choices regarding the ordering of society, the variety of strategies available for accomplishing or guaranteeing the same fundamental value, the possibility of different interpretations of the basic principles of political theory, and the technical complexity of many political problems". This explains why Catholics might belong to several different political parties.[71] I will not rehearse my arguments from my previous paper for my reading of both the encyclical and the moral tradition upon which it builds, as these matters will be further explored by Finnis and Harte later in this volume.

---

[69] In Fisher, "Some problems…" I asked: "What are the reasons that might persuade a pro-life parliamentarian to engage in such material cooperation?" I suggested than these might include saving lives (of the unborn, handicapped or dying) and helping others (*e.g.* pregnant women). But I also suggested that politicians must consider all the relevant downsides of such material cooperation which I listed at some length.

[70] CDF, *Catholics in Political Life*, 2002.

[71] *Ibid.* §3.

3. Some fundamental issues raised by these examples

These several examples, and the responses to them, suggest six fundamental issues worth further consideration.

3.1. *The human act*

How one views the human act is central to these questions. In *Evangelium Vitæ* John Paul defines as formal cooperation "an action, which either by its very nature or by the form it takes in a concrete situation, can be defined as a direct participation in an [evil] act ... or a sharing in the immoral intention of the person committing it."[72] There is a great deal packed into the words "by its very nature", "direct participation" and "sharing in the intention" – far more than I can explore in this paper. *Veritatis Splendor* makes it clear that "the object rationally chosen by the deliberate will" is what is at issue and that this way of characterising human acts excludes the accounts of situationists, proportionalists and other subjectivists.

The encyclical would seem to allow, however, at least two accounts of the human act: a "natural meanings" account and an "intended acts" account. This has been at the heart of debates between orthodox Catholics about matters as diverse as the gravamans of sterilization, abortion and euthanasia, whether and what imperfect legislation one might support, ovulation-suppression after rape, vaccines grown on foetal cell-lines, craniotomy and what to do when someone is trapped in the mouth of a cave obstructing the exit of people suffocating behind him.[73] I think it is also at the heart of why in my earlier examples some commentators thought the cooperators were co-conspirator principals or at least formal cooperators, while others thought them material cooperators only, and some thought them not cooperators at all.

---

[72] John Paul II, *Evangelium Vitae*: §74. The example the Pope uses of an intrinsically evil act here is of killing the innocent.

[73] John Paul II, *Veritatis Splendor*: Encyclical on Certain Fundamental Questions of the Church's Moral Teaching, 6 August 1993: §78: "The morality of the human act depends primarily and fundamentally on the 'object' rationally chosen by the deliberate will .... In order to be able to grasp the object of an act which specifies that act morally, it is therefore necessary to place oneself in the perspective of the acting person. The object of the act of willing is in fact a freely chosen kind of behaviour .... By the object of a given moral act, then, one cannot mean a process or an event of the merely physical order, to be assessed on the basis of its ability to bring about a given state of affairs in the outside world. Rather, that object is the proximate end of a deliberate decision which determines the act of willing on the part of the acting person."

Each of these writers might claim to find support in the encyclical and elsewhere in the tradition for their understanding of the human act.[74] But some acts that, on the natural meanings account, are implicit formal cooperation in evil, whatever the agent says or believes he/she intends, are only material cooperation on the intended acts account; likewise some acts that are only immediate material cooperation on the natural meanings account are formal cooperation on the intended acts account. To advocates of the natural meanings account those who support an intended acts account look subjectivist, and the encyclical's warnings against intentionalism seem very telling; to the second group the first look physicalist, and the encyclical's insistence on the perspective of the acting subject seems most telling.[75]

This in turn raises issues for the traditional casuistry of cooperation in evil. Is there, for instance, such a thing as an "implicit" intention – central to the idea of "implicit formal cooperation" and possibly to the ideas of both

---

[74] Kaveny, *op. cit.* p. 288 points out that the manualists increasingly adopted an account of human action at odds with Aquinas' agent-centred approach: "They began to formulate their description of human actions by assuming an external viewpoint that emphasized the physical structure and causal consequences of the action, not by empathetically adopting an internal viewpoint that described it in terms of the agent's purposeful activity. They *ascribed* intentions to agents based on external descriptions of their actions...."

[75] In *Evangelium Vitæ*, John Paul II distinguishes the withdrawal of burdensome treatments and the giving of pain relief from an act of euthanasia on the basis of the intended ends and means of the agent, not the private motivations or external appearances of the act. To remove a treatment *because* it is futile or too burdensome and to give enough analgesia in order effectively to relieve pain is not homicide unless there is also an intention to hasten death.

This has not always been as clear as it could be. In its 1980 *Declaration on Euthanasia* the CDF defined suicide as "intentionally causing one's own death". But when it came to describing euthanasia the Congregation said: "By euthanasia is understood an action or an omission which of itself or by intention causes death, in order that all suffering may in this way be eliminated. Euthanasia's terms of reference, therefore, are to be found in the intention of the will and in the methods used." Pain relief, the Congregation went on to explain, is permitted as long as "death is in no way intended or sought, even if the risk of it is reasonably taken; the intention is simply to relieve pain effectively, using for this purpose pain-killers available to medicine". But the definition of euthanasia, if taken by itself, seemed to suggest that an action could be euthanasia "of itself" without any intention of causing death – which would make a nonsense of the distinctions between withdrawal of burdensome life-sustaining treatments and/or the giving of appropriate but possibly life-endangering pain-relief on the one hand, and euthanasia or other homicide on the other. Thus in *Evangelium Vitæ* John Paul II, while citing the 1980 document, is careful to amend the "or" to read "and": "Euthanasia in the strict sense is understood to be an action or omission which of itself *and* by intention causes death, with the purpose of eliminating all suffering."

immediacy and proximity in material cooperation – and if so, what precisely does each mean? What is the difference between implicit formal cooperation and immediate material cooperation – categories often used interchangeably by the manualists[76] but unknown to contemporary philosophy, and ones which, for reasons I have explored previously, are of uncertain value?[77]

3.2. *The intended end*

Even if we resolve what precisely we mean by end and/or intention and what its importance is in the human act, *identifying what precisely is intended* in any particular act or proposal may itself be far from easy. Some will adopt a sanguine description of the object of a sterilisation operation or an agreement between a Catholic provider and a non-Catholic partner for the latter to perform sterilisations for the former's clients as "institutional survival under duress". Some will call the object of condom information "satisfying people's right to know", "educating grandmothers and catechists" or "protecting the common good". Some will say that the object of drug injecting rooms is "to promote a drug-free life-style". Such act-descriptions incline the agent to a very different judgment about the admissibility of those acts to the judgments of the magisterium noted above. Sometimes one suspects pre-disposition colours description. But even without such pre-judgments, identifying intentions can be extraordinarily difficult. It can be all the more difficult when intentions come in chains of multiple means and ends, or complex configurations of intentions, motives and wishes, or multiple agents (such as institutional owners, managers and clinicians) with diverse powers and responsibilities.[78]

---

[76] Keenan, "Prophylactics..." 216 suggests that "cooperation is immediate when the object of the cooperator is the same as the object of the illicit activity" – as when a surgical nurse actually performs the abortion herself. But that is surely not immediate *material* cooperation but formal cooperation or, indeed, acting as the principal agent of the evil-doing. Keenan also uses as examples of immediate *material* cooperation a servant who, instead of assisting his master to engage in illicit sexual acts by bringing the ladder to the target's window instead performs the illicit sexual acts himself, and of a wife who, instead of pressing a less dangerous weapon upon her violent husband takes part in the beating herself. But these are surely examples not merely of material cooperation, nor even merely of formal cooperation, but of being the principal agent of an evil.

[77] I think "immediate" material cooperation either reduces to formal cooperation or relies upon a misconception of the human act: see Anthony Fisher OP, "Co-operation in evil". XLIV (3) (Feb. 1994) *Catholic Medical Quarterly*: 5–8.

[78] On this matter see Elizabeth Anscombe, *Intention*. Oxford: Blackwell 1957; and the long line of important writing on intention which has followed from writers such as Joseph Boyle, John Finnis, Germain Grisez and Ralph McInerney.

3.3. Duress

A third matter which we might consider is *the relevance, if any, of pressure* of a financial or other kind. Despite the appendectomy of the 1994 US *Directives,* Keenan and Kopfensteiner continue to assert that duress gives hospitals lee-way to decide whether or not to cooperate in sterilization and other wrongful activities.[79] Of course there is hardly any bioethical question upon which the Church has a position for which there is not pressure upon hospitals to behave to the contrary. Is there therefore "lee-way" on all matters? For the reasons mentioned above, I think "the duress exception" is based upon a misunderstanding of moral responsibility.[80]

3.4. Pluralism

Another "exception" proposed by, for instance, Lewis, is that if there is a difference of opinion amongst theologians or conscientious health profes-sionals there must be latitude for practitioners and patients to decide for themselves.[81] Yet on almost every bioethical teaching of the Church there are theologians or practitioners who disagree. As early as the 1975 *Declaration* the CDF saw this coming and made the point that widespread theolo-gical dissent from the Church's teaching on a matter such as contraception or sterilization has no doctrinal significance in itself. Theologians do not offer "a theological source which the faithful might invoke, forsaking the authentic magisterium for the private opinions of theologians who dissent from it."[82]

---

[79] Keenan, "Collaboration..." 171: "Immediate material cooperation is always wrong, except in very rare occasions of duress.... To capitulate or not is a question that the CEO, the bishop and others must consider. The principle gives them some lee-way to decide...". Similarly Kopfensteiner, *op. cit.* 2003.

[80] Lewis (*op. cit.* p. 159 n. 1, following Peschke *op. cit.* pp. 251–2) suggests that breaking-and-entering under threat of death looks like implicit formal cooperation but is actually immediate material cooperation because "this kind of cooperation is not performed with real consent, a necessary condition for formal cooperation". But in what sense is "consent" used here? A person acting under duress may not consent in the sense of concurring in the evil ends or bad will of the principal agent. But to the extent that he/she is free that person consents to his/her own act of material coopera-tion. To the extent that the agent is *not* free his/her responsibility for the act of cooperation is diminished or even entirely vitiated. Either way, this does not bear on whether the person's cooperation is formal or material, immediate or mediate.

[81] Lewis *op. cit.* p. 162.

[82] CDF, *Quaecumque sterilizatio*: §2. See also CDF, *Instruction on the Ecclesial Vocation of the Theologian* (1990).

3.5. Reasons to cooperate and not to cooperate

There are lots of good reasons to cooperate materially in any particular evil. There is the good aimed at in the cooperator's own chosen purpose. There are the spin-offs in terms of keeping one's job or position in the healthcare world, such as the opportunity to do all the other good things which the job or position allows (e.g. saving, healing and caring for others); the income this brings, thereby supporting a reasonable life-style for oneself and one's dependents or a reasonable margin for the institution to focus on its mission; the friendship with the others with whom one works; and so on. When considering whether to engage in an action which has the foreseeable effect of assisting someone else's wrongful purposes, we must ask ourselves: how important are the benefits expected from this action, how probable, how lasting, how extensive and for whom? What kind of loss or harm would result (and how serious, and for whom . . .) from foregoing this proposed action? People with dependents, for instance, have more to lose from refusing to take part in certain procedures, than do people with no dependents. People who can readily get another good job will be freer to say no. Someone who cannot readily fulfil some important responsibility, except by agreeing to cooperate materially, will have more reason to do so than someone with a ready, morally acceptable alternative.

On the other hand, for reasons which I will explore in the next part of my paper, there are strong reasons not to cooperate in many cases. Given the risks to self and others both of material cooperation in evil and of foregoing acts which materially assist someone else's evil acts, *what would count as relevant and sufficient and even decisive reasons* to take such risks or permit such evil foreseen side-effects? To cooperate materially in evil a more serious reason is required:

- the graver (or more probable or more lasting or more extensive or less preventable) the evil of the principal agent's act in itself;
- the graver (or more probable or more lasting or less preventable) is the harm which may be caused to the principal agent, e.g. by helping and even apparently encouraging him/her to engage in a wrongful act and possibly further wrongful acts, with all the moral and spiritual consequences of that for the principal agent;
- the graver (or more probable or more lasting or more extensive or less preventable) is the harm which may be caused to third parties, especially the innocent, e.g. by assisting or apparently encouraging the principal agent to do something which damages third parties or their interests, perhaps giving the impression that, on the cooperator's view, the wrong done is trivial; or by engaging in activity which may foreseeably corrupt third party observers;

- the graver (or more probable or more lasting or less preventable) is the harm which may be caused to the cooperator him/herself, e.g. by inclining the cooperator to do similar acts in the future and worse; by gradually corrupting him/her; by compromising the cooperator's ability to give witness to true values; by damaging his/her relationship with God, the Church and fellows;
- the harder it is to protest the evil and/or to avoid or minimize scandal in both the ordinary sense and, more importantly, in the theological sense of leading people into sin;[83]
- the more easily the same good could be achieved by another course of action without similar or worse side-effects; and
- the more difficult it would be for the principal agent to proceed without the cooperator's involvement.[84]

Some writers would add immediacy and proximity to this list of factors. But for reasons I have explored previously, the most important factors in determining the reasonableness of a particular instance of material cooperation will only sometimes correlate with immediacy and proximity.[85]

All these matters are in fact difficult to assess and usually incommensurable with each other and with the goods hoped to be achieved by the cooperator's act. After appropriate moral reasoning and discernment, two

---

[83] See Griese *op. cit.* pp. 414–6 on "Dissipating the appearances of evil in scandal situations".

[84] Grisez *op. cit.* Vol. 3 (1997), p. 883: "In considering bad effects … one must take several different measures of magnitude into account. How extensive is the damage? … How lasting is it? … How greatly will the damage disrupt the person's life? … In regard to adverse effects on the cooperator's feelings and dispositions, the extent of injury depends on the likely seriousness of their negative effect on his or her subsequent actions. In regard to moral detriment to the wrongdoer, occasions of sin for the cooperator, and scandal to third parties, the extent of injury to the person adversely affected depends on whether the sin is or would be venial or mortal, less or more grave, more or less likely to be repented. In regard to tensions with victims of wrongdoing, the bad effect can be a more or less serious impediment to a good relationship that should be more or less central to the lives of those involved. In regard to impairment of the cooperator's witness and other obstacles to fulfilling his or her vocation, the bad effects can be a more or less serious detriment to serving goods whose service is more or less central to a person's vocation …"

[85] Fisher, "Co-operation in evil." As Grisez (*op. cit.* Vol. 3 (1997), p. 890) points out, "involvement in others' wrongdoing usually is more likely to impede a cooperator's witness, be an occasion of sin to him or her, have bad moral effects on the wrongdoer, and scandalize others if it is immediate material cooperation than if it is mediate, and, when mediate, if it is proximate than if it is remote. Still, closeness of involvement is morally insignificant unless correlated with some factor that affects the strength of a reason not to cooperate."

people of good will and right reason might come to a different judgment. In this situation, instead of high-blown polemic and name-calling, respectful dialogue is required and possibly some judgment from a competent authority.

3.6. *Different moral worldviews*

Furthermore, the principles of cooperation highlight a difference in moral worldview. For some there are moral absolutes, such as that against formal cooperation, which cannot be compromised in any weighing exercise, and even merely material cooperation in another's wrongdoing is a serious matter requiring justification.[86] Morality on this account is part of the vocation to human perfection or holiness under grace, and the (rebuttable) presumption is *against* cooperating even materially, unless there is a sufficiently strong reason to warrant proceeding.[87] Such an approach seems to underlie the various magisterial judgments outlined in the first half of this paper.

There are, however, a good many "tax-lawyer" moralists who seem to regard the moral law as a series of constraints on human freedom and happiness, rather than the roadmap to both. On this approach the role of the moral adviser is to help people find a way around the moral law or at least a way of sailing as close to the wind as possible without falling in the water. Preference fulfilment and social acceptability are paramount; conversion and self-sacrifice have little place here. Using traditional casuist categories,[88] more 1970s situationism[89] or

---

[86] Grisez, *op. cit.* Vol. 3 (1997), p. 871: "insofar as doing anything facilitates or contributes to another's wrongdoing, it cannot serve an authentic common good. If one is unjustifiably involved in another's wrongdoing, one is doing evil, and that cannot serve good or build up genuine community even with a wrongdoer; if one is justifiably involved in another's wrongdoing, community is prevented or damaged insofar as the other's bad will and one's good will are opposed, at least with respect to that matter."

[87] Amongst the authors one might associate with such an approach are John Paul II, Benedict Ashley, Joseph Boyle, Romanus Cessario OP, Augustine di Noia OP, Robert George, Germain Grisez, William E. May, Ralph McInerney, Livio Melina, Servais Pinckaers OP and Janet Smith.

[88] *E.g.* Keenan, in the several places cited.

[89] Lewis *op. cit.*, for instance, presents the principles of cooperation as tools which should not be applied in a "narrow and blinkered way" but transcended as required in the quest for "better and more creative solutions in particular circumstances". He suggests that individual conscience must have primacy and that the serious obligation to respect the freedom of others means that one should be willing in some cases to cooperate in what is objectively evil but not so considered by the principal agent. Where this leaves the conscience of the cooperator is far from clear...

proportionalism,[90] or the new (and otherwise very attractive) talk of virtue and narrative,[91] these writers end up reducing almost all cases of cooperation in evil to material not formal cooperation and almost all cases of material cooperation to permissible cooperation. Duress, probable opinion, proportionate reason, the common good, prudence and epikeia – such very traditional-sounding labels are attached to these novel schemes for paying less moral tax. And those who come to conclusions in line with the magisterium are quickly dismissed as "scrupulous", "conservative" and "inhuman".

I do not mean to suggest that there are the only two moral worldviews or that everyone (or anyone) fits neatly and clearly into one or the other. Rather I am suggesting that two polarities are particularly evident in the scant literature on cooperation and that this might help to explain why two people can describe and judge the same example of cooperation so differently. While the range of moral approaches at one pole offers a "line of best fit" for the several recent Church documents considered above, those gathered around the other pole can offer no such account and so tend to dissent on many issues. This might in turn help explain why the "debate" over such issues so often generates more heat than light.

---

[90] The second of St Alphonsus' conditions for the moral acceptability of material cooperation is that the cooperator have in view as his end a reason that is "just" and "proportioned" to the gravity of the wrongdoing to which his action contributes and the moral proximity of that contribution to the wrongful deed. Grisez (*op. cit.* Vol. 3 (1997), p. 878) has explored well some of the deficiencies of this formulation of what makes some material cooperation licit and other material cooperation illicit and has proposed a more precise analysis which I, for one, find persuasive. Grisez explains that the only real issue of "proportion" here is the necessary comparison between reasons for engaging in the act of material cooperation and reasons for not doing so. The graver the evil assisted and the more closely the cooperator is involved, Alphonsus might be read to suggest, the more serious would the cooperator's reasons have to be for going ahead with his own action. Fair enough. But, as Grisez points out, there will be other reasons not to cooperate which are not well captured by Alphonsus' formulation: the "psychological" effects on oneself and effects on one's future options; the effects on the instigator and the cooperator's relationship with him or her; the effects on third parties and the cooperator's relationships with them. "The magnitude of the various bad side effects, how likely they are to occur, and how much confidence the cooperator has in his or her own judgments also can affect the strength of the reasons to forgo an act that would constitute material cooperation."

[91] In his passionate defence of *The Many Faces of AIDS* Keenan praises the "new and profoundly challenging ideas" that are replacing the old categories of cooperation in evil and the like. "Attempts to replace duties with virtues, the classical with the historical, the object with the acting person, the normative with the narrative are emerging." (Keenan, "Prophylactics..." 219).

4. Why it matters so much

4.1. *Cooperation, the love of God and the Christification of the human person*

I want to conclude this paper by suggesting three reasons why the question of the permissibility of cooperation in evil matters so much and why one would be reluctant to engage in even material cooperation in serious evil unless there were very persuasive reasons to do so.

First, *we must love the Lord our God* with all our minds and wills.[92] The goal of human life is the pursuit of holiness – becoming lights to the world, more and more conformed to Christ, living stones of God's house and temples of his Holy Spirit, perfect like our Heavenly Father.[93] As John Paul II wrote in *Veritatis Splendor*:

> The new evangelization will show its authenticity and unleash all
> its missionary force when it is carried out through the gift not
> only of the word proclaimed but also of the word lived. In
> particular, the life of holiness which is resplendent in so many
> members of the People of God, humble and often unseen,
> constitutes the simplest and most attractive way to perceive at
> once the beauty of truth, the liberating force of God's love, and the
> value of unconditional fidelity to all the demands of the Lord's
> law, even in the most difficult situations. For this reason, the
> Church, as a wise teacher of morality, has always invited believers
> to seek and to find in the Saints, and above all in the Virgin
> Mother of God "full of grace" and "all-holy", the model, the
> strength and the joy needed to live a life in accordance with God's
> commandments and the Beatitudes of the Gospel... The life of
> holiness thus brings to full expression and effectiveness the
> threefold and unitary *munus propheticum, sacerdotale et regale*
> which every Christian receives as a gift by being born again "of
> water and the Spirit" in Baptism...[94]

Yet so often we fail not just to reach but even to pursue this goal. Instead of offering a distinctively Christian form of witness to the life of God's kingdom, even to the point of martyrdom, we settle for more comfortable collaboration with the powers of this world. As Paul puts it so graphically, rather than lifting up Christ and his Church to God we take them down

---

[92] Mt 22:35–38; Lk 10:25–28.

[93] Mt ch. 5; Lk 6:36 etc; Rom 12:1–2, 11–14; ch. 6; 1 Cor 2:16; 3:10, 16–17; 6:19–20; 12:27; 2 Cor 6:3–10; Eph 2:19–22; Phil 1:27; 3:17–21; Col 3:12–17; 1 Thess 5:5–11; 2 Thess 3:13. See also Vatican II, *Lumen Gentium* on the universal call to holiness.

[94] John Paul II, *Veritatis Splendor*: §107.

into the bed of the prostitute.[95] In so doing we damage our relationship with God, making God a cooperator in evil, for it is only by God's power that we are supported in being and by God's permissive will that we are free to do what ill we do. We also compromise our ability to give witness to the true and the good as *alteri Christi*, and so undermine the progress of the Gospel. A keen sense of the privilege that it is to be apostles and prophets, saints and even martyrs, and a deep commitment to the new evangelisation, will give us a greater sensitivity to the issues of cooperation in evil than any purely secular account which sees the principles of cooperation as, at best, useful action guides and, at worst, hindrances to human freedom and happiness.[96]

4.2. *Cooperation, the love of neighbour and mission to others*

In addition to and as an expression of whole-hearted love of God *we must love our neighbours.*[97] This is a large part of the reason for the presumption *against* material cooperation in evil as it is for the case *for* material cooperation. Out of love of our neighbours we desire to help them and to help them do good. We need a very serious reason indeed to do anything that foreseeably helps them to do serious evil, given the potential moral and spiritual consequences for them. But cooperation in evil, especially by "good" people and especially when "successful", can reassure sinners and encourage obduracy.[98] Innocent third parties such as unborn children can also be harmed. And onlookers can be misled. What we do will inspire and educate or else mislead others; it will encourage those who imitate us to acquire virtues or vices. The example that healthcare administrators and senior clinicians give to juniors can, for example, elevate or corrupt those

---

[95] 1 Cor 6:15–17.

[96] Catholic Health Australia, *Code of Ethical Standards*... §8.17: "Material cooperation may also compromise one's ability to witness to certain values or principles. Catholic facilities and their professionals share in the Church's "prophetic" calling to witness to the truth of the Gospel, and so they will be wary of doing anything which might compromise the mission of the facility or the Church more broadly. The reasons which would justify cooperation by institutions sponsored by the Church are usually required to be more stringent than they need to be in the case of individuals, since institutions have a higher public profile and a correspondingly greater prophetic responsibility. The best way to avoid compromising that witness is for the facility or individual to explain their basic commitments clearly and publicly, and to testify to them in ways which help to ensure there is no misunderstanding that they have lessened their commitment to those values."

[97] Mt 22:39–40; Lk 10:27–37; Rom 12:9–10.

[98] Grisez, *op. cit.* Vol. 3 (1997), pp. 880–881.

juniors.[99] Thus Eleazar declared that he would rather die painfully than lead the young to disobey God's holy law,[100] Our Lord inveighed against those who corrupt others[101] and Paul counselled caution lest we scandalise our brothers even at table.[102]

---

[99] Thus Grisez, *op. cit.* Vol. 3 (1997), p. 881: "Third parties can be scandalized by someone's material cooperation. This can happen in various ways. Sometimes the fact that 'good' people are involved makes wrongdoing seem not so wrong and provides material for rationalization and self-deception by people tempted to undertake the same sort of wrong. Perhaps more often the material cooperation of 'good' people leads others to cooperate formally or wrongly, even if only materially. Thus, if medical residents, compelled to choose between giving up their careers and materially cooperating in morally unacceptable procedures, give in to the pressure, their example may lead other health care personnel, who could resist without great sacrifice, to cooperate materially when they should not. This bad effect might suffice to require the residents to forgo what otherwise would be morally acceptable material cooperation."

[100] "Now they tried to make the elderly and noble Professor Eleazar eat pork. But he preferred an honourable death to a tainted life and was determined never to break God's law. So he spat out the meat and freely submitted to torture. His long-time friends amongst those in charge of the unlawful sacrifice took him aside and urged him to save himself by bringing along some meat of his own choosing and pretending it was the meat of the pagan sacrifices. But Eleazar had lived virtuously since childhood, had earned his grey hairs with distinction and had faithfully followed God's holy Law. Making a high resolve, worthy of such a man, he declared himself quickly, saying he'd rather go to hell. "Such dissimulation would be unworthy of someone my age," he said. "What if the young should think that in my ninetieth year I've changed to some alien religion. It would defile my life and disgrace my old age if just for the sake of living a little longer I should lead the young astray by my pretence. In any case, even if I can evade the punishment of men for a time, I can never escape the grip of the Almighty. Better for me to submit manfully now, act my age and leave to the young an example of how to live and die well." He was led to execution and those who had only a little while ago conspired to save him now turned against him, because they thought his words sheer madness. And so he died, leaving us all an example of virtue and fortitude." (2 Macc 6:18–31)

[101] "If any man therefore sets aside even the least of the Law's demands and teaches others to do the same, he will be least in the kingdom of heaven" (Mt 5:19); "Woe to the world because of the things that cause sin! Such things must come, but woe to the one through whom they come." (Mt 18:7 *cf.* Lk 17:1–2); "Better to have a millstone tied around your neck and be thrown into the sea than to cause one of these little ones to be led into sin" (Mt 18:16); "Woe to you scribes and pharisees, you hypocrites! You shut the door of the kingdom of heaven in men's faces" (Mt 23:13); "Woe to you scribes and pharisees, you hypocrites! You travel over seas and land to win a convert and then make him twice as fit for hell as you are yourselves"(Mt 23:15).

[102] 1 Cor 8:10–13; 10:25–29; Rom 14:1–3, 15, 20–21. Cf. *CCC* 2284 and 2287: "Scandal is an attitude or behaviour which leads another to do evil... Anyone who uses the power at his disposal in such a way that it leads others to do wrong becomes guilty of scandal and responsible for the evil that he has directly or indirectly encouraged."

All these concerns, it seems to me, depend for their bite upon two things. First, a strong sense of moral solidarity with others: that we are, contrary to Cain, our brothers' and sisters' keepers; that our example does, as the Maccabean heroes saw, impact upon those around us; that as Jesus commanded we must always be lights to the world, trying to draw people into the life of God's kingdom and wary of ever being an obstacle to their entry; that our actions, as Paul insisted, do affect the whole body of Christ. The contemporary secular writer on complicity, Mark Sanders, has likewise been concerned to show that a rich sense of human "folded-together-ness" will yield a much broader sense of co-responsibility for evils than will an individualism which focuses only upon personal blame, especially for grave acts of commission.[103] For this very reason, concerns about material cooperation in evil are likely to be less keenly felt in cultures strongly affected by Dutch-Calvinist or Anglo-American individualism. But recent philosophical work on the role of community and tradition in the formation of moral character and theological work on original and social sin suggest that we ignore the social dimension of our personal choices at our peril.[104]

Furthermore, these concerns depend for their piquancy upon a high sense of the moral possibilities of one's neighbour. I have suggested above that, all too often, "harm minimisation" programmes at least implicitly amount to giving up on the other party as beyond anything better.[105]

---

[103] Sanders, *op. cit.*

[104] Amongst those who have written about the communitarian basis of human valuing and choice, Alasdair MacIntyre, Charles Taylor and Michael Sandel are best known. On original and social-structural sin see: John Paul II, *Reconciliatio et Paenitentia*: Apostolic Exhortation on Confession, 2 December, 1984: esp. §16 and John Paul II, *Sollicitudo Rei Socialis*: Encyclical on Social Concerns, 30 December, 1987: §46.

[105] "Harm minimization" has become the catch-phrase for all sorts of programmes, including the nudge-nudge-wink-wink strategy of some parents, schools and pastors who tell their charges (perhaps cynically, perhaps well-meaningly) "if you can't be good, be careful". Beginning with "if you can't" falsely implies that the particular behaviour – sexual promiscuity, abortion, substance abuse, speeding – is somehow unavoidable. Grisez (*op. cit.* Vol. 3 (1997), pp. 98–102) shows that this is not only incompatible with sound philosophy but also with defined Catholic teaching. Of course addicts are in a different category to those who simply choose to take drugs, and youthful sexual experimenters in a different category to predatory adults. There are degrees of gravity, and in some cases personal responsibility may be reduced. But reverence for the human person, hope even amongst great difficulties and faith in the power of divine grace counsel against despairing of anyone, even adolescents and addicts. Many people do in fact overcome vices and addictions, but that is only likely to happen if we as a community continue to hold out the

Catholic healthcare agencies must always seek to offer our society witness to the dignity of the human person as a free and responsible agent made for greatness and therefore worthy of our high expectations and our best care.

4.3. *Cooperation, the love of self and authenticity of life*

Christ commands that we *love* our neighbours as *ourselves*. Appropriate self-love includes an abiding concern for the kinds of persons we become as a result of our choices. Much reflection upon the nature of the human act, virtue, and implicitness, immediacy and proximity in cooperation reflects a sharp awareness of the reflexive effects of human choice and habit, and of how corrupting cooperation can be. As Cathleen Kaveny has pointed out:

> The Catholic moral tradition is agent-centred. According to this tradition, the most significant aspect of a human action is the way in which it shapes the character of the person who performs it. Thus, according to traditional Catholic doctrine, individuals who engage in deliberate evildoing harm themselves far more than they do those who suffer injustice at their hands.... Agents who engage in actions [foreseeably but unintentionally resulting in the death of a human being], particularly if they do so repeatedly, can accustom their minds and hearts to causing the death of another human being, albeit unintentionally.... The experience of causing the death of a fellow human being can be brutalizing, even if it is justified. While not sinful in itself, it can make sinning in the future far easier.[106]

---

hope (and provide the support) that make this possible. If, on the other hand, we class people amongst the "moral incurables", best dealt with by damage limitation measures, then we may only confirm the despondency that drives or maintains many in their tragic situation. It is hard to see how condom counselling and injecting rooms can avoid communicating the message to the users, especially young people: "To be honest we don't have much faith in you, and we do not really expect you to give up sex/drugs. It would be nice if you did, and we'd help you if you showed willing. But since you probably won't, we'll at least help you avoid harming yourself or others."

[106] Kaveny, *op. cit.* pp. 303–4 citing Vatican II, *Gaudium et Spes* §27.

This consciousness of the self-creative effects of choice and thus of the burden of personal responsibility[107] and integrity[108] helps explain Christ's apparently extreme exhortations – to cut off from ourselves everything that might cause us to sin and enter heaven disabled rather than hell with all our limbs; to avoid sexual promiscuity, violence and acquisitiveness not just of action but even of the mind; and to be ever conscious of that which emerges from the deepest recesses of the human heart.[109] A keen sense of who we are, of our Christian identity and vocation, is essential to moral discernment in all difficult cases. But a healthy resistance to occasions of, temptations to, and habits of sin is especially necessary when discerning whether to cooperate materially.[110] Sometimes this will require sacrificing our personal preferences, our desire to get on well with others, our

---

[107] John Paul II, *Evangelium Vitae*: §74: "Formal cooperation in evil... can never be justified either by invoking respect for the freedom of others or by appealing to the fact that civil law permits it or requires it. Each individual in fact has moral responsibility for the acts which he personally performs; no one can be exempted from this responsibility, and on the basis of it everyone will be judged by God himself (*cf.* Rom 2:6; 14:12)."

[108] Kaveny, *op. cit.* p. 306 notes that "unless the cooperator exercises great vigilance, the principal agent's description of that action could 'seep' into the cooperator's moral identity, by affecting the self-conception of the kinds of acts of which he or she is capable.... Particularly if working in very close quarters with the principal agent, it is very difficult for a cooperator not to get swept up into the principal agent's project in such a way that he or she wills its success."

[109] Mt ch 5; 12:33–35; 15:10–20; 18:8–9; 23:25–28; Mk 7:20–21; Lk 12:34.

[110] One bad side-effect of some material cooperation is the temptation to cooperate formally. There are two ways this might happen. First, one may so often, repeatedly, habitually and unreflectively engage in some act of material cooperation that one becomes blasé about it, dulled to the evil side-effects, and happy enough to admit them as one's intention. Second, cooperation often involves engaging in a team relationship with the principal wrongdoer(s) and can thus lead to deeper involvement, including a sharing of purposes. Thus, merely material cooperation can easily become the occasion of formal cooperation. This might explain why the traditional advice has been that the more remote the cooperation, the easier it is to justify. Grisez (*op. cit.* 1997, pp. 879–880) observes: "In materially cooperating, one's very accepting of the action's primary bad side effects – its contribution to another's wrongdoing and that wrongdoing's bad effects – can have bad effects on oneself. One's feelings can be adversely affected.... Performance, especially repeated performance, tends to become habitual; interaction with wrongdoers tends to generate psychological bonds and interdependence. Thus, cooperation often leads to opportunities and temptations to engage in further cooperation. Even if the initial cooperation otherwise is morally acceptable material cooperation, the further cooperation may be formal or, though still material, morally unacceptable. In this way, material cooperation often is an occasion of grave sin."

institutional commitment, or even the great goods that our actions might otherwise achieve.

5. Conclusion

I opened this paper with a reference to Sanders' recent book, *Complicities*, which suggests that many South African thinkers during the era of apartheid colluded with that system. I said that we might consider the extent to which Catholic intellectuals and professionals have likewise cooperated with evils that the Catholic bioethical tradition opposes, including the very cases of formal and wrongful material cooperation repudiated by the magisterium in recent years.

In the second half of my paper I have suggested some reasons for this. Some go to the heart of action theory and other aspects of fundamental morality. Some ways of reading the human act allow almost any cooperation in evil to which the moralist is already inclined (upon other grounds) and empty the categories of cooperation of their usefulness. Some "tax-lawyer" and secular-individualist approaches to morality present moral law, tradition and community as enemies of human fulfilment. On this view the function of ethics advice is helping healthcare managers and professionals avoid being caught engaging in flagrant violations of "Church law" while sailing as close to the wind as possible. This will orient us in a particular way to questions of cooperation. A contrasting orientation to morality sees life as the pursuit of perfection or, in Christian terms, the wholehearted commitment to the holy love of God, neighbour and self – a far from easy undertaking, even under grace, and one that will make the agent much more sensitive to issues of cooperation in evil. The apparently arcane subject of this book therefore matters not just in itself but also for what it says about the whole project of the moral and spiritual life.

4

Tax lawyers, prophets and pilgrims: a response to Anthony Fisher

M. Cathleen Kaveny

What should be our basic stance toward questions of complicity with evil? In the concluding paragraph to his paper, Bishop Fisher presents us with a clear choice: we can be "tax lawyers" dedicated to finding the loopholes in the moral law that will allow us to do what we want while preserving a patina of moral righteousness. Or we can be prophets, seeking Christian perfection and pursuing "the wholehearted commitment to the holy love of God, neighbour and self."[1]

We owe a debt of gratitude to Bishop Fisher for framing the issue in this way. Most discussions of complicity with evil, particularly within the Roman Catholic context, immediately descend to, and happily remain at, the level of detailed case analysis. The application of the scholastic categories used to analyse cooperation not only demands both precision and rigour, but also permits vigorous and frequently inconclusive debate. As Bishop Fisher notes, at least one weary participant in the debate has concluded that in the entire field of moral theology, there is no question more difficult than cooperation in evil.[2]

---

[1] Fisher, 64.

[2] Fisher, *op. cit.,* 28, citing Henry Davis SJ, *Moral and Pastoral Theology.* Vol. 1. London: Sheed & Ward 1958: 342.

But why is the debate so important? What, really, is at stake in questions of complicity with the wrongdoing of others?[3] Unfortunately, the authors of the moral manuals have been far too reticent on this question. In this context, Bishop Fisher helpfully reminds us that complicity problems involve not only judgments about what we *should do*, but also judgments about who we *should become*. Our actions affect not only the external world, they also affect our very selves: every act we perform and every choice we make shapes our moral character. In turn, our character – our moral personality – significantly determines the set of actions we will never choose to perform, those we will choose to perform under certain circumstances, those we will perform gladly, and those (such as acceptance of martyrdom) that we hope we will have the grace and strength to perform, should it be God's will for us to do so.

This reciprocal relationship between an agent's character and his or her actions holds true, of course, with respect to *each and every* action that we perform. What, then, is so special about complicity with evil? Does it make a moral difference that my action contributes to or makes use of the wrongful action of another, and thereby in some sense "intertwines" with the wrongful will of another? I agree with Bishop Fisher that it does make a difference.[4] By performing an action that we know will be intertwined with the wrongful act of another person, we run the risk that their description of our action (given from the perspective of someone who views us as a component in their wrongful plan) will "seep" into our own description of the act, and that we will deceive ourselves about the evolution of our own attitudes toward the wrongdoing of the other party. This problem is particularly dangerous in cases of ongoing cooperation.

---

[3] I have argued elsewhere that the broad topic of complicity with evil includes two foci. First, we need to consider situations in which an agent believes that his or her action (or its fruits or by-products) will be used by another agent in committing a wrongful act. This, of course, is the situation considered by Roman Catholic manualists under the heading of "cooperation with evil." Second, we need also to consider situations in which an agent is contemplating making use of the wrongful act (or its fruits or by-products) of another agent in performing his or her own action. In my view, a new category of "appropriation of evil" needs to be developed in order to deal with this set of cases, which includes such issues as whether or not it is permissible to make use of tissue obtained from electively aborted fetuses. See M. Cathleen Kaveny, "Appropriation of Evil: cooperation's mirror image". 61 (2000) *Theological Studies*: 280–313.

[4] I do not mean to deny that this question merits far more rigorous theoretical attention than it has thus far been given. It seems to me that Grisez's theory would deny that there is anything special involved in complicity *per se* that cannot be accounted for in a double effect analysis. See his appendix on cooperation in Germain Grisez, *The Way of the Lord Jesus, Vol. 3: Difficult Moral Questions*. Quincy, IL: Franciscan Press 1997, pp. 871–98. But this is a question for another day.

For example, a secretary typing a series of blackmail letters for her boss may initially describe her role as nothing more than "typing every letter my boss puts in my inbox." She may hope that his blackmail plans will fail, or at the very least, she may be entirely indifferent to their success. But over time, her attitude toward her boss's illicit scheme may change. She may begin to want it to succeed, perhaps because of the new prosperity that it brings to the office. Since her own immediate behaviour will not have changed at all from the beginning of the process (she is still doing nothing more than typing the letters), it would not be difficult for her to deceive herself about the evolution of her own intentions, or to fail to recognise the shift in her moral identity until long after it had occurred, if she ever recognises it at all.

When viewed in this broader perspective, it is clear that Bishop Fisher is quite correct to force us to pay attention to fundamental questions of who we want to become, and to the way in which complicity in the wrongdoing of others may shape our character. Let us look more closely, therefore, at the two fundamental options with respect to character that Bishop Fisher presents for our consideration.

1. Catholic Tax Lawyers

According to Bishop Fisher, those who fall under the label of Catholic Tax Lawyers believe that "the role of the moral adviser is to help people find a way around the moral law or at least a way of sailing as close to the wind as possible without falling in the water."[5] In order to achieve this objective, the first task of Catholic Tax Lawyers is to ensure that the desired cooperation falls into a category that is not deemed always impermissible (*i.e.*, formal cooperation), or highly problematic apart from special circumstances (*e.g.*, immediate material cooperation). Bishop Fisher writes that Catholic Tax Lawyers "end up reducing almost all cases of cooperation in evil to material not formal cooperation and almost all cases of material cooperation to permissible cooperation."[6]

What means do Catholic Tax Lawyers use to achieve their objective? According to Bishop Fisher, their basic strategy is to manipulate traditional casuistical categories used to analyse cooperation cases. For example, he claims that they attach "traditional-sounding labels" such as "[d]uress, probable opinion, proportionate reason, the common good, prudence and *epikeia* ... to these novel schemes for paying less moral tax."[7] Fisher also

---

[5] Fisher, 56.
[6] Fisher, 57.
[7] *Ibid.*

contends that they defend their lax approach by drawing upon moral theories popular in the 1970's (such as proportionalism or situationism) or in the contemporary discussion (such as virtue theory or narrative theory).[8]

Why do Catholic Tax Lawyers approach cooperation problems in this manner? Fisher's answer reflects his perception of the close connection between acts and character; in his view, what Catholic Tax Lawyers do both reflects and confirms what they value and how they choose to constitute their moral identities. More specifically, he claims that Catholic Tax Lawyers "seem to regard the moral law as a series of constraints on freedom and happiness, rather than the roadmap to both."[9] Consequently, they strive to get around that law, rather than to probe its requirements more deeply. The values they promote indicate that for them, "[p]reference fulfilment and social acceptability are paramount."[10] Fisher fears that "conversion and self sacrifice have little place" in their framework for living.[11]

2. Prophetic Witnesses for the Kingdom

Turning away from the framework of the Catholic Tax Lawyer, Bishop Fisher encourages us to view our lives – and the problems of complicity with evil that we encounter in the course of them – through an entirely different conception of human flourishing, which is found in the lives of Prophetic Witnesses for the Kingdom of God. He suggests that "[t]he goal of human life is the pursuit of holiness – becoming lights to the world, more and more conformed to Christ, living stones of God's house and temples of his Holy Spirit, perfect like our Heavenly Father."[12] Fisher maintains that this fundamental orientation toward the purpose of life will dramatically affect our attitude toward questions of complicity with evil. He writes:

> A keen sense of the privilege that it is to be apostles and prophets, saints and even martyrs, and a deep commitment to the new evangelisation, will give us a greater sensitivity to the issues of cooperation in evil than any purely secular account which sees the principles of cooperation as, at best, useful action guides and, at worst, hindrances to human freedom and happiness.[13]

---

[8] Fisher, 56–57.
[9] Fisher, 56.
[10] *Ibid.*
[11] *Ibid.*
[12] Fisher, 58.
[13] Fisher, 59.

Bishop Fisher maintains that a specifically Christian understanding of the nature and purpose of life will give us special perception, or as he puts it, "greater sensitivity" concerning problematic aspects of cooperating in the evildoing of another. It is not entirely clear to me what he means by this claim. He could be merely affirming the traditional Catholic claim that faith gives us greater insight into the universal moral law, which is binding upon all persons, believers and non-believers alike.[14] Yet it seems to me that he wishes to say something more; it seems to me that he wants to claim that questions of cooperation with evil raise special issues for those who have received the gift of faith, issues which do not arise for all persons of good will and solid moral character.[15] In other words, he seems to be asserting that Christians, called to be prophetic witnesses to the kingdom of God, are bound by certain distinctive role-related obligations, the fulfilment of which may be threatened or compromised by cooperating with evil.

What distinctive obligations, what distinctive values, does Fisher believe are threatened by cooperation? On my reading of his essay, the threatened obligations and values seem to revolve around preserving a type of purity for Christian persons and institutions, which is primarily characterized by clear separation from the activities of an unredeemed, sinful world. For example, consider Section 4.1 of his paper, which is entitled "Cooperation, the love of God and the christification of the human person," and which is the first of three sections in which he considers why cooperation is problematic from a Christian perspective. In my view, it nicely encapsulates his basic position. Bishop Fisher worries that "instead of offering a distinctively Christian form of witness to the life of God's kingdom, even to the point of martyrdom, we settle for more comfortable collaboration with the powers of this world."[16]

What are the dangers of this "comfortable collaboration"? Significantly, Bishop Fisher does not emphasise the possibility of being drawn into evildoing oneself, or of becoming hardened to the continuing existence of sin in the world. Instead, he identifies a different set of dangers, which have to do with preserving a type of spotless purity for the Christian as a member of the Church, which is defined by its distance from evildoers and evildoing. In his analysis, moral purity seems to be entwined with cultic purity.

---

[14] See *e.g. Catechism of the Catholic Church*, para. 1960.

[15] Obviously at issue here is the general question of the distinctiveness of Christian ethics, a topic which has long been hotly debated in Roman Catholic circles. In my view, the best overview of the issue (which in fact involves a number of distinct sub-issues) is Vincent MacNamara, *Faith and Ethics*. Washington DC: Georgetown University Press 1985.

[16] Fisher, 58.

First, he argues that cooperation contaminates the Church, writing that "As Paul puts it so graphically, rather than lifting up Christ and his Church to God we take them down into the bed of the prostitute."[17] Second, he suggests that we dishonour God in cooperating, by bringing his power and generosity into contact with evil. "We damage our relationship with God, making God a cooperator in evil, for it is only by God's power that we are supported in being and by God's permissive will that we are free to do what ill we do."[18] Third, he suggests that cooperation taints us, thereby destroying our religious and moral credibility. "We also compromise our ability to give witness to the true and the good as *alteri Christi*, and so undermine the progress of the Gospel."[19]

3. A stark choice

Bishop Fisher thus presents us with a stark choice. We can either be Catholic Tax Lawyers or we can be Prophetic Witnesses. It is clear that for him there is no choice; we must be prophetic witnesses for the kingdom of God. But his clarion call for prophetic witness forces us to face a radical question. Why not view each and every case of cooperation with a jaundiced eye? Why not say that the preservation of purity is paramount? It is impossible, of course, to avoid all cooperation with evil; our actions contribute to the actions of others in ways we cannot foresee, even if we engage in some amount of investigation prior to acting. But why not impose a positive duty upon Christians to perform due diligence before acting, and adopt a norm prohibiting all reasonably foreseeable cooperation with evil?

When Bishop Fisher's paper is reviewed as a whole, the pressing nature of these questions becomes apparent. More specifically, his analysis of cooperation with evil in the context of his discussion of the Prophetic Witness can be characterized as negative in its focus, in two significant respects. First, he spends comparatively little time in his paper sympathetically considering the positive reasons *why* morally upright agents typically enter into situations involving cooperation with the wrongdoing of another. He acknowledges, of

---

[17] Fisher, 58–59.

[18] Fisher, 59. This point is not entirely clear to me. If we wrongfully cooperate with evil, we are using our God-given freedom to "do what ill we do." But if our cooperation is morally permissible, we are by definition not doing evil. Our action is, however, being used to further the wrongdoing of another party. Does it dishonour God for me to engage in permissible cooperation? If so, does this rule out all cooperation with evil, or does the dishonour to God count as one of a number of factors that must be weighed in determining whether cooperation is permissible?

[19] *Ibid.*

course, that they do so not because they value cooperation in and of itself, but rather because they want to realize a good or avoid an evil that cannot be achieved or avoided in any other way.[20] Nonetheless, in my judgment, the considerations that would justify cooperation are not presented in as vivid or sympathetic a way as the considerations that render it morally problematic. Second, Bishop Fisher's account of the shape of a Christian life of prophetic witness is largely *negative* in its concern; we are told in some detail what it does *not* consist in (*i.e.*, contamination by close connection to the evildoing of others or immersion in situations in which there is significant potential for doing evil oneself), but we are not told in similar detail about what such a life *positively* involves.

Unfortunately, because his concerns are negative in their focus in the twofold manner just described, Bishop Fisher does not address a certain set of hard questions that I believe are of great importance. More specifically, he does not consider whether and when one's positive obligations, articulated and understood in light of one's specifically Christian commitments, might entail some cooperation with the actions of evildoers. For example, consider Section 3.5, his basic discussion of "Reasons to cooperate and not to cooperate." Without exception, the examples of licit cooperation he provides involve lay individuals struggling to meet their obligations to their family and maintain a decent lifestyle. Bishop Fisher does not characterize the obligations of any of these individuals in specifically Christian terms, and does not adduce specifically Christian (or even broadly religious) reasons in support of their decision to cooperate. By contrast, his discussion of the reasons against cooperation liberally draws upon specifically Christian theological language and imagery.[21]

In my view, this differential treatment of reasons in favour of cooperation and reasons against cooperation is worrisome in several respects. First, the disparity in treatment does not seem to be justified by reference to the source discussions in the moral manuals, which were not particularly concerned with distinctively Christian obligations in any aspect of their

---

[20] Seven of the seventeen "traditional examples" Bishop Fisher gives are of permissible material cooperation. Six are of formal cooperation, which is always impermissible; four additional examples are of impermissible material cooperation (Fisher, 33). In Section 3.5, entitled "Reasons to cooperate and not to cooperate," about one-third of the text is devoted to the former set of reasons and two-thirds to the latter set. Of the five contemporary examples discussed (Fisher, 33–49), four involve impermissible cooperation, while one involves permissible cooperation.

[21] The considerations Bishop Fisher offers in favour of cooperation are confined to Section 3.5. In contrast, he not only develops a general set of considerations against cooperation in Section 3.5 but also devotes the remainder of the paper to the specifically theological considerations against cooperation.

discussion of cooperation.[22] Second, Bishop Fisher is surely to be commended for introducing such concerns with reference to his discussion of the reasons against cooperation: he is drawing upon the insights of Germain Grisez, Servais Pinckaers and other post-Vatican II moral theologians who have long strived to integrate the Good News of the Gospel into their moral reflection. Yet there is no theological or logical reason that a discussion of the reasons in favour of cooperation should not be recast and updated in a similar way. Third, and most important, I fear that the disparity in treatment will lead an unwary reader of Bishop Fisher's paper to mistakenly conclude that Catholic morality is two-tiered: persons of ordinary goodness may on occasion cooperate with evil, but the more saintly course of action is always to refrain from cooperating.

But Bishop Fisher's paper does suggest the possibility of a *tertia via*, a way of understanding cooperation within an explicit stance toward the Christian life that is neither that of a Catholic Tax Lawyer nor a Prophetic Witness.[23] Bishop Fisher notes, for example, that while some traditional authors set up a presumption "*against* cooperating, even materially, in evil unless there is a sufficiently grave reason to warrant proceeding," others "thought that the presumption should be *in favour of* the cooperator's chosen good or neutral act, unless the foreseen effects of unintentionally assisting someone else's evil acts are so grave that one should abstain from so acting."[24] If the only available stances toward the Christian life are the two described by Bishop Fisher, how can we account for the second group of moralists? They do not seem to fall into either the category of the Catholic Tax Lawyer or the category of the Prophetic Witness. How could they legitimately support a presumption in favour of proceeding with the good or morally neutral act, despite the fact that it would contribute to someone else's wrongdoing?

In the remainder of this response, I would like to flesh out the theological dimensions of the *tertia via* to which Bishop Fisher's paper only alludes. In

---

[22] Persons of public authority in the Church faced special questions involving scandal, but they do not seem to me different in principle from those faced by persons of public authority in general.

[23] Bishop Fisher seems to explicitly allow for this possibility, but then immediately denies its relevance with respect to the debate over cooperation: "I do not mean to suggest that there are only two moral world views or that everyone (or anyone) fits neatly and clearly into one or the other. Rather I am suggesting that two polarities are particularly evident in the scant literature on cooperation and that this might help to explain why two people can judge the same example of cooperation so differently." (57) As I argue below, the fundamental trouble with this typological polarity is that it tends to assume that all positions evincing a deep skepticism about cooperation are theologically and morally legitimate, and that all positions more sympathetic toward cooperation are theologically and morally suspect.

[24] Fisher, 31.

essence, I will attempt to recast the presumption in favour of cooperation in theological terms, just as Bishop Fisher has done for the presumption against cooperation. First, by drawing upon *Lumen Gentium*, I will attempt to give this *tertia via* a name. In my view, the path it describes is neither that of the Catholic Tax Lawyer nor that of the Prophetic Witness for the Kingdom. Instead, it is that of the Pilgrim on the Way to the New Jerusalem. Second, I will argue that those who fall in this category do not necessarily fall prey to the key moral defects that Bishop Fisher associates with the Catholic Tax Lawyer approach, which I believe is best viewed as a distorted form of the Pilgrim on the Way approach. Third, I will suggest that the Prophetic Witness approach is also haunted by its own distorted form, which can be as destructive of the new evangelisation as the distortions entailed by the Catholic Tax Lawyer approach. I call this distorted form the Celestine approach.

4. Pilgrims on the Way to the New Jerusalem

Like Bishop Fisher, I agree that the stance of the Catholic Tax Lawyer is unacceptable. I also agree that there is a strong monastic strand in the theological tradition that has honoured the importance of a radical witness to the values of the inbreaking kingdom of God. For centuries, the role of prophetic witness to the values of the inbreaking kingdom was associated almost exclusively with religious life. For example, Aquinas recognized that it would not be "fitting" for clerics to kill evildoers, because it is inconsistent with the values of the New Law, the law of the kingdom inaugurated by Christ.[25] In the twentieth century, however, it became more and more apparent that the vocation of prophetic witness was not limited to members of the clergy. Chapter V of *Lumen Gentium* recognizes that "all Christians in any state or walk of life are called to the fulness of Christian life and to the perfection of love, and by this holiness a more human manner of life is fostered also in earthly society."[26] As the life of Dorothy Day and the history of the Catholic Worker Movement in the United States demonstrates, for some members of the laity, their particular call to holiness means an uncompromising commitment to the values of the kingdom of God.

But there is another way of conceptualizing the tenor of our earthly lives, also a legitimate option, also rooted in the tradition, also expressed in the documents of the Second Vatican Council: some Christians legitimately understand their calling not as Catholic Tax Lawyers, nor even as Prophetic Witnesses, but instead as Pilgrims on the Way to the Heavenly City. They too

---

[25] *S. Th.*, II-II, q. 64 art. 4.

[26] *Lumen Gentium*, chap. 5, para. 40, in Austin Flannery OP (ed) *Vatican II: The Conciliar and Post Conciliar Documents* (New Revised Edition). Dublin: Dominican Publications 1996: 397.

are called to holiness, but their call takes a different form, which emphasizes an appropriate sensitivity to the degree to which the kingdom of God is yet incomplete in our midst. The timbre of this approach is captured in chapter 7 of *Lumen Gentium*:

> Already the final age of the world is with us (*cf.* 1 Cor. 10:11), and the renewal of the world is irrevocably under way; it is even now anticipated in a certain real way, for the Church on earth is endowed already with a sanctity that is real though imperfect. However, until there be realized new heavens and a new earth in which justice dwells (*cf.* 2 Pet. 3:13), the pilgrim Church, in its sacraments and institutions, which belong to this present age, carries the mark of this world which will pass, and she herself takes her place among the creatures which groan and travail and yet await the revelation of the sons of God (*cf.* Rom. 8:19–22).[27]

In my view, the sensibilities of Pilgrims on the Way are best articulated in the writings of St. Augustine. These Pilgrims know that they are presently sojourning in the City of Man, even as they are striving to reach the Heavenly City. In their sojourns, they know that they will come in contact with saints and sinners; they will often know not which is which. They are concerned to do the will of God, but not to secure for themselves complete insulation from those who are wrongdoers. As Augustine tirelessly repeats, separating the wheat from the chaff is God's job, not ours; it will therefore be achieved in God's time, in the end of time, not before.[28]

What is the difference between those who view the task of Christians to be Prophetic Witnesses and those who view that task as being Pilgrims on the Way? The basic theological difference, in my view, revolves around the question how Christians are to live with the realization that the Kingdom of God has already been inaugurated, but is not yet fully instantiated.[29]

---

[27] *Lumen Gentium*, chap. 7, para. 48.

[28] See, *e.g.*, St. Augustine, *Answer to Letters of Petilian, Bishop of Cirta*, in Philip Schaff (ed) *Nicene and Post-Nicene Fathers: Vol. 4*. Grand Rapids MI: Eerdmans 1979, 519–628, book 1, chaps. 18–20.

[29] The stand one takes on the appropriateness of Christian participation even in a just war also frequently depends on which pole of the tension one emphasises. See *e.g.* National Conference of Catholic Bishops, *The Challenge of Peace: God's Promise and Our Response*. Washington DC: United States Catholic Conference 1983, para. 58: "Christians are called to live the tension between the vision of the reign of God and its concrete realization in history. The tension is often described in terms of 'already but not yet': *i.e.*, we already live in the grace of the kingdom, but it is not yet the completed kingdom. Hence, we are a pilgrim people in a world marked by conflict and injustice. Christ's grace is at work in the world; his command of love and his call to reconciliation are not purely future ideals but call us to obedience today."

The advocates of the Prophetic Witness place priority upon pure and unambiguous witness to the values of the inbreaking Kingdom; as Bishop Fisher has suggested, avoiding association with evildoers is a key component of this witness.

In contrast, the stance of the Pilgrim on the Way places priority upon the need to respond to those suffering the effects of the sin that is still in our midst, especially to secure justice and mercy for those vulnerable to the wrongdoing of others. On occasion, promoting these goals may require some amount of cooperation with individuals and institutions perpetuating wrongdoing. It is by reflecting upon the requirements of neighbour love in a sinful world that Augustine justified the participation of Christians in the machinery of government, including in the waging of war.[30] These activities, in Augustine's time no less than in our own, brought Christians into close proximity with evildoers, and doubtless on many occasions resulted in the conscription of the fruits or by-products of the activities of the Christians into the wrongful plans or purposes of others.[31]

The Pilgrim on the Way is very concerned to address certain questions that the Prophetic Witness stance tends to sideline. More specifically, as described above, Bishop Fisher's description of the Prophetic Witness stance focuses primarily on *what must not be done* so as not to compromise that witness, rather than on *what must be done* in order to realize the Kingdom. In contrast, the Pilgrim on the Way stance emphasizes the urgent necessity of building up the Kingdom, of performing the corporal and spiritual works of mercy in this world that still "groans and travails" with sin and its effects. Consequently, while the Prophetic Witness emphasizes the risks and dangers of cooperating with evil, the Pilgrim on the Way highlights the good that it can accomplish – and more importantly, insists upon seeing this good not merely as a "secular" or "natural" good, but also as a crucial part of the evangelical mission of the Church.

For example, Bishop Fisher writes that "sometimes this [salutary resistance to cooperating with evil] will require sacrificing our personal preferences, our desire to get on well with others, our institutional commitment, or even the great goods that our actions might otherwise achieve."[32] Pilgrims on the Way would worry that this general description does not sufficiently recognize the specifically Christian values that weigh in favour of a decision to cooperate.

---

[30] See Paul Ramsey, *War and the Christian Conscience*. Durham NC: Duke University Press 1961, chaps. 2–3.

[31] "And then how do you dare to say to Christians, "What have you to do with the kings of the world?" because Daniel suffered persecution at a king's hands, and yet not look back upon the same Daniel faithfully interpreting dreams to kings, calling a king lord, receiving gifts and honors from a king?" St. Augustine *op. cit.*, book 2, chap. 212.

[32] Fisher, 63–64.

Their worries would be intensified by an examination of Section 2.1 of Bishop Fisher's analysis, which considered the question of when and whether it is permissible for American Catholic hospitals to cooperate in sterilization procedures. Unfortunately, Bishop Fisher does not elaborate in any detail the reasons why many American Catholic hospitals found themselves in the position of discerning whether or not to cooperate in sterilization procedures, or what specifically religious values or goods militate in favour of cooperation. He mentions them only in connection with a comment on the recent revision to the Ethical and Religious Directives binding on American health care facilities, stating that because of this revision, "no longer can a Catholic institution claim that financial, political, or other pressure justifies cooperation with sterilisation."[33]

To someone sympathetic to the stance of the Pilgrim on the Way, however, it would be important to articulate the specific concerns that prompted American moral theologians to dust off the concept of cooperation with evil in order to analyse issues involving the affiliation of Catholic and non-Catholic health care facilities. In the early 1990's, the health care financing and delivery system in the United States underwent extensive restructuring, largely in order to respond to increasing pressures to control the spiralling costs of health care. Most hospitals found themselves scrambling to participate in "integrated delivery networks" that frequently involved two or more hospitals, several physician groups, and ancillary services such as laboratories or x-ray facilities. Hospitals that did not participate in such networks would quickly find themselves squeezed out of existence, because they could not compete for contracts to provide a whole range of services to groups of patients whose costs were covered by insurance companies, the government, or employers. Catholic hospitals, which accounted for about 15% of all community hospital admissions in the nation, and which constituted the largest single group of not-for-profit hospitals, were not immune from these new pressures.[34]

Obviously, the best course of action would be for Catholic facilities to join together to form their own integrated delivery networks. In some cases, that course of action was followed. In other cases, however, it was not an available option: the available partners included only non-Catholic health care facilities. What then? Some, like Germain Grisez, have suggested that the Catholic sponsors should simply refuse to cooperate with institutions that provide services inconsistent with Catholic teaching. Instead, such facilities should voluntarily go out of business: they should sell their hospitals, and put

---

[33] Fisher, 38.

[34] Current statistics can be found in Catholic Health Association, "Role and services of the Catholic Health Association". Available online at http://chausa.org/aboutcha/chamiss.

their financial resources and energies into caring for marginalized groups, such as women facing crisis pregnancy and the elderly.[35] The benefits of this strategy flow from the fact that it avoids moral dangers involved in cooperating with evil identified by Bishop Fisher on behalf of the Prophetic Witness Approach, including the real possibility of scandal. Pilgrims on the Way, however, would be concerned about several drawbacks that would follow from entirely eliminating a Catholic institutional presence from the heart of the American health care financing and delivery system.

What are those drawbacks? Pilgrims on the Way might identify several. First, eliminating a Catholic institutional presence could mean the loss of the crucially important insight that health care is best viewed as a corporal work of mercy, not as a commodity to be provided in the most cost-effective manner possible. With the increasing influence of for-profit health care, along with financial pressures of third-party payers such as insurance companies and employers to control costs, the counterweight provided by the powerful and articulate voice of Catholic health care facilities may be absolutely essential to protecting vulnerable populations.[36] For example, compassionate care for those who suffer from chronic, serious disabilities with no prospect of improvement is extremely difficult to justify on the increasingly prominent view of health care as a commodity to be provided as efficiently as possible in a way that achieves measurable results. In contrast, it is the central case for health care viewed as a corporal work of mercy.[37]

Second, and relatedly, the presence of Catholic values in mainstream American healthcare may serve as a bulwark against the erosion of commitment to certain negative moral absolutes that are under sustained attack in our culture. For example, in many Western countries, the pressure to legalize euthanasia and physician assisted suicide has been considerable in the last fifteen years. In my view, that pressure cannot effectively be counteracted by abstract arguments against the taking of innocent life or on behalf of the dignity of every human person, no matter what his or her state of dependence. Instead, the three-dimensional fears of pain, diminution of autonomy, and vulnerability, to which the pro-euthanasia activists appeal so effectively, can only be countered by the three-dimensional witness of

---

[35] Grisez, *op. cit.*, 401–402.

[36] Some, like Grisez, have suggested that Catholic health care facilities have not done a particularly good job with regard to these tasks. In my view, the proper response to that suggestion is for Catholic health care facilities to strive to do a better job, not to abandon the task entirely.

[37] For a discussion of some of the threats to vulnerable populations arising from changes in the health care financing and delivery system, see M. Cathleen Kaveny, "Managed care, assisted suicide and vulnerable populations". 73 (1998) *Notre Dame Law Review*: 275–310.

the corporal works of mercy, which reveal the truth about the intrinsic values of caring for the dying, and dying well oneself, even when faced with an inexorable illness such as Alzheimer's Disease or terminal cancer. Furthermore, this witness to the true meaning of health care must not be cabined off into Catholic hospices entirely separated from mainstream services obtained by millions of Americans every day. We must demonstrate that our treatment of the terminally ill is continuous with our vision of *all* health care as a work of mercy.

To take another example, the ongoing presence of Catholic health care may have helped reduce the availability of abortion in the hospital setting, even while making positive ways of dealing with crisis pregnancy more available within the community. Not infrequently, a Catholic partner has been able successfully to convince a potential non-Catholic partner to cease all provision of abortion services as a condition of the affiliation – a fact that has not escaped the critical attention of Planned Parenthood and other family planning associations.[38]

Third, the values generally at stake in maintaining a powerful Catholic presence in the American health care system are frequently instantiated in particular affiliations. Sometimes, for example, the only way certain populations in rural areas or in inner cities will continue to receive the health care they need is if a Catholic health care institution affiliates with a non-Catholic institution: neither institution may be fiscally strong enough to "go it alone." The concern expressed in the Gospels for the weak and the vulnerable, as well as Jesus's own injunction that "whatsoever you do to the least of my brothers, that you do to Me" (Mt 25:40), can furnish a powerful motivation for a Catholic health care provider not to abandon a population in need.

Ideally, therefore, the kind of person that a Pilgrim on the Way aspires to be is someone who is animated by the virtue of mercy, which, citing Augustine, Aquinas defines as "heartfelt sympathy for another's distress, impelling us to succour him if we can."[39] Aquinas maintains that the virtue of mercy is the highest of all virtues through which we relate to our neighbour,[40] and states that the "sum total of the Christian religion consists in mercy, as regards external acts."[41] Someone who approaches cooperation problems animated by the Christian vision of mercy seems to me to be very far from Bishop Fisher's Catholic Tax Lawyer, whose only aim is to pay as little moral tax as possible.

---

[38] A group called "Merger Watch" tracks and publicizes this phenomenon. See http://www.mergerwatch.org.

[39] *S. Th.*, II-II, q. 30, art. 1.

[40] *S. Th.*, II-II, q. 30, art. 4.

[41] *S. Th.*, II-II, q. 30, art. 4, rep. ob. 2.

I do not mean, of course, to deny the dangers of cooperating with evil in the health care context. Nor do I mean to suggest that the considerations adduced above can be invoked automatically to justify any and every affiliation proposed for a Catholic health care institution. Each case needs to be examined on its merits; in particular, the complicated legal and financial relationships entailed by an affiliation need to be evaluated according to the norms governing formal and material cooperation. My concern has simply been to stress that the goods to be gained (and evils to be avoided) by the maintenance of a Catholic presence in the American health care system are not merely secular in nature, but touch upon matters intimately connected with the Gospel message. It is these matters that are of acute concern to the Pilgrim on the Way, and it is these matters that can make factors supporting a decision to cooperate very difficult to ignore for someone trying to grow in the virtue of mercy.

5. The Catholic Tax Lawyer: a distorted form of the Pilgrim on the Way

What is the relationship of the Catholic Tax Lawyer stance to that of the Pilgrim on the Way? In my view, the former is best viewed as a distorted form of the latter. While analysing the relevant distortions in detail is beyond the scope of this response, my diagnosis is that the Catholic Tax Lawyer has failed to hold on to both prongs of the tension between "Already" and "Not Yet" with respect to the instantiation of the Kingdom of God in our midst. Instead, it has let go of the first prong, the "Already" prong. Consequently, it proceeds as if the values of that Kingdom are entirely irrelevant to the manner in which we conduct our lives here and now. On this distorted view of the moral life, as Bishop Fisher sketched, minimizing pain and maximizing personal autonomy are frequently the only values that actually count.

To the extent, therefore, that any moralists actually hold to the propositions Bishop Fisher attributes to the Catholic Tax Lawyer, they are legitimately criticized. But in my view, the same criticisms are not applicable to the stance of the Pilgrim on the Way to the New Jerusalem. Despite its emphasis on the "Not Yet," the Pilgrim on the Way stance does not entirely let go of the "Already." It does not act as if the values of the Gospel are entirely irrelevant in this fallen world. In particular, as I describe below, it refuses to dismiss the negative moral absolutes as unworkable, and does not fail to recognize that they protect and support important positive values (*i.e.*, the dignity of each human being).

According to Bishop Fisher, the Catholic Tax Lawyer stance frequently entails a commitment to a proportionalist methodology in evaluating human acts. In contrast, precisely because it does not let go of the "Already," the Pilgrim on the Way stance entails no such commitment. A Pilgrim on the Way can and should believe that: (a) there are intrinsically evil acts, (b) that it is never morally justifiable to perform an intrinsically evil act, and (c) that it is never permissible to perform any evil action (whether it is wrong by reason of its object or because of its circumstances) in order that good may come. Furthermore, as a specification of these commitments, a Pilgrim on the Way can and should believe that it is never permissible formally to cooperate in the wrongdoing of another.

This does not mean, however, that there will be no disagreement about what actions, concretely, qualify as intrinsically evil acts, and what actions, concretely, qualify as formal cooperation in evil. But this sort of disagreement need not be attributed to the fact that the advocate of the apparently more "lax" position belongs to the party of the Catholic Tax Lawyers. It may simply be the sort of good faith disagreement about particular applications of the natural law that is to be expected this side of the eschaton.[42]

Bishop Fisher levies an additional criticism against the Catholic Tax Lawyers: he charges them with the corrupt practice of manipulating casuistical categories in order to achieve a desired result.[43] One might reasonably conclude that he is charging the Catholic Tax Lawyers with being "jesuitical," which is commonly used pejoratively to mean being "designing; cunning; deceitful; crafty." This is a serious and painful charge; as Bishop Fisher well knows, from the time of the Reformation, it has frequently been levelled by Protestants against any Catholic attempt (by Dominicans as well as by Jesuits) to use the tools of casuistry to sort through difficult moral issues. Yet in the face of Protestant polemics of this sort, the Church has rightly defended the merits of the Catholic casuistical tradition. Its strength, its honour, and its worthiness to be embraced by honourable and faithful Christians can be found in its effort to take into account the values or goods at stake in a particular situation, in all their diversity, complexity, and even ambiguity.

It is true, of course, that casuistical categories can be manipulated or abused by those acting in bad faith, or misunderstood and misapplied by those acting in good faith. Bishop Fisher is right to highlight the dangers of abuse and misapplication, just as the Protestant reformers were right to criticize instances where casuistical tools were in fact cynically manipulated by Catholics in order to achieve a result desired on other

---

[42] Bishop Fisher acknowledges this type of disagreement with respect to the dispute between advocates of the "natural meanings" approach and advocates of the "intended acts" approach to action theory, discussed below.

[43] ...er, 56–57.

grounds. Nonetheless, I think it is important to place these dangers in some perspective, in two ways.

First, I think it is crucial to differentiate between an abuse of casuistical tools, on the one hand, and a use of those tools that is based on legitimately different perceptions of the moral reality of a situation, on the other. Sometimes, those differing perceptions can pertain to the appropriate moral description of an action. For example, Bishop Fisher has noted that those who advocate a "natural meanings" account of intention would not describe some actions (such as a craniotomy performed on an unborn child lodged in its mother's birth canal) in the same way as those advocating an "intended acts approach."[44] It may be that in time, one or the other approach to action theory is decisively shown to be mistaken. At this point in time, however, both approaches are consistent with Christian moral reflection.

Alternatively, the difference could simply involve strategic judgment regarding the best way to promote the Gospel message in this culture. One person, for example, might be sympathetic to the Pilgrim on the Way approach in principle, or as applied in other times and places, but nonetheless believe that successful evangelization today requires Christians to present a clear, forceful and uncompromising alternative to the cacophony of postmodern culture. Such a person would adopt the attitude toward cooperation attributed by Bishop Fisher to the Prophetic Witness stance as a matter of strategy, not a matter of principle. In contrast, another person might believe that the best strategy for evangelization is active engagement with others. For example, such a person might think that the best way of opening hearts and minds to the full message of the culture of life would be to make common cause with people of good will, attempting to show how their own truest insights are best accommodated within a Catholic Christian framework regarding the nature and purpose of life. Such a person would be drawn to the Pilgrim on the Way approach as a matter of strategy, rather than as a matter of principle.

Second, I think it is important to recognize that *no* philosophical or theological tool or method or stance is immune from abuse or misapplication, *including* a denunciation of casuistical abuse accompanied by a call for prophetic clarity. For example, many of those favouring legalized euthanasia have suggested that the doctrine of double effect is precisely the sort of manipulative or bankrupt intellectual tool denounced by Bishop Fisher in his discussion of the Catholic Tax Lawyers. Issuing their own call for prophetic clarity, these advocates of legalized euthanasia have argued that it is casuistical hair-splitting to differentiate between (1) a physician who withdraws treatment from a patient foreseeing, but not intending, the

---

[44] Fisher, 50.

death of that patient, and (2) a physician who withdraws treatment with the purpose of causing that patient's death. On this basis, they contend that euthanasia is morally justified, and should be legalized.[45]

But this line of argumentation is specious. It is, in fact, the abuse of the criticism of casuistical abuse. To reject the distinction between intended consequences and merely foreseen consequences in the context of medical–moral decision-making is both unsound and dangerous. It is unsound because it fails to account for a key aspect of the character-constituting aspects of choice: we stand in a different relationship to the effects we intend in our actions, either as an end or as a means, than we do to their foreseen-but-unintended side effects. It is dangerous because it renders people unable to distinguish between morally different types of actions, making them more likely to approve impermissible actions (*e.g.* euthanasia by omission) on the basis of their superficial resemblance to actions that they realize are clearly permissible, and may even be required for the benefit of the patient (*e.g.* withdrawal of extraordinary means, fore-seeing but not intending death).[46]

In my view, then, the Pilgrim on the Way can and must avoid the moral distortions endemic to the Catholic Tax Lawyer approach. That does not mean, of course, that there will not continue to be painful disagreements between Pilgrims on the Way and Prophetic Witnesses about how to analyse a particular situation involving cooperation with evil, or how to assess the relative values at stake within it. It does mean, however, that these disagreements should be viewed as disagreements within the family of faith, not as disagreements that tear our faith asunder.

6. The Celestine: a distorted form of the Prophetic Witness

I have suggested that the Catholic Tax Lawyer stance should be viewed as a distorted form of the Pilgrim on the Way – distorted not because it gives priority to the "Not Yet," but because it entirely lets go of the "Already" with respect to the instantiation of the Kingdom of God in our midst.

---

[45] See, *e.g.*, the opinion of the United States Court of Appeals for the Second Circuit in *Vacco v. Quill* (1996). 80 F.3d 716 (2nd Cir.), *reversed by* Vacco v. Quill, 521 U.S. 793 (1997).

[46] The cumulative force of Ronald Dworkin's rhetoric in *Life's Dominion* (New York: Knopf 1993) is calculated to encourage readers to make this move. Most of his powerful examples involve decisions to withhold or to withdraw life-prolonging treatment, which could have been made in a way consistent with Catholic teaching pertaining to end-of-life decision making. Without explicit argument, Dworkin equates these decisions with decisions that involve intentional killing of the patient, suggesting to the unwary reader that all medical decisions that foreseeably hasten the patient's death are to be viewed as morally the same.

I would now like to consider the possibility that the stance of Prophetic Witness is plagued by its own distorted form, which is the mirror image of the distortions plaguing the Pilgrim on the Way. I will call this distortion the stance of Celestine, in order to evoke its vivid sense of the complete (or nearly complete) presence on earth of God's heavenly kingdom. The stance of the Celestine is distorted not because it gives priority to the "Already" (as does the stance of the Prophetic Witness) but because it entirely lets go of the "Not Yet." This distortion has been present in numerous sectarian movements that have arisen throughout the history of Christianity, which are premised on the belief that by cooperating with the grace of God, the righteous can fully instantiate the Kingdom of God on this earth, or at least on a well-bounded portion of it.

In my view, the dangers to authentic Christian faith and life posed by the Celestine are no less severe than those posed by the Catholic Tax Lawyer. In fact, it seems to me that many of the dangers of the former are mirror images of those of the latter. More specifically, just as the Catholic Tax Lawyers' functional obliteration of the "Already" leads them to pay too little attention to negative moral obligations, particularly negative moral absolutes, so the Celestines' functional obliteration of the "Not Yet" leads them to pay too little attention to the positive moral obligations entailed by the corporal works of mercy.

How and why does this come about? First, it seems to me that in a world that is still marked by sin and brokenness, the only way one can hope to preserve the illusory sense of being untouched by its effects is to focus nearly exclusively on negative moral obligations. The negative moral absolutes bind always and everywhere; it is therefore always possible to comply with their requirements. It is impossible, however, to fulfill each and every positive moral obligation in each and every circumstance. We may have one loaf of bread and two hungry families to feed. We may have enough time to visit either the criminal in prison or the person dying in the hospital, but not to visit both. For this reason, positive obligations, including the obligation to perform the corporal works of mercy, are frequently called "imperfect" obligations. They are morally binding only under certain conditions, including suitability of time and place, and adequacy of resources.

It is important to remember, however, that the term "imperfect" does not mean that they are somehow flawed or second-rate obligations. Looking at the Latin roots of the term, one could say that it means they are unfinished or uncompleted.[47] The fact that it is impossible for us to meet the needs of each and every needy person is a result and a sign of the perduring effects of

---

[47] The Latin verb "perficio, perficere, perfeci, perfectum" means "to finish" or "to complete."

sin in this world. Those effects cannot be ignored by those who grapple seriously with their positive obligations to perform the corporal works of mercy, and who realise that nothing they can do will ever be enough to meet the crying needs of every person made in the image and likeness of God. Such persons will not sin in failing to meet the needs of others for legitimate reasons. They will however, experience sorrow, and pray more intensely for the full realization of God's kingdom in our midst.

In contrast, reconceptualizing the shape of a well-lived life exclusively in terms of preserving one's own purity, largely by complying with a set of negative moral obligations, allows one to minimize, if not entirely avoid, a necessary existential confrontation with the "Not Yet" dimension of the Kingdom. One can not only avoid sin, but fully and successfully comply with the requirements God has set for us, if those requirements are exhaustively understood in terms of avoiding the commission of certain acts.[48]

If one's sense of oneself as living a flourishing Christian life is defined only or primarily by compliance with the negative moral absolutes, a clear strategy emerges. Avoid each and every occasion of sin, never put yourself in a position where you might conceivably be tempted to violate the moral law, and create for yourself an environment that reinforces your convictions and will-power in every respect. But a major difficulty with this strategy is that it renders it extremely difficult to meet positive obligations which, although they are not binding always and everywhere, are binding here and now. The Celestine may look for ways to minimize positive moral obligations, or perhaps may suggest that a positive moral obligation cannot be an absolute obligation if it involves any temptation to wrongdoing whatsoever.

In addition, the quest for purity, when taken to an extreme, may directly militate against performing the corporal works of mercy. We feed the hungry, clothe the naked, comfort the broken-hearted. But we cannot control what they do with their full bellies, warm bodies, and restored wills. A doctor may save the life of two young gunshot victims whom she suspects will continue selling illegal drugs while becoming increasingly involved in gang activity. Even if customary analysis of the problem of cooperation does not extend so far, the fact remains that we have in some way been the "but-for" cause of the evildoing of those whom we help in this way: it would not have occurred but for our assistance. The only way to be certain to avoid helping other people who will go on to do evil is to forswear helping

---

[48] Many moral theologians writing after the Second Vatican Council, both so-called "liberals" and so-called "conservatives," have criticized the moral manuals for "legalism." By this they generally mean a reduction of the Christian moral life to refraining from the commission of certain sins, primarily those that directly violate the commandments of the decalogue.

other people entirely, or at least people who do not entirely share our worldview. In this light, it is not difficult to see why many Celestines have advocated a form of sectarianism throughout the ages.

Looking at the mind-set of the Celestine from a theological perspective, it seems to me that there are several fundamental problems. First, it may be possible to avoid all cooperation with evil by living a very constricted life, dealing only with people one believes are upright, and interacting as little as possible with those one believes to be sinful. Even a very cursory glance at the Gospel tells us, however, that a life spent shrivelled by the fear of violating a negative moral obligation, and blind to one's positive obligations in love and in justice to oneself and to others, is in no way a model Christian life.

Second, it wrongly suggests that the absolute nature of negative moral norms entails the claim that their violation is always a more serious sin. But a moment's reflection suggests that this is not the case. For example, Aquinas teaches that telling a lie may be only a venial sin, while failing to give alms under certain conditions may be a mortal sin.[49]

Third, it wrongly suggests that the absolute nature of some negative moral norms (*i.e.*, one is never permitted to violate them, even in order to achieve a good end) translates into an absolute (or nearly absolute) obligation to avoid any temptation to violate these and other negative moral norms. Clearly, that cannot be the case; we know, after all, that Jesus was subjected to (and allowed himself to be subjected to) temptation in the desert at the end of forty days of prayer and fasting.[50] Moreover, such a posture tacitly undercuts belief in the power and day-to-day effectiveness of the sacramental framework that Catholics believe was divinely given to the Church in order to allow the members of the Body of Christ to grow in faith, hope and charity.[51] Through the sacraments of baptism, confirmation and the Eucharist, the faithful are provided with the moral and spiritual strength to go forth and evangelize the world, recognizing its goodness even while they resist its temptations to wrongdoing.

---

[49] *S. Th.*, II-II, q. 110, art. 4 ("Whether Every Lie Is a Mortal Sin") and II-II, q. 32, art. 5 ("Whether Almsgiving Is a Matter of Precept").

[50] Mt 4:1–11, Mk 1:12–13, Lk 4:1–13.

[51] "The sacraments are efficacious signs of grace, instituted by Christ and entrusted to the Church, by which divine life is dispensed to us. The visible rites by which the sacraments are celebrated signify and make present the graces proper to each sacrament. They bear fruit in those who receive them with the required dispositions." *Catechism of the Catholic Church*, para. 1131. In my view, the necessary renewal of moral theology called for in the wake of the Second Vatican Council cannot succeed if it is carried out in separation from systematic theology and liturgical theology. Unfortunately, Bishop Fisher's clarion call to living a radical commitment to holiness in Christ Jesus does not mention the Church's sacramental framework, a primary means by which God communicates divine grace to the members of the Church.

Fourth, the Celestine position seems particularly to minimize the nature and function of the sacrament of penance in the ongoing life of the Christian. Not only does this minimization undermine the importance of the sacraments in the way described in the preceding paragraph, it also assumes that Catholics are living their lives without a "net" – that the commission of a serious sin will irretrievably destroy their relationship with God. Yet this is not the case. Divine forgiveness, mercy, and renewed grace are constantly available to us through the sacrament of penance, which participates in the decisive act of God's life-giving mercy in his death and resurrection. The "net" provided by the sacrament of penance constantly reminds us that the point of forgiveness and mercy is freedom for new life, which requires freedom from crippling fear. The "net" provided by the sacrament of penance is not an excuse for a Christian to fall into sin deliberately or with callous negligence, any more than the net in the centre ring is an excuse for a master circus performer deliberately or negligently to fall off the high wire. Rather, in both cases, the purpose of the net is to set one free to act in a way that most fully expresses who one is called to be.

What is the upshot of these reflections on the theological problems with the stance of the Celestine? In my mind, there are two. First, they suggest that we cannot approach cooperation problems with the tacit assumption that there are no dangers involved in drawing the boundary around impermissible cooperation *too broadly*, in the attempt to create a moral demilitarized zone whose purpose is to give us a sufficient buffer against enemy attacks. Bishop Fisher and I are no doubt in agreement that the enemy is sin and the associated suffering it causes; one can sin by failing to meet one's actual positive obligations, as well as by violating one's negative obligations. Drawn too broadly, the boundary around impermissible cooperation impedes the fulfilment of positive obligations; drawn too narrowly, it impedes the fulfilment of one's negative moral obligation not to contribute to the wrongdoing of others. The boundary around impermissible cooperation, therefore, needs to be drawn in just the right place.

Second, I think it is important to bear in mind the true and intimate relationship between negative moral obligations and positive moral obligations. Negative obligations should be viewed as the foundation and necessary precondition of positive obligations: compliance with them is not an end in itself.[52] More specifically, we must not do evil because so doing renders

---

[52] In my view, one of the contributions of enduring importance made by Pope John Paul II in *Evangelium Vitae* is its clear-sighted recognition of the intimate relationship between negative moral obligations and positive moral obligations. The "culture of life" called for by the Pope does not merely reject practices such as abortion and euthanasia, it also calls for active protection of the weak and vulnerable.

us unfit to fulfill the positive obligations of the Gospel: to preach the Good News of Christ's death and resurrection and to practise the corporal works of mercy toward all of those created in God's image and likeness, in the manner of the Good Samaritan. We must not cooperate too closely with the evildoing of others for precisely the same reason. Too intimate involvement with the wrongful acts of others, particularly acts that violate the basic dignity of human beings made in the image and likeness of God, will render us unable to recognize the corporal works of mercy we are called on to perform, and will leave us badly equipped, both morally and psychologically, to perform them.

These final two points, of course, are equally telling against the stance of the Catholic Tax Lawyer. The tension between the "Already" and the "Not Yet" is an ineliminable feature of our lives; it can be a fruitful tension, provided that neither pole is entirely relinquished. The emphasis of the Prophetic Witness for the Kingdom on the "Already" is a gift to the entire community of the faithful, to the degree that it does not entirely let go of the "Not Yet." At the same time, the emphasis of the Pilgrims on the Way on the "Not Yet" contributes its own wisdom to the degree that it does not entirely let go of the "Already." By contrast, the distortions created by the willingness of the Catholic Tax Lawyers to let go of the "Already" and by the willingness of the Celestines to let go of the "Not Yet" mean that both will ultimately lead us away from the full truth of our redemption in Christ Jesus.

7. Conclusion

I would like to conclude this essay, not with a statement, but with a question. Is it possible that the disagreements over cooperation with evil in most or all of the case studies described by Bishop Fisher can fruitfully be analysed in terms of the differences in emphasis favoured by Prophetic Witnesses, on the one hand, and Pilgrims on the Way, on the other?[53] Bishop Fisher rightly notes that "[o]ne of the side-effects of cooperation in evil not identified in the traditional manuals is the academic controversy it can occasion, including a great deal of uncharitable *ad hominem*."[54] In my view, this defect in charity is not limited to one side of the discussion. Perhaps we

---

[53] The sections dealing with these examples are entitled "Sterilisation in American Catholic hospitals," "Condoms against HIV," "Drug injecting rooms in Australia," "Counselling pregnant women in Germany," and "Support for improving abortion laws."

[54] Fisher, 40–41.

will all be able to minimize instances of academic uncharitableness if we let our attention linger upon the broader theological values that our conversation partners are attempting to protect in their analysis of specific cooperation problems, before we turn to the theological values we fear that their analysis might sacrifice.

5

Cooperation with past evil and use of cell-lines derived from aborted fetuses[1]

Alexander R. Pruss

1. Introduction

The production of a number of vaccines involves the use of cell-lines origin-ally derived from fetuses directly aborted in the 1960s and 1970s. Such cell-lines, indeed sometimes the very same ones, are important to on-going research, including at Catholic institutions. The cells currently used are removed by a number of decades and by a significant number of cellular generations from the original cells. Moreover, the original cells extracted from the bodies of the aborted fetuses were transformed to produce the cell-lines, since otherwise they would be incapable of the kind of culturing that is required.

It is generally acknowledged by ethicists, including many Catholic ones generally considered to be orthodox, and by the U.S. bishops, that the use of the cell-lines in connection with the production of vaccines is morally permissible. It does not appear that there is a relevant qualitative difference between use of the cell-lines in vaccines and in research. One might argue that there is certainty of benefit from a vaccine, while the benefits of research are uncertain. However, in any given case of the administration of a vaccine to an individual, it is far from certain that such administration will be of benefit to that individual. After all, the individual might never come in contact with someone infected with the disease in question, particularly if

---

[1] This article was first published in the *Linacre Quarterly* (71 (2004): 335–350) and is reprinted here with some stylistic revisions.

the disease is now uncommon in the individual's locale. Yet it is morally certain that *some* of the administrations of the vaccine will be beneficial. This is parallel to the fact that while any one research project might not be beneficial, the history of biomedical research makes it extremely probable, indeed morally certain, that *some* project involving the use of such cell-lines will be beneficial. There may, of course, be quantitative difference between the cases – the probabilities and benefits may not be equal – but the difference does not seem to be a qualitative one. Therefore, if one accepts use of the cell-lines in vaccines, one should accept their use in research in at least some conceivable and perhaps actual circumstances.

The main argument I am interested in in favor of use of these fetal cell-lines proceeds by first granting that the initial abortion and extraction of cells from the now dead fetus was morally gravely illicit. However, the connection between the currently used derived cells and the abortion and original derivation is sufficiently remote that the use becomes licit. Not all fruit of a poisoned tree is poisoned: it can be morally acceptable to profit from a remote evil act. The currently used cells are temporally and generationally far removed from the originally extracted cells. Moreover, they are ontologically removed by the initial transformation which rendered them capable of the unlimited growth needed for culturing. Furthermore, at least in the case of some of the research projects, though perhaps not in the case of some of the vaccine projects, neither the individuals nor the companies involved in the initial illicit act profit economically from the continuation of the research. Those making use of the cell-lines may be quite unaware of their origin, or may have been unaware at the beginning of the use thereof, and hence cannot be said to be tacitly or overtly approving the illicit source. Finally, it can be argued that as a matter of fact the continued use of these cell-lines, unlike perhaps the use in other cases of stem-cell lines, does not increase the market demand for new cell-lines, and therefore does not encourage further illicit acts.

The arguments in favor of use of these cell-lines are powerful and I believe largely convincing. But nonetheless, those who have a strong belief in the illicitness of the initial abortion and cell-line derivation feel a *discomfort* with the use of the lines, even if they are convinced by the arguments. For instance, Dr Edmund Pellegrino, in conversation, talked about the need for us to sometimes "get our hands dirty". Yet it appears that if the arguments are sound, the hands of the researcher need not get at all dirty: the researcher is doing something morally quite unobjectionable, it appears. Any discomfort thus appears to be mistaken and irrational, a confusion between an arguably rational disapproval of the initial illicit acts of abortion or derivation and an irrational distaste for the use of biological material ultimately produced by these acts.

It is this discomfort that I wish to analyze in this paper. I will argue that there is indeed a rational source for the discomfort. Now, there are two radical positions one can hold vis-à-vis the use of cell-lines as described. First, one might think that such use is intrinsically wrong, and hence cannot be tolerated no matter what the benefits or distance from the original illicit activity. This is the "radically restrictive" position. Second, one might think that given the distance from the initial derivation, current use of the cell-lines is permissible for *any* beneficial purpose, no matter how small, providing that such use does not lead to other bad results. This is the "radically permissive" position. Obviously, anyone who holds that the initial abortion and derivation were morally licit will take the radically permissive position, but it appears that by the above arguments *everyone* should take this position. And indeed there are Catholic ethicists convinced of the grave wrongfulness of the initial acts who take the radically permissive position. The qualifier that the use does not lead to other bad results is there in part because these ethicists may, however, think that knowing about some uses of the cell-lines may cause a third party unjustifiedly to come to the mistaken belief that, say, abortion is morally permissible.

I will argue, however, that both of the extreme positions are mistaken. The right position is that one may use the cell-lines for *sufficiently beneficial* purposes but not for other purposes. I will argue for this claim without making use of the "scandal" argument that use of the cell-lines may cause people to come to mistaken beliefs about, say, the morality of abortion or be encouraged to commit that or other illicit acts. Neither am I interested in arguments that such use of cell-lines may create a demand for more cell-lines in the future. My lack of interest in these arguments is purely analytic: these arguments may indeed be sound for all I know, in which case a more restrictive position is appropriate. What I would like to examine, however, is what we can say *solely* on the basis of the facts about cooperation with past evil.

Moreover, while there are very important bioethical issues at stake in the concrete issue of cell-lines, what interests me most is not the actual case but the general issue of cooperation with past evil. It is by analyzing cooperation with evil that I shall arrive at my "moderate" position. Moreover, surprisingly, this analysis may throw light on what *prima facie* seems a completely different but no less thorny issue: the problem of the justification of retributive punishment.

2. The radically restrictive position

I take it for granted, both for the purposes of the argument and *in persona propria*, that intentional abortion is a morally illicit act of killing a juridically innocent human person. Moreover, one can argue that extracting tissue or organs from the body of a dead person is only permissible with the permission of that person or of a responsible proxy – this is because appropriate respect for the bodies of deceased persons is called for. An aborted fetus does not give implicit or explicit permission for such extraction. On the contrary, one might argue that one can always presume non-cooperation between the non-willing victim of an illicit killing and the person involved in the killing. If so, then even without considering the question of proxies, we might argue that no one complicit in the killing would be permitted to extract the tissue.

And in any case, no one complicit with the abortion counts as a "responsible proxy" if abortion is an illicit killing of a human person. For instance, our society rightly takes a parent to lose his or her parental rights after intentionally attempting to inflict grave harm on a child. Since abortion is such a grave harm, those parents complicit in the abortion cannot count as responsible parties, and hence their permission for the use of tissue or organs would be irrelevant. Furthermore, there does not appear to be any other responsible party around to authorize such extraction. The two exceptions would be a case where either the mother is coerced into undergoing the abortion and consents to the use of the tissue or organs, and a case where the father disapproves of the abortion and consents to the tissue or organ extraction. Nonetheless, I am not aware of any evidence that any of the cell-lines generally under discussion originate in one of these two exceptional circumstances. Thus, it seems, the initial extraction was wrong. Moreover, this extraction was almost surely done in close cooperation with the person performing the abortion, and that gives further reason to think it wrong, and indeed seriously so.

But it does not follow from the fact that something is the product of a gravely illicit action that we are not permitted to make good use of it. One can licitly live in a building originally built by slave labor. If an ethnic group were entirely wiped out through genocide, there would be no moral imperative to keep their land vacant until the end of history. A policeman only makes a living because of the immoral actions of criminals.

Now, one might make a specific argument that in the case at hand, the use of the cell-lines is illicit. For instance, if one believes that the end-result of the derivation process is still a part of the body of the deceased fetus, then one may think that the argument that prohibited the derivation continues to prohibit use of the cell-line. However, such reasoning would be incorrect. First, as has been pointed out by Kevin Fitzgerald,[2] the cells have been

---

[2] Kevin Fitzgerald sj, panel discussion on research on cell-lines derived from aborted fetuses, Georgetown University, 2004.

biologically transformed after the extraction, and we do not consider tumor-cells, being similarly transformed, to be a part of the body of the individual. Second, if an organ is transplanted from one person to another, new cells grown from the organ in the body of the recipient are surely no longer the donor's cells.

The only other argument that comes to mind here is that each human being has some special right, perhaps akin to "copyright" or "patent right", to his genetic code. And indeed laws to that effect have been passed in some locales and there are societal attitudes that might make this somewhat plausible. Thus many people would object to the research use of DNA extracted without the person's permission from items that are no longer a part of the person's body and indeed are no longer even the person's property, such as hair clippings left behind in the hair-dresser's shop. The one exception they might make would be in the case of DNA thought to possibly originate from a guilty party, such as DNA extracted from items left at a crime scene. I must confess that I do not have a convincing response to this argument apart from the autobiographical statement that it has little traction on me. I see no reason why I should have ownership over the information contained in my DNA, if this is information that neither was created by me nor was created by someone else who has ceded title to me. My parents did not create my DNA in the way that an artist creates a painting: the process involved apparent randomness. The only candidate for a creator of the DNA is God, and I have no evidence that God has ceded ownership over this information to the individuals in whom it is embodied, or, for that matter, that God prohibits the use of this information.

3. The poisoned tree

3.1. Formal and material cooperation with evil

Traditionally, cooperation with evil is divided into the formal and the material.[3] You formally cooperate in someone's illicit action provided the achieving of the same illicit object of activity is a part of your action plan. Here, I am assuming that agents have action plans that stipulate both final goal and intermediate sub-goals, each of which I call an "object", and each of which is something intended, either as an end or as a means. An action is said to be "intrinsically wrong" provided some object of it – say, someone's being humiliated (as opposed to humbled, which would be a good thing) – is such that it is always wrong to intend it. One formally cooperates with an

---

[3] E.g., Dominic M. Prümmer, *Handbook of Moral Theology*, transl. G. W. Shelton. London: Collins Roman Catholic Books 1957, Section 233.

illicit action if and only if one cooperates in such a way that one intends to achieve that object which is illicit. Any other kind of cooperation is material. It analytically follows from the above that formal cooperation in an intrinsically wrong action is intrinsically wrong, since it involves intending a goal the intending of which is intrinsically wrong.

Cooperation in evil can be understood in many ways. We can understand it as helping the agent achieve his illicit goal, or we can understand it as being "an accessory after the fact", say, by praising the agent or by helping the agent avoid the just consequences of the action. Each of these can be formal or material: on the formal side we can praise the agent in such a way as to express our standing behind his illicit intention, or on the material we can praise the agent in a more general way, for instance by saying: "I respect your character." Finally, we are only interested in cases of *conscious* cooperation: if I leave a broom outside my door for five minutes and you use it to break a window, typically I will not have cooperated in any morally interesting way.

Now we have a fairly clear handle on what merely material cooperation before the agent's action is like: it is engaging in activity that I know helps the agent do his nefarious deeds, even though I do not intend to help him do the nefarious deeds *qua* nefarious. Thus, if I own a cutlery store and know that some tiny percentage of customers will use the knives for immoral violent purposes, I am materially cooperating with evil. But as this example shows, material cooperation need not be wrong. However, observe that there is a *presumption* against such cooperation. One needs a sufficiently serious reason to engage in it. If the only licit use knives had was something completely trivial, I would not be justified in such cooperation with evil. But there are many important morally licit uses of knives, and so I am justified.

Material cooperation after the fact is a much more hazy affair. Helping a criminal escape may count as such. Again, note that such cooperation can be licit. For instance, if a child has stolen a candy bar in a state that punishes every theft with death, I would be justified in helping the child escape punishment. (Note that the alternative of imposing punishment myself would not be available if I wasn't authorized by the child's parents.) The cooperation would be merely material unless thereby I expressed my sharing in the child's illicit intention. Nonetheless, there would be a presumption against such cooperation. One would need to have a sufficiently good reason for it.

3.2. Profiting from evil

Almost everything I said so far is well-known material. But it is now that things get interesting. The question before us is whether *profiting* from the effects of an evil act counts as cooperation with evil after the fact. I shall assume that the profiting does not constitute *formal* cooperation. The cooperation is not a part of a plan of action of one's own that includes the same intended illicit goal as the evildoer had.

Consider five cases of profiting from evil:

THE VIOLINIST.   You are a world-famous violinist and need a new kidney to survive. One of your fans, without consulting you, kills Jones, whom he knows to be a good genetic match for you and to have signed an organ donor card. The murderer is caught. The hospital finds that Jones's kidneys match you and only you. No one but you would benefit from Jones's kidney and so you accept the kidney.

THE POLICEMAN.   You became a policeman in order to make money for your family. You would not make enough money for your family were there no crime, since as it happens being a policeman is the only job you would be able to get.

THE TOURIST.   You walk on pavement in Rome originally built by slaves.[4] It would be less comfortable to walk on bare earth, and so you profit from the fact that ancient Romans forced people into slavery.

THE HISTORIAN.   Using historical records, you reconstruct the dynamics of prisoner–guard interaction at Auschwitz, and on that basis you come up with a new sociological theory that explains many things, and has application to making our society a better one.

THE TYPHUS RESEARCHER.   You discover that some of the gravely immoral typhus experiments done at Auschwitz produced data that is scientifically valuable. You use this data in your own research, building on it.

I think that in each of these five cases, the actions described are defensible. Nonetheless, I believe that there are significant differences between the cases. I believe that the cases of THE VIOLINIST and THE TYPHUS RESEARCHER trouble us most. The case of THE TOURIST may trouble us: we may and I believe should feel a discomfort walking on the paving stones and thinking of the blood of the slaves killed while building Rome. But I think that neither THE POLICEMAN nor THE HISTORIAN needs to trouble us at all. You may not share these intuitions, but they appear quite plausible to me. I hope you will find these intuitions even more plausible when I finish.

Now, we could say that the discomfort felt about the cases of THE VIOLINIST, THE TYPHUS RESEARCHER and THE TOURIST is simply due to confusion. The people feeling the discomfort have not been able to

---

[4] This example is due to William May, panel discussion on research on cell-lines derived from aborted fetuses, Georgetown University, 2004.

internalize the fact that *clearly* by accepting the organ, using the data and treading on the pavement they are not in any way contributing causally to the bad things done or expressing approval for them. Or perhaps transference is at fault: we transfer the moral disapproval of the building of the pavement onto our walking on that pavement, albeit in attenuated form. But the idea that the discomfort is confused is not plausible, I believe. Arguments that imply that it is confused are missing an important moral dimension that really is there.

I think it is fairly clear that the Aristotelian prudent agent *would* feel discomfort about THE VIOLINIST, THE TYPHUS RESEARCHER and THE TOURIST. But not about THE POLICEMAN and THE HISTORIAN. Yet all five cases are cases of profiting from evil actions in the past. Observe, too, that the distance that the evil actions are removed from the present is not what makes for the difference between the problematic and unproblematic cases. After all, the policeman and the violinist both deal with very recent evils, while our historian and typhus researcher both profit from an evil that is equally far back. And the paving stones are much older than the crimes the policeman solves or the structure of institutionalized evil that the historian studies.

Rather, the difference, I submit, is that our violinist, tourist and typhus researcher all profit from evil in more or less the way that the malefactor intended for the evil to be profited from. The violinist's fan killed Jones in order for the violinist to have Jones' kidney. The "owners" of the slaves intended to build a pavement that people could walk on, maybe even hoping it would be part of the appeal of an "eternal" city. It is plausible that the Nazi doctors did research on typhus in part to promote the scientific understanding of the disease (and in part to further the war effort on the Eastern Front). But the criminal rarely commits crimes in order to encourage us to employ policemen, and Rudolf Höss certainly did not serve as the commandant at Auschwitz in order to provide historians with a case study of a radically unjust society. I think this difference is significant. And I hope to soon show why.

3.3. Frustrating evildoers

There is a particular satisfaction people get from seeing evil punished and an indignation at seeing the wicked prosper. Traditionally, the problem of evil included *both* the sufferings of the innocent *and* the apparent good fortune of the wicked. The latter is no longer felt to be as problematic nowadays – such a concern is felt to be too "vengeful". Nietzsche offered us the idea that the satisfaction we got from seeing people suffer was what made sense of retributive punishment: Fred has hurt Bob and since Fred cannot undo

Bob's pain he repays Bob by giving him the joy of seeing Fred suffer. Nietzsche is wrong, I think. If he were right, then society would sufficiently do justice by lying to Bob that Fred is suffering, and surely that is not sufficient for justice.

I think there is *something* right about the feeling that it is appropriate that the wicked should be punished, that they should suffer, not just *pour encourager les autres*, but that justice may be done. It is a feeling too deeply tied to our notions of justice to go away. The main argument against this is simply that the idea is too vengeful for it to be appropriate for us, that there can be no rational justification for it. I will argue that there *is* a rational justification that has a surprising connection with our attitudes towards profiting from evil, though I am aware that my story does not exhaust what is to be said about retributive punishment – I know that there are cases where the story is insufficient.[5] As a general methodological point, when we have a deep-seated affective ethical intuition, one not obviously rooted in a vice but connected with a virtue (in this case, that of justice), there is a presumption in favor of a project of justifying rather than explaining away this intuition.

Observe that it is not just *any* suffering of the wicked, or just any suffering that is causally connected with the crime, that gives the most satisfaction. We want an eye for an eye and a tooth for a tooth, but not a tooth for an eye or an eye for a tooth. This need not be judicially imposed for us to be satisfied. If the fan goes deaf shortly after killing Jones in order to save the violinist's life and therefore can never hear the violinist's music for the sake of which he killed Jones, we consider this "poetic justice." If the plantation goes broke while the slaves are employed, we find this deeply appropriate, though we sympathize with the slaves who will bear the brunt of this failure.

If Nietzsche were right, it would be the greatest possible degree of suffering in the evildoer that would satisfy our instinct for justice. But, rather, it is the greatest possible *appropriateness* of the malefactor's suffering that satisfies us. And it appears that we take it to be very appropriate when the malefactor suffers by being deprived of precisely that which he sought to achieve: the fan who wanted to listen to more music and committed murder who goes deaf and the exploiter who loses money. Observe, interestingly, that we find the second case rather satisfying even though the sufferings of the slave "owner" through bankruptcy are incomparably smaller than those that he had imposed on the slaves. We may feel that justice demands *more* suffering from the master, but the appropriateness of the suffering imposed is indisputable. This, I think, is sufficient to show that our notion of "poetic

---

[5] The case below of the slave master who goes broke is one.

justice" is not just vengefulness. Appropriate retributive justice *does* seem to restore the order of the universe.

If I am right, then one rationale for retributive justice is that it *frustrates* the intentions of the malefactor. She wanted money: she gets bankruptcy. He wanted music: he never hears any anymore. This is true even when the frustrated intentions of the malefactor are *good* ones. After all, it is good that a person enjoys music, and the more people enjoy music the better it is, in so far as this goes. Conversely, we are indignant when an evildoer achieves that goal for which he did the illicit action – the professor who becomes famous because of a paper plagiarized from an obscure third-world journal, the fan who kills to be able to hear the violinist's music and who spends the rest of his life enjoying the violinist's concerts, the slave "owner" who grows in wealth.

This suggests that it is *prima facie* a good thing to frustrate an evildoer's designs, to disrupt his action plan, and it is *prima facie* a bad thing to cooperate in the action plan of which the illicit action is an integral instrumental part. Now one can cooperate in the action plan long after the illicit action was done, by promoting that goal which the malefactor wanted promoted and promoting it in the way in which he wanted it promoted, indeed when one's action was implicitly or explicitly a part of that malefactor's action plan. This is cooperation in evil, and it is opposed to the *prima facie* good, a good of justice, of disrupting the action plan. Note that it need not count as cooperation in evil *at all* when one promotes the same goal that the malefactor had by a means *different* from those the malefactor intended. There was no *prima facie* wrongness in acting for the amelioration of the condition of the German people in the aftermath of the First World War, even though this was the same goal Hitler had set for himself, as long as one proceeded by causally independent means. Likewise, if those philosophers and theologians who claim that in some way each person always seeks beatitude in every action as an ultimate end are right, it does not follow that it is wrong to help the evildoer achieve *that* part of his illicit action plan, but we would like to depart from his planned means for achieving this end.

If this is right, then the same kinds of consideration that show up when analyzing our intuitions about retributive justice are relevant to the question of profiting from evil. Plainly, the policeman is acting to *frustrate* the action plans of the criminals, and the money he receives enables him to make a vocation of doing so. There is no presumption of any sort against this.

If, however, I were a temporarily unemployed fireman and a colleague set fire to a forest not to benefit herself but to benefit *me*, there would be a presumption against my profiting from this. Nonetheless, the *prima facie* badness of cooperating materially in this evil would be easily overridden by my need to cooperate in fighting off the bad effects of my colleague's action.

On the other hand, it was part of the action plan of the builders of Rome that people should enjoy the pavement, that they should admire the might of Rome, and so on. The tourist by doing this is materially complicit. Again, this is a defeasible consideration. In this case, as in that of the fireman, it is a consideration defeated in a particularly powerful way by aspects of the situation closely connected with the evils done. Despite not being justly compensated for their labor and not being given a choice about the work, the slaves were *workers*. They did good work. In enjoying the fruit of their labor after many centuries, one is showing respect to their solid workmanship. Tearing up the pavement would, on the other hand, be disrespectful to these workers.

Go back to the case of THE TYPHUS RESEARCHER. There *is*, I think, a *prima facie* badness in her use of the Nazi research data, insofar as the research was done to further the state of science, and hence the researcher's actions were implicitly a part of the action plan of the Nazi doctors. They intended to produce scientific data (and by and large failed in this, but let us assume that this is a case where they succeeded) that would be used by future scientists. One is playing their game by using the data. Nonetheless, the cooperation is only material. One is furthering some of the Nazi doctors' goals, but this consideration against one's action is defeasible by the significant medical benefits that the data, I am supposing in my fictional case, make possible.

Consider a variant case. Suppose you are a Soviet doctor and you helped liberate Auschwitz. You come upon the data. You realize that you can use the data in order to strengthen the war effort against Nazi Germany, both by a better understanding of the weaknesses of soldiers afflicted with typhus and by ameliorating the condition of Allied soldiers at the front. And so you use the data precisely for this purpose. Here, I think, there should be no discomfort. On the contrary, there should be a just satisfaction that one is acting in a way that the malefactors did not intend and by doing so frustrating one of their intentions for their evil action – helping the German war effort.

An agent's intentions may extend beyond his natural lifespan. Someone who gathers scientific data may do so for the sake of posterity. It is possible to promote or frustrate the goals of a malefactor even after he is dead. There is a *prima facie* reason to frustrate these goals by not going along with his action plan, by not being a pawn in his game.

Note, too, how the intuitions here go along to some degree with the intuition that temporal distance from the agent matters. For, apart from megalomaniacs and the truly great (whether for good or evil), our plans peter out in the future. People may have plans for their children and grandchildren and maybe great-grandchildren. Someone might have the intention of producing a continuous line of descendants or of attaining eternal life through religious means, but apart from these kinds of cases the horizons of our intentions are short. The further we are removed from the evil deed, the less likely that we are doing what the malefactors intended us to do.

4. The cell-line research case

In the case of cell-line research, the researchers illicitly extracting the cells probably saw themselves as *scientists*, as people promoting future scientific research. Insofar as one is scientifically building on their work, one may well be doing exactly what they intended one to do. One is being a cog in their action plan, and hence one is cooperating materially with evil. There is a presumption against that: it is a *prima facie* bad thing to do, assuming of course, as I do, that the initial activity was illicit.

The National Catholic Bioethics Center when asked to comment compared the research to two cases. The first is that of receiving organs from a murder victim. We can now see that this analogy is ambiguous between an unproblematic case where the person is killed for a reason independent of the organ donation, in which case the murderer's action plan is not at all furthered by use of the organs, and there is no *prima facie* consideration against, and the problematic case of the violinist. The second comparison case was that of anti-abortion advocates using pictures of aborted fetuses. For the pictures to exist a prior abortion had to have occurred. However, this fails as an analogy now that we see the most serious problem with profiting from the proceeds of an evil. For clearly the use of the pictures does not further any action plan that the abortionist has, but on the contrary is meant to counter the action plans coming from the general maxim that the abortionist was acting on. Thus there may even be argued to be a *prima facie* presumption in favor of such use if it *frustrates* the illicit goals of the abortionist. (Of course I leave aside the question whether the use of such pictures is prudent and helpful.)

Therefore, not every positive reason suffices to justify research on cell-lines derived from abortions. One needs a *proportionately strong* reason. In the case of vaccine production, this strong reason is almost surely present – assuming one is doing the best one can to find alternatives to the use of the illicitly derived cell lines. In the case of research, this has to be analyzed on a case by case basis. If the research is on how to cure a mild form of acne and is extremely unlikely to yield a cure, it seems wrong – apart, of course, from the general wrongness of wasting research resources. If, however, the research is very likely to yield a cure for a fatal form of cancer, then it seems acceptable.

I have no idea what to say about the in-between cases, nor how to draw the line. In general, there are no mathematical formulae for weighing costs and benefits, for weighing different kinds of consideration, though such formulae do exist in specific cases (for instance, if the cost is the doing of an intrinsically wrong action, the cost is always too high). But nonetheless I think that when one does something that has a presumption against it – that is *prima facie* bad – one has usually reason to feel a certain discomfort. This discomfort is a recognition of the fact that something objectively bad comes from one's action, even though one is not intending it to do so.

For instance, while the researcher is not, I shall assume, intending to promote the action plan of the malefactor *qua action plan of the malefactor*, such promotion is a side-effect of his work: the evildoer is in fact being rewarded, though such rewarding *qua rewarding* is not the researcher's intention. For, intuitively, it rewards someone to causally promote his action-plan – even if the person rewarded does not know this has occured. Perhaps this is another area for the Principle of Double Effect. The good effect is the benefits of the research; the bad effect is the unintended rewarding of evil.

Whenever Double Effect is in play, one can only act for a *sufficiently strong* reason. Hence, the radically permissive view is wrong, just as the radically restrictive view is.

5. Objections

(i) Extraction of cells from fetuses not aborted for research purposes is not wrong. One might argue that the requirement of consent for organ donation is not a moral requirement, though it is politically prudent in an individualistic society. Our society's distaste for non-consensual organ transplants should not deceive us into thinking that such transplants are actually wrong.

If this objection succeeds, then my argument in Section 2 for the wrongness of the extraction of fetal cells fails. Note that such extraction need not constitute either formal or material cooperation with the abortion after the fact if the extraction was not one of the reasons for which the abortion was done. Therefore, the rest of my argument would seem to be inapplicable, and revisions of accepted current Catholic medical ethics standards would be called for. Nonetheless, my general analysis of cooperation after the fact would, I think, have plausibility, even if it lacked application to the case at hand.

Two responses are possible. The first is that while such extraction *need not* constitute cooperation, in practice it often does. The researcher has some kind of a formal arrangement with the abortionist or with a go-between, and it is unlikely that this arrangement is such as to communicate to the abortionist anything other than approval of the abortion.

Secondly, we should not be unduly sceptical of our moral intuitions about non-consensual use of other people's organs. A human body after death is still something that calls for a respect akin to that which a living body receives, albeit expressed differently. Even a corpse should not be treated as a mere thing, given its intimate connection with the living body of the person. Now, it is acceptable for a person to give himself to another bodily and it is acceptable for the other to receive that gift, e.g., on personalist grounds that say that the nature of a human person is to be a gift. But it is arguably not acceptable for a person to simply *take and use* another person. And a similar kind of respect is called for the body of the person even after death: it is not a thing to be merely taken and used, though it may be received as a gift.

(ii) This analysis implies that it does not matter whether the cells currently used for research are ontologically removed from the original cells. On this analysis, all that matters, it seems, is the "distance" measured relative to the original malefactor's intentions. Yet when people who were originally opposed to such research find out that a genetic modification took place in the cell-line, their opposition tends to weaken. Thus my analysis, it seems, does not correctly capture the moral issues involved.

At least four responses are possible. The first is simply for me to dig in my heels. The ontological modification indeed does not affect things. We may *feel* it does because usually significant changes in the things produced from evil also distance the effects from the intentions of the original male-factor. However, in this case, this is only an illusion, akin to that whereby a physically smaller item may seem to be further away, since the original malefactor's intentions included this transformation.

Secondly, one might argue that the greater the number of steps leading to a given point in a malefactor's plan of action, with only the first step in the plan being intrinsically wrong, the lesser the presumption against cooperation at that point. This, however, seems implausible. For on the account I have given, it is the distance vis-à-vis the malefactor's intentions that matters. And the malefactor may just as much intend things many steps away as things closer to himself. Indeed, surely, the malefactor intends the end, which is many steps removed, just as much as he intends the means.

Thirdly, and perhaps most satisfyingly, one might note that there are multiple moral dimensions along which an action can be measured. Thus when I lie to someone that an unsound bridge is sound, I do wrong both by lying and by potentially causing physical harm. It may be that the notion of ownership of one's body and of the genetic descendants of that body is not *completely* flawed. While this is not ownership *simpliciter*, there may be something sufficiently analogous to ownership to produce certain presumptions against use of the descendant material without the person's permission. This may even be connected in some way to the rights of parents with respect to children. If so, then genetic modification weakens the link to the original person, and hence weakens the presumptions. Note that this would also strengthen the response to (i), by giving another dimension to the badness of the original derivation, namely the dimension of something analogous to theft.

However, to work out the details here is a difficult, and perhaps impossible, task. Suppose that details cannot be worked out and that in the end there is no analogy between one's relationship to one's genetic descendant material and one's relationship to one's property. Nonetheless, there clearly is at least the *appearance* of an analogy, and this appearance would be enough to explain our intuition that genetic modification decreases wrongness, though without justifying this intuition. Our moral feelings can, after all, go wrong.

6. Applications

Are there any practical consequence of this view? There may well be. I do not have a story about how one weighs the benefits of a given research project over and against the *prima facie* badness of cooperating materially with a past evil. The decision probably needs to be made on a case-by-case basis by an Aristotelian *phronimos*: a person of practical reason. At the same time, it is essential that the *phronimos* when making the decision should be informed by the correct theory of why the cooperation is *prima facie* bad and precisely what is bad about such cooperation. The account given will contribute to such a moral education of the agent.

Moreover, because there is something *prima facie* bad about such cooperation, there is thereby positive reason to pursue methods, whether of producing of vaccines or of doing research, that avoid such cooperation. It might be possible, for instance, to seek sympathetic private donors to fund such activities, and this is the sort of thing that research institutions have a reason to pursue.

Finally, because the decision needs to be made on a case-by-case basis, an argument could be made that strong informed consent doctrines require that persons receiving any treatment that involves such cooperation, or proxies of these persons, be informed of the ethical issues involved. This may mean that parents need to be informed about the ethical issues in the case of vaccinations, which currently apparently they are not. Given the lack of an objective rule for weighing the issue, especially in the case of vaccinations for diseases that are generally unlikely to be life-threatening, it might be necessary for the individual parent to make the decision. Of course one might think, on paternalistic grounds, that public health considerations override the need for informed consent, and so it is sufficient for the medical personnel to make the decision. Weakening informed consent requirements in favor of public health leads to a dangerous slippery slope, however, and so probably should only be done when absolutely necessary.[6]

[6] I am grateful to Dr Edmund Pellegrino and Fr Kevin Fitzgerald for enlightening discussions, as well as to my audience at the Works in Progress series at the Center for Clinical Bioethics, Georgetown University Medical Center, for many helpful comments and criticisms. Most of Section 5 is based on that discussion, and I apologize for not individually attributing the views, pro and con, I make use of there.

6

Cooperation problems in science: use of embryonic/ fetal material

Neil Scolding

He that planted the ear, shall he not hear?
he that formed the eye, shall he not see? . . .
He that teacheth man knowledge, shall he not know?
Psalm 94:9–10

The Church has a great esteem for scientific and technological research . . . it is a
service to truth, goodness and beauty
Pope John Paul II, May 2000

Behold I am sending you out as sheep in the midst of wolves. . . .
. . . so be wise as serpents and innocent as doves
Matthew 10:16

1. The medical need for cells

In the whole of the last decade, few areas of science or medicine have gener-
ated as much excitement, press coverage or debate as that of embryonic stem
cells. In order to understand why these cells have provoked such interest and
such controversy, and why many scientists and clinicians worry about the
extent to which they may cooperate or collaborate with those who work
with these cells, it is necessary first to understand what these cells are, and
why future medical therapies might require cells with their properties – if
not their provenance.

We should therefore consider first the medical needs that advocates of
embryonic stem cells hope these cells will meet, in order to understand the

background to the debate. The key lies in the limitations of conventional medical (pharmacological) or surgical treatments. Whilst these are variably successful in dealing with an enormous range of infectious, inflammatory and malignant disorders, they are unable to generate replacement tissue when organs or parts of organs have been destroyed, whether by trauma, degeneration or some other cause.

Perhaps the most obvious examples may be found in neurological (and especially neurodegenerative) diseases such as Parkinson's disease, Alzheimer's disease, and multiple sclerosis. In all these disorders, populations of brain cells die for various reasons. These are at present incurable diseases – the degenerative processes cannot be halted, and the brain cells, once lost, cannot be replaced. Decades or longer of conventional medical research has had as its aim the prevention of these diseases, so far without success. This research continues, but in addition the last 10–15 years has seen the emergence of a new field of therapeutic research: *regenerative medicine*. Whilst its advocates acknowledge that prevention is better than cure, and that research designed to yield preventative treatments must and will continue, they recognise that many years may yet pass before such treatments are established, and that even then they may be only partially successful. *Regenerative medicine* seeks to restore function to diseased tissues by replacing or regenerating lost cells, usually by some form of direct injection of cells into the damaged area.

There are, of course, many different types of brain cell which different diseases affect, and which therefore might need replacing. Furthermore, *regenerative medicine* is not limited to neurological disease: in fact, almost every major organ has its own common but incurable disorders – the heart (myocardial infarction or "heart attack"), the pancreas (diabetes), muscles (muscular dystrophy) to name but a few. One key property of cells potentially usable in regenerative medicine is therefore the ability to turn into a wide range of different cell types. The second crucial requirement is for large numbers of cells: the repair of one area of damaged tissue in just a single patient is likely to require many millions of cells. Therefore a pronounced capacity for proliferation is also vital.

It is these two fundamental requirements of any potential reparative cell that first focussed attention on the embryo. The embryo, after all, originates in just a single cell – the fertilised ovum. Cells in the very early embryo must constitutively exhibit these very properties to perfection, so as to produce a fully developed individual with a huge spectrum of highly specialised cells in vast numbers. Scientific work in experimental animals unsurprisingly but nonetheless excitingly confirmed that cells could be isolated from the early embryo which showed these properties – *pluripotentiality* (the ability to turn into a whole host of specific cell types – brain cells, heart cells, etc) and an almost endless capacity for *proliferation*. These were embryonic stem cells.

Developing therapies for patients, however, requires the use of human cells – transplanting pig or other animal cells into humans remains fraught with complications. Further research quickly (and again unsurprisingly) established that human embryos too contained embryonic stem cells, and speculation that cell therapies for diseases could realistically be developed thence mounted rapidly. Yvette Cooper, then Health Minister of the British Government, encapsulated (or fed) the feverish excitement, proposing that "Embryonic stem cells [are] ... the Holy Grail in finding a cure for cancer, Parkinson's disease, diabetes, osteoporosis, Alzheimer's and multiple sclerosis".[1]

From an ethical perspective, the difficulties, therefore, are obvious. Embryonic stem cells can only be had from human embryos, or so it would appear. Formerly, there were only two sources of human embryos: abortion and IVF, which produces many "surplus" embryos, and some purpose-made for research. (Almost) by chance, at approximately the same time that human embryonic stem cells were discovered, a third potential source of embryos was also found: cloning. Scientists in Edinburgh reported the first cloned mammal, Dolly the sheep, removing any serious doubt that human embryos could not similarly be cloned. Uniquely in the UK, new laws allowing the development of human cloning techniques specifically to permit their use as a source of stem cells were enacted.

At this point it is worth emphasising two fundamental facts: first, that all three sources of human embryos require that the embryo be destroyed if stem cells are to be extracted for use or study. Second, later experimental studies revealed that the developing human individual is not the only source of potentially useful stem cells: developed tissues also contain such cells.

2. Pressure to cooperate

The establishment position (both political and scientific, and not just in the UK), is that embryonic stem cells are, as indicated by Yvette Cooper, a medical "Holy Grail". Those reluctant to engage in or support research whose raw material is the deliberately destroyed human embryo are therefore obliged to resist a certain pressure from a number of quarters.

The enthusiasm from Government that this research be pursued has been articulated already, and comes not only from the hierarchy of the Department of Health, but from the Prime Minister Tony Blair himself, who has

---

[1] *The Times*, 16 December 2000.

said on this question "Let us get to the facts and *then* judge their moral consequences. Our conviction about what is natural or right should *not* inhibit the role of science in discovering the truth" (my italics). The main-stream scientific journals, in their editorial content and commentating role, have consistently given prominence to every apparent advance in embryonic stem cell research – and equal prominence only to every suggested setback in adult stem cell science ["these findings are a reality check for those hoping to use adult stem cells for clinical purposes"; "the *hyped* ability of adult stem cells to sprout replacement tissue types" (my italics)[2]].

No less important from a practical perspective, the principal UK research funding bodies have declared a position of marked enthusiasm for human embryonic stem cell research, as have prestigious and influential scientific bodies in the UK – for example, the Royal Society and the Academy of Medical Sciences.[3] Lay Patient Groups, such as the Parkinson's Disease Society, have adopted a position of explicit opposition to those questioning the need for or ethical propriety of human embryonic stem cell research. Adopting this latter position whilst working within a community of scientific peers, however personally amicable they may be, is also hardly free from perceived if not overtly applied pressure.

3. Persuasion to cooperate

When they are articulated, what are the arguments used by those defending the use of human embryos as a source of stem cells? The positive arguments – the potential for new therapies – have been mentioned above, and we will consider some weaknesses of these arguments shortly. A number of negative arguments aimed at discrediting opponents of destructive human embryo research are employed.

Perhaps the most common is that the human embryo is no more than a "ball of cells" – to describe such a cluster of a few cells as "a person" is worthy of ridicule: only a "callous Luddite" would wish to confer full human rights on this cell clump "in order to" prevent this potentially life-saving research which could "spare millions from misery".

Of course, the question whether the early embryo can semantically be termed a "person", whilst not without interest or indeed importance, is hardly in fact central. What is central is that the embryo has three attributes which are unquestionable: it is alive; it is human; it is an individual. It is

---

[2] *Nature Science* update, 14 March 2002.
[3] The Royal Society, *Stem cell research and therapeutic cloning* 2000.

therefore quite literally *a human being*. Deliberately to destroy a human being, regardless of the (potential) material benefit to humankind is, for many of us, indefensible. (And the "ball of cells" description is hardly useful: both the author and (for example) the Prime Minister are now, and will remain as long as they both shall live, balls of cells.)

Moving on to the next argument, proponents assert that human embryonic research will be "tightly regulated". The UK *Human Fertilisation and Embryology Authority* (HFEA) is a widely esteemed and highly professional body which can, under its terms of reference, permit scientists to engage in such research, including human cloning, "... only when there is no alternative". Likewise the US *National Bioethics Advisory Council* (NBAC) could authorise such work "... only if no less morally problematic alternatives are available". The *Polkinghorne Report*[4], which defines the circumstances under which human embryos/fetuses may "acceptably" be used for research in the UK (apparently) adopts a position of respectable caution: such research is only acceptable providing there is proper separation of the abortion procedure from the researcher. All is therefore carefully regulated and considered, and anxious scientists should rest assured that greater experts than they have pondered these deep questions and found themselves able to pronounce in favour of such research.

Sadly, anxious scientists cannot rest: the history of science offers repeated examples (which need no rehearsal here) confirming that scientists must consider these matters for themselves. The Polkinghorne Report, for example, has been seriously criticised.[5] It includes such extraordinary contradictions as permitting destructive embryo research while stating "*The live fetus, whether in utero or ex utero, ... should be treated on principles broadly similar to those which apply to ... adults and children*", and "*With the exception of abortion ... intervention on a living fetus ... should carry only minimal risk of harm*". The degree of care and rigour with which the HFEA performs its duties has also been seriously called into question.

Next, advocates of embryo research claim their position is built on the "special status, and special respect" due to the human embryo, phrases possibly first offered by Dame Mary Warnock, but re-capitulated by many of the established bodies mentioned above. The key here is the use of the adjective "special". It suggests, of course, a positive and respectful position, but in fact as a simple qualitative term can always be out-flanked. Therefore the "huge benefits" of HES research (of course) outweigh this "special

---

[4] J.C.C. Polkinghorne, *Review of the guidance on the research use of fetuses and fetal material.* London: HMSO 1989.

[5] J. Keown, "The Polkinghorne Report on Fetal Research: nice recommendations, shame about the reasoning". 19 (1993) *Journal of Medical Ethics*: 114–120.

status". The general benefits to society and to the sick may now be *balanced* against the now defined and qualified status of the human embryo.

This is a distraction: of course the embryo is "special", but it is far more than this – it is a human being: the rights of one individual human being (a human embryo) must not be "balanced" against the good of other human beings. This imposition of a new mode of describing the embryo is arbitrary and cannot therefore be accepted at face value.

The novelty of these arguments is illustrated by reference, for example, to the *Nuremberg Code* of 1947 and subsequent *Declaration of Helsinki* of 1964, the latter a code of medical ethics (otherwise) still very much used today to inform questions and judgements of ethics in medicine and medical science. These codes assert – in entirely unqualified language, "...experiments performed on an individual must be of benefit to the individual, not just benefit society", and in other parts specifically define the individual, and human life, as "human life *from the time of conception*" (my italics). Generations of medical scientists have formerly adopted the position that the potential wider benefits never justify unethical research; individual autonomy must not be compromised. Extraordinarily in many ways, even the 2000 revision of the Helsinki Declaration emphasises that "In medical research on human subjects, considerations related to the well-being of the human subject should take precedence over the interests of science and society."

Yet further attempts are made to justify abandoning this historical position. Abortion "would happen anyway"; IVF procedures will always generate spare embryos – these otherwise would only be destroyed: surely in both cases it is better to use this tissue positively than let it uselessly disappear? How can it be wrong to rescue some good from that which may well be less than morally perfect? And then regarding the third source of tissue, cloning, then yes, of course it is right and proper to ban *reproductive cloning*, the production of babies, but *therapeutic cloning* is fundamentally different and can only do good: it is the opponents of embryonic stem cell research who are morally compromised by not recognising this fundamental difference and proposing recklessly to ban both procedures.

Yet again, these arguments cannot bear detailed interrogation. There is a genuine question to be asked of the assertion that an abortion "would occur anyway". One study of women who said that they would consider an abortion if they were pregnant found that 17.2% would be more likely to have an abortion if they could donate tissue for fetal tissue transplants, while 19.7% were uncertain.[6] (An additional ethical argument concerns the question of valid consent. All accept the need for such consent when

---

[6] D.K. Martin *et al.*, "Fetal Tissue Transplantation and Abortion Decisions: A Survey of Urban Women". 153 (1995) *Canadian Medical Association Journal*: 545–552.

research is to be performed on human tissue, but who can give real consent for so using the aborted embryo? For a minor, the parent or guardian ordinarily does this, "acting in the best interests of the child" – surely the mother, who has first consented to the abortion procedure, cannot fulfil this role? And if the procedure is performed within a National Health Service, neither can the State.)

Finally there is the question of *cooperation*. In practice, the researcher cannot obtain this tissue without close cooperation with the executor of the abortion: there is clear and undeniable complicity.

Such close cooperation is not, however, required respecting the *acquisition* of IVF embryos, particularly if frozen embryos are used for research, but here there is more than complicity, in that the scientist performing the research is he or she who destroys the embryo. Even if a scientist should use an already ("freshly") dead embryo, clear complicity of timing would be required, and in any case, it would surely be inconsistent and even scandalous to adopt the position that one was fundamentally opposed to the destruction of human life implicit in IVF *as it is currently practised*, and yet willing to exploit the product. Surely the only properly respectful way of approaching the frozen or thawed embryo is as one would approach a doomed or dying adult: avoiding destructive intervention during life; respectful disposal after death.

Lastly: *reproductive* and "*therapeutic*" cloning. These depend, of course, on what is technically precisely the same process, the only difference being in the fate of the cloned embryo so made. In the former it is implanted in a uterus to be grown to birth; in the latter it is destroyed to obtain stem cells. Life has been created – manufactured – purely as an instrument. (That serious biological problems are now reported in the scientific literature concerning the stability and safety of cloned cells[7] is technically not relevant to this ethical argument.)

To summarise, almost all arguments in favour of destructive human embryo research have their origin unsurprisingly in claims of the massive benefit that may accrue to patients. It hardly needs reiterating that no such benefits are apparent for the embryo, which fact alone is sufficient wholly to undermine the case for such research.

4. Any allies?

Moving quickly on from this rather adversarial dialogue, it is important to emphasise that those objecting to destructive human embryo research

---

[7] J.S. Draper *et al.*, "Recurrent gain of chromosomes 17q and 12 in cultured human embryonic stem cells". 22 (2004) *Nat. Biotechnol.*: 53–54.

would be wrong to conclude that the whole secular world was in a state of perpetual and constitutional opposition to their view.

The lay press has not been slow to explore the emerging discrepancy between the claims made for therapeutic research using human embryos and its achievements, and indeed the potential hazards that might be associated with the clinical use of human embryonic brain cells [*Guardian* 13 March 2001: *"Parkinson's miracle cure turns into nightmare"*] or stem cells [*Guardian* 19 April 2002: *"What went wrong with the cloning dream?"*]. Some scientific journals have adopted a more principled stand – the *Lancet*, for example, in an editorial commentary entitled "Stem cell research: drawing the line" declared (of cloning) that "...the creation of embryos solely for the purpose of producing human stem cells is not only unnecessary but also a step too far".[8]

Finally, although senior UK politicians appear to suggest that ethics should play no role in governing decisions about the pursuit of research goals, the same cannot be said of politicians elsewhere. Taking the opposite line, George Bush has stated "Even the most noble ends do not justify any means ... human life is a sacred gift from our Creator."

5. Positive stem cell science

At the level of purist medical ethics, the rightness or wrongness of such activities as human embryonic stem cell research hardly depends on whether or not a valid alternative exists. At a more practical and day-to-day level, it is enormously valuable that there are such alternatives.

Let us briefly diverge and return to science, and in particular, to the disease multiple sclerosis. In this disorder, the cells responsible for making the electrical insulating material in the brain (*myelin*), called *oligodendrocytes*, become damaged and irreversibly lost. The aim of regenerative medicine in this disease is therefore to replace, possibly by direct injection into the brain, human oligodendrocytes. However, animal model studies indicate that in fact, replacing mature oligodendrocytes results in rather inefficient and unsuccessful myelin repair.

Far more successful repair occurs following the injection of cells that turn into oligodendrocytes, *oligodendrocyte progenitors*, not least because these cells, unlike their mature counterparts, have a pronounced ability to divide and repopulate damaged areas of the brain. It was originally thought that these oligodendrocyte progenitors were only found in the developing brain (and could therefore only be obtained for research from the developing

---

[8] Anon, "Stem-cell research: drawing the line". 358 (2001) *Lancet*: 163.

brain). Rather surprisingly, however, it emerged that the adult brain – including the human adult brain – also contains oligodendrocyte progenitors.[9]

Scientific research then moved quickly on. It soon emerged that a cell type with limited stem cell-like properties – a *brain stem cell* – also existed in and could be prepared from the adult brain, as well as the developing brain.[10] (A *brain stem cell*, like conventional stem cells, has an enormous capacity for proliferation, but is less versatile than a true stem cell in that it can turn itself into all of the many cell types found in the brain, including oligodendrocyte progenitors, but not into muscle, kidney and other non-brain tissues.) When first reported, the discovery of brain stem cells raised the possibility that, in order to help treat diseases like multiple sclerosis, it might be possible operatively to remove a small sample of an MS patient's brain, grow brain stem cells from it and expand them to produce very large numbers of cells, turn these in the test tube into oligodendrocyte progenitors, and then re-inject them into damaged areas. Whilst in principle this is of considerable interest, in practice it is difficult to see such a (relatively) hazardous procedure as a realistic way forward.

The basic research continued, however, and most surprising of all was the later demonstration that the adult brain (again, including the human brain) in fact also does contain cells not just with brain stem cell properties, but which in fact resemble true stem cells more closely. They are able not only to expand or proliferate almost endlessly, but can turn into both the various brain cell types and into non-brain cells. One of the cell types yielded by adult brain-derived stem cells was the bone marrow cell, and very rapidly the reverse experiment was performed, and it became clear that cells isolated from the bone marrow could turn themselves into brain cells.[11]

It is now well established that adult human bone marrow does contain a population of cells which have undeniable stem cell-like properties. Their discovery has quickly led to the emergence of a whole new field of research into spontaneous tissue healing.[12] It is clear that, in normal health, a small number of such cells is continuously released into the bloodstream and

[9] N.J. Scolding, P.J. Rayner, J. Sussman, C. Shaw and D.A.S. Compston, "A proliferative adult human oligodendrocyte progenitor". 6 (1995) *NeuroReport*: 441–445.

[10] B.A. Reynolds and S. Weiss, "Generation of neurons and astrocytes from isolated cells of the adult mammalian central nervous system". 255 (1992) *Science*: 1707–1710; S. Weiss *et al.*, "Multipotent CNS stem cells are present in the adult mammalian spinal cord and ventricular neuroaxis". 16 (1996) *J. Neurosci.*: 7599–7609.

[11] Y. Jiang *et al.*, "Pluripotency of mesenchymal stem cells derived from adult bone marrow". 418 (2002) *Nature*: 41–49.

[12] M. Korbling and Z. Estrov, "Adult stem cells for tissue repair". 349 (2003) *New England Journal of Medicine*: 570–582.

circulates around the body. When an organ is damaged – as with the heart, for example, during myocardial infarction – the damaged tissue releases specific chemicals which first increase the number of these cells released by the bone marrow, and second attract them from the circulating blood to the area of damage. Here, acting under further signals from the surrounding tissue, they turn into the "correct" and required cell type, and contribute to repair.

This remarkable and only very recently described system has important implications for regenerative medicine. If one settles on the adult bone marrow stem cell as a candidate for therapeutic cell implantation, then it could be argued that all one is asking of this cell is that it perform its normal function in life, enhanced by the far greater numbers one might experimentally generate before injection. This might theoretically give the therapeutic scientist far more grounds for optimism than, for example, using embryonic stem cells – whose "normal" function in life is to help produce a developing organism, not to relate to and repair tissue in an adult cellular environment.

There is therefore considerable excitement in many quarters regarding the prospect for developing cell therapies based on adult human bone marrow-derived stem cells. Bone marrow cells have been used medically, of course, for many decades, and physicians therefore know already the best techniques for obtaining them from consenting donors, storing them, and injecting them into patients. We know also that these are basically very safe techniques, again in contrast to embryonic stem cell injection, which carries the serious and thus far unaddressed hazard of tumour development.

Animal studies have confirmed that when bone marrow cells are injected into areas of damage (in the spinal cord) which model the type of damage seen in multiple sclerosis, successful myelin repair does occur. Outside the area of neurological disease, clinical trials have already commenced in diseases such as myocardial infarction, following small pilot studies – in patients, not experimental models – indicating that bone marrow cells, taken from patients suffering myocardial infarction a few days after the event and re-injected later directly into the damaged heart – do appear to lead to significantly better recovery of cardiac function.[13] Translating such work in cardiology to various neurological diseases will undoubtedly commence in the very near future, again in marked contrast to embryonic stem cell therapies which are, even according to their most enthusiastic

---

[13] B.E. Strauer *et al.*, "Repair of infracted myocardium by autologous intracoronary mononuclear bone marrow cell transplantation in humans". 106 (2002) *Circulation*: 1913–1918.

scientific advocates, still 10–15 years away (not least because of some of the hazards mentioned).

6. Specific cooperation questions

Having therefore considered both the background to this debate, the arguments and pressures applied, and the alternatives, let us now consider – extremely briefly – whether this allows us to address some specific questions of cooperation: questions which may daily confront clinical scientists interested in regenerative medicine.

(A) *What of direct collaboration using fetal/embryonic material?*

This question has, the author hopes, been answered adequately already. Even the rather common "better than the tissue being wasted" argument has been shown not to be valid. To oppose in principle the destruction of the live human embryo, and yet in practice condone or engage in research which closely depends on this destruction, is surely not a sustainable position.

(B) *Can one work, performing what one considers to be ethically robust work, within the "system" at all? If (in the UK, for example) the NHS, the Universities, the principal research-funding bodies, and most scientific journals have declared a stance in favour of destructive embryonic research, and such research constitutes a core part of these bodies' activities, is it the case that one is complicit in this wrongdoing simply by being part of – a paid employee of – this system?*

There is an attractive if daunting logic to this question. The author has taken the view that it would be simply impossible to engage in any ethically robust work at all independently of the system, and yet it is important that this work be done. To work for a UK university, performing research using money from an organisation that also funds destructive embryonic research, is not to give tacit support to such research, any more than to pay one's taxes can be taken to imply that one supports every use to which this revenue is put.

(C) *What of working within a Unit where others use fetal material?*

This situation will almost inevitably face any researcher wishing to pursue stem cell research but to work with stem cells from non-embryonic sources (or even from spontaneous abortion (miscarriage) – derived tissue). In many ways, however, it is *Question B* writ small. One is in no position to prevent colleagues from pursuing their (legal and sadly officially sanctioned) research, and to work in such a unit, and to meet and engage with individuals pursuing ethically dubious research on a daily basis, is by no means necessarily to condone their research. Any measure of positive witness offered by those pursuing ethically sound research in this situation should also not be forgotten.

(D) *What of directing a Unit where others use fetal material?*

This is a little different. Authority naturally carries responsibility: one in such a position cannot therefore permit ethically dubious research to continue in his or her unit without accepting complicity.

(E) *What of research using fetal material derived elsewhere?*

At first glance, this is what Homer Simpson might call a "no-brainer". Plainly, if tissue has been obtained by means the researcher regards as unethical – by the destruction of a human embryo – then whether the destruction has taken place next door or a continent away, a few hours previously or a generation ago, does not alter the principle of moral culpability or complicity.

A number of European countries have, however, adopted policies which implicitly fail to recognise this tolerably obvious assertion. Germany is just one example of a country which recently has declared a ban on destructive embryonic research, but indicated that research using imported embryonic stem cells could proceed.

One should perhaps exercise some caution, however, before condemning any perceived illogicality in making distinctions of "closeness" which are based on (for example) the passage of time. On the subject of certain childhood vaccinations which have depended absolutely for their development on the use (a generation ago) of abortion-derived human embryonic material, the declared Catholic position appears to be that current doses of the vaccine are sufficiently far removed from the use originally of human embryonic material, and the potential benefits so great, that parents (in this instance) can in good conscience put their children forward for such vaccination, at least in the absence of alternative vaccines.

(F) *What about cooperative Grant Applications and collaborative experiments?*

Superficially, this is the same in principle as Question C, and the answer might therefore immediately be assumed to be in the affirmative. But here there is a direct and close working relationship. Does this not imply an acceptance of – and even therefore complicity in – ethically dubious research? I think it can be argued that it need not. In the current funding environment, it may well be that the only realistic approach to succeeding in obtaining grant funding is through scientific collaboration with those seeking funds for destructive embryonic research. Insofar as the likelihood of such (unethical) research successfully acquiring funding is not enhanced (probably rather the opposite) by one's addition of an adult stem cell component, one is not assisting the embryonic stem cell researchers in the sense of helping them be more effective in achieving their goal. The problem remains that one may still be intending the joint application to succeed – unless one is simply intending that if any project is approved, one's own morally justified project will be approved (ideally, on its own). If one contributes to a joint application without approving the unethical research, without directly engaging in it, and whilst continuing to set an example of ethically robust work, is this acceptable – or is it an unacceptable degree of cooperation in evil?

(G) *What about referring patients to clinicians for treatments which use embryonic stem cells?*

At present there are, as far as the author is aware, no such therapeutic trials, at least in the UK. They may emerge in the future, but in the meantime the ethically identical question is being posed to clinicians. Various Neurology Centres around the world are currently assessing treatments for incurable degenerative brain disorder Huntington's and Parkinson's Diseases which involve injecting embryonic brain cells (not stem cells) into the patient's brain. Nowadays, with alert patient-centred charities and the internet, relatively few patients are unaware of such therapeutic trials. Not rarely, they will directly ask for referral to Centres where such procedure are being carried out.

This is directly analogous to the question, dealt with elsewhere in this volume, of patients asking to be referred by their Family Doctor for an abortion. The solution might be to explain to the patient why one takes the view that the procedure is wrong in principle but then, if the patient persists in his or her demands, indicate that one can no longer continue looking after the patient, and provide him or her with information (referral centres or other primary care physicians) allowing the patient to change doctors if he or she so wishes. Whilst carrying the disadvantage of appearing obstructive in setting a tortuous path for the patient, it may be the only way of avoiding the hypocrisy of referring the patient directly to an individual one knows may carry out an objectionable procedure.

7

Medical training: cooperation problems and solutions

Charlie O'Donnell

1. Introduction

This article is meant for those who want to struggle to be perfect (i.e. to fall in love with Jesus Christ, because that is what Catholicism is all about). Jesus Christ taught us that there are three good reasons to be perfect: to get to heaven ourselves, to help others get to heaven, and to make this world a better place.

I have tried to make the article "user friendly" and therefore suitable for the busy medical student and junior doctor with little time for the complexities of theology or philosophy. It goes without saying, of course, that I am indebted to those who generously spend their lives immersed in the depths of philosophy and moral theology to provide a "hands on" amateur like myself with the opportunity to write a clinically focused summary. My own particular thanks must be given to the staff of the Linacre Centre for showing me the way to truly love Jesus Christ as an imperfect medical student, an imperfect junior doctor and still to the present day a far from perfect Consultant.

2. Principles of legitimate cooperation in evil

It is impossible to live in society and not interact with others. The Principles of Cooperation recognise that we are often legitimately involved in the actions of others yet must try to do good and never deliberately do evil so that good may come. Jesus Christ gave us the template. The Principles of Cooperation are a practical application of the commandment to love God,

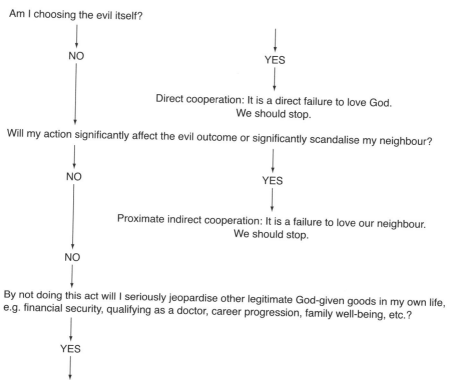

Am I choosing the evil itself?

NO

YES

Direct cooperation: It is a direct failure to love God.
We should stop.

Will my action significantly affect the evil outcome or significantly scandalise my neighbour?

NO

YES

Proximate indirect cooperation: It is a failure to love our neighbour.
We should stop.

NO

By not doing this act will I seriously jeopardise other legitimate God-given goods in my own life,
e.g. financial security, qualifying as a doctor, career progression, family well-being, etc.?

YES

Permissible remote indirect cooperation. If we did not proceed it would be a failure to love
ourselves as we should. We should continue.

Fig 1. Types of cooperation and our response

to love one's neighbour and finally to love oneself. The hierarchy of
questions that one must ask oneself go through love of God first and
foremost followed by love of neighbour and finally love of self. This
obviously presupposes that we have informed our consciences in the
light of the teaching of the Church so as to know what is truly good (see
Figure 1).

The nature of direct/deliberate cooperation in evil is relatively clear, i.e.,
one is responsible for mutilation, murder, lying, contraception etc. Conversely, indirect/material cooperation be it proximate or remote is more a
matter of degree, and of judgement according to a sincerely informed
conscience.

These facts are very important since in the case of indirect cooperation it is
for the individual to inform him or herself and decide. Dr O'Donnell is not
writing a treatise on how to make heavy burdens for his junior colleagues!
Others may, I believe, in good conscience consider what I have judged to

be proximate indirect cooperation, especially when I was a medical student, remote indirect cooperation.

3. Medical student cooperation problems

The following are common issues that may arise:

1. Being requested to clerk patients for morally wrong procedures, e.g. abortion or sterilisation.
2. Being requested to attend theatre for morally wrong procedures.
3. Teachers asking your opinion about treatments that are standard in the UK yet morally objectionable to you.
4. Patients asking your opinion about treatments where you are likely to disagree with your Consultant on moral grounds.

4. Solutions to medical student cooperation problems

The aim is to be perfect and introduce others to a life seeking perfection whilst at the same time avoiding looking for trouble, appearing to be a complete idiot, failing to qualify as a doctor or showing an inability to know when to open one's mouth or keep it shut! The life of St Thomas More serves as a very good lesson in the latter strategy. He was a man who knew that the primary aim of life is to fall in love with God (i.e. become a saint) and get others to do likewise. Yet he also knew that providing one loves God and neighbour one can also love oneself. He tried his best to avoid the executioner by keeping silent about his belief in the indissolubility of King Henry VIII's marriage and the authority of the Pope. As a medical student one is not faced with the possibility of execution but one is faced with the possibility of disruption of one's medical career – which is some-thing worth preserving if possible!

Overall I can see four general strategies that are acceptable methods of coping with problems of cooperation one faces as a medical student. One may need to use all four at different times:

1. Pre-emptive strike
The pre-emptive strike involves recognising that there are still three sacro-sanct objective principles in the medical profession that a medical student can use to his or her great advantage. These are: the belief in the rights of conscience, the belief in the best interests of patients and the belief in the anathema of imposing one's morality on another individual. It is this last point that can very rapidly make life extremely difficult, for example, with the nursing staff on a gynaecology ward if it is not turned around to your advantage. The commonly held assumption is that Catholics will impose

their morality upon others. The pre-emptive strike is to write a letter to your supervising Consultant prior to starting with the firm. It means playing the PC game. My own letter went something like this:

Dear Professor,

I am about to join your firm for my 12-week Obstetric and Gynaecology medical student attachment. I am very much looking forward to it.

Before I start I thought that it was important and courteous to inform you that I have a conscientious objection to therapeutic abortion, artificial contraception and methods of infertility management not involving normal sexual intercourse. I sincerely feel that these treatments are not in the best interests of patients and therefore I wish to be excused from any involvement in their pre-operative or operative management.

Obviously, I am well aware that I am in no position to force my morality on patients. At the same time, I am sure you will agree, it would not be right for my teachers to impose their morality on me.

I realise that I must become theoretically competent in these subjects and I shall endeavour to be a hard-working student.

Thank you for your consideration.

With your letter and the Professor's response in hand (i.e. "OK") you can pick and choose your activities and any problems can be dealt with by saying "Sister/Doctor... I will not do this because Prof... has agreed – please read this."

2. Duck and Dive

The Duck and Dive strategy is one where you keep a low profile and just try to avoid challenging situations. It is fine to use this technique: there are many ways to evangelise and not everybody is called to stand on Hyde Park Corner. The technique involves keeping busy, being a good medical student, deflecting any problems by changing the subject, seeking an alternative, morally neutral path or looking for potential areas of conflict before they arise and avoiding them. The only problem is that occasionally you may find yourself in a corner where you are morally obliged to show your true colours.

The Duck and Dive strategy is certainly a very useful and effective means of defusing potentially explosive situations. Also, there are some points of Christian teaching that cannot be adequately explained in a soundbite and any attempt at providing a soundbite will come across as uncharitable and judgemental.

Therefore, Duck and Dive methods which can help you to do the most amount of good and avoid doing evil are often essential. For example, you may be asked by your Consultant during a busy clinic with the patient sitting in front of you: "Do you think IVF is the treatment to offer this patient?" Since IVF is never morally licit you must not say yes: that is a lie. You could say the truth in black and white. The problem is that this may not go down well with your audience and you will not have the time or opportunity to explain your position, which, although it is actually the most charitable, sounds as if you have zero consideration for the pain of infertility, or respect for your teachers, who are probably involved in IVF out of a sincere (albeit misplaced) sense of concern for the infertile. Some form of Duck and Dive may be a better overall strategy. You could answer in one of the following ways:

1. "This is a complex decision on which there are two schools of thought, both of which recognise the pain associated with infertility. Those who agree because... those who disagree because...." If you are asked which side of the fence you stand on then after these introductory compassionate remarks you must declare your true colours.
2. Another method is to do what I call the Arthur Scargill Trick. Arthur Scargill was the communist leader of the Miners' Union during the 1980's who led the miners out on strike without holding a ballot of his members. Leaving aside the rights and wrongs of the dispute, Arthur was often confronted by the media for this perceived lack of democratic decision-making and asked time and time again "why didn't you have a ballot?" Undoubtedly fully aware that such a question cannot effectively be answered in a soundbite, Arthur would deflect the subject by saying "what I will say is..." and then bring into the conversation subject-matter of his choice (workers' rights, questionable management strategies etc). It is often the case that in day-to-day clinical teaching in response to a question a student can legitimately say "would it be possible before I answer that question for you to explain to me the various investigations a patient such as Mrs Smith would have gone through up until this point in her management since I find it all quite confusing?" You will be surprised how easy it is to seduce/flatter a Consultant away from his or her own questioning: students do it to me all the time!

Another very important principle to remember which is part of most people's Ducking and Diving is that we are always meant to tell the truth but not all of the truth all of the time. This is especially the case when as a student you are dealing with vulnerable and sensitive patients. For example, a patient may ask you as a medical student during your psychiatry placement: "Do you think that I should move in with my boyfriend? He is very supportive when I am suffering with my mental illness." Premarital cohabitation is not in the patient's best interests although most people (your Consultant included) may beg to differ. Telling the patient this in black and white runs very great risks for a medical student. The greatest risk is one of misinterpretation of your words: "Your student said that I should not live with my boyfriend – he made me feel cheap and nasty and his attitude was very judgemental". The second greatest risk is annoying your Consultant who may perceive you as an interfering puritan. All of this will not help your patient, your final assessment or your chances of becoming a doctor. If it is a choice between your word or the word of a patient, the patient will usually win. It is vital to remember that unwitnessed conversations on controversial matters can easily be distorted. Possible strategies therefore include:

1. Simply say: "I am just a medical student and at present I should not comment on how your life-style decisions would influence your treatment".
2. Get a witness whom you can trust and then in a charitable way explain the reasons why you think it is not in the patient's best interests to live with her boyfriend.

3. All guns firing
All guns firing is the St Bishop Fisher method. If St Thomas More was the Duck and Dive expert, Bishop Fisher let Henry VIII have it straight down the line. Henry VIII was an informed Catholic and therefore it was a good strategy with a fair chance of success in bringing him back to the truth. The souls that one is dealing with in our hospitals by and large are not like Henry and therefore perhaps this strategy may not be the most prudent or efficacious. But it is undoubtedly a courageous method and occasionally it is the best thing to do; for example, in the lecture theatre when our Catholic faith is being directly misrepresented.

4. Just say No
Of course the simplest method is what we hopefully do in other aspects of our lives all of the time: just say No. The problem with such a relaxed attitude is that in the day-to-day busy schedule of a medical firm an unexpected human spanner in the works may be perceived as a troublesome, inconsiderate individual who lacks the courtesy to inform colleagues about his/her conscientious position in advance yet expects colleagues to courteously furnish him/her with the privileges due to a conscientious objector at the drop of a hat. Telling your Consultant two minutes before a vasectomy where you are scheduled to assist that you will not do so is good at the level of better late than never but it lacks a degree of charity. This perhaps is not the best of advertisements for our faith.

If one does opt for this strategy it is important to say No discreetly and politely. This is because embarrassing patients and your teachers are not good things to do, both because you may not pass your assessment and become a doctor and more importantly because your Consultant and the patient have souls that need to be cherished.

5. Cooperation problems for junior doctors

The same principles of discerning one's level of cooperation apply when working as a junior doctor. Opportunities to be directly or proximately indirectly involved are, however, more likely to come up than during life as a medical student. Common problems that face junior doctors are:

1. You are asked to prescribe or perform something morally objectionable by your boss.
2. You are asked to prescribe or perform something that is usually considered to be routine by a patient but you consider it to be morally objectionable.
3. You are asked by your boss to refer a patient for something that you consider to be morally objectionable.
4. You want to get appointed to jobs where your conscientious position is respected.
5. You want to become a Consultant in Obstetrics and Gynaecology in the UK.

6. Solutions to cooperation problems for junior doctors

Whilst all of the four strategies I recommend above to medical students have a place in the life of the junior doctor there are five more strategies I have found to be invaluable. These are as follows:

1. Turn the question of referral into a strength rather than a weakness
By this I mean that one of the common misunderstandings of both patients and one's supervising Consultant is "OK, I can understand that you have a conscientious objection to... so just call the registrar to do it instead." This is actually moral stupidity. It means saying "I do not think this treatment is in your best interests so I am not prepared to do it myself, but I know a man I can send you to!" Rather than just your own soul being stained with sin you have potentially got another soul into trouble as well.

The way to turn the issue of no referral into strength is to communicate the consistency of your position. For example, talking to a patient in the A/E Department who has presented for post-coital contraception: "Miss Smith, I will not prescribe this for you, I have a conscientious objection to this medication. I sincerely believe that it is not in your best interests. I know that you may not agree with my position; however, I am sure that you would agree that it would be very wrong if I were to do something to you that I felt could be harmful, and that is the situation I find myself in at the moment. You obviously have the right to consult another doctor, though I hope you will not consider that necessary. In any case, I will not refer you since it would be crazy to get somebody else to do a job that I will not do because of my concern for your well-being." Obviously this discussion is more conversational in reality than the summary of the salient points given here, and has to include the reason for one's objection. A similar approach can be used to inform one's boss about the issue of referral. The GMC insists that the patient is made aware of their right to another opinion and that you do not obstruct the patient in this venture. That is fine, there is nothing wrong in telling patients their rights, it does not mean you agree with them: they have a legal right to go to another Hospital, GP, Private Clinic etc.

2. Keep the boss happy
It is vital to be a hard-working competent doctor. Nobody will take a Catholic seriously in matters of cooperation if that individual shows no concern for the equally important standard of using our talents to the best of our ability for the honour of God's name and the well-being of patients. In fact all of the human virtues need to shine out so your boss is pleased to have you on the firm.

Keeping the boss happy also means being honest with him or her before you start the job. How one goes about this needs a bit of prudence. The aim is to get your prospective boss to think: this is the doctor I want to work for me. This is not the forum for me to say how to sell yourself, but you need to know how to do this. After applying, I would suggest that you come clean either in writing once you have been short-listed but before the interview or at the end of your interview before any decision is made about whom to appoint. This needs to be done applying the principles of the "pre-emptive strike."

3. Have a witness during conversations with patients about your conscientious objections
It is vital that your conversations with patients are a compassionate presentation of your beliefs with a witness present. After the conversation (which may result in an unhappy patient) the details of the conversation should be recorded in the notes, including the statement that you informed the patient that he or she has the right to seek the opinion of other doctors. Both the witness (usually a nurse) and you should sign the notes. The nurse will be happy to sign the notes if you write: Staff Nurse Smith witnessed this conversation. Also, the entry in the notes should clearly stress your respect for the patient and the non-judgemental content of the conversation.

The statement that a patient has the right to seek an opinion elsewhere is not cooperating in evil since you are merely telling someone the law in this country, albeit a law that can at times lead to immoral decisions being taken. By saying this you provide yourself with a further degree of protection against the charge of "imposing your morality".

4. Local solutions to universal problems

Find out the logistics of patient flows in the hospital that you are applying for. You may find the particular moral dilemma that you are concerned about does not exist in that unit. For example, you may be "pleasantly" surprised that all so-called "safer sex" advice is given by someone else in the team and is not your responsibility as an SHO in HIV medicine (you can get on with the medicine side of things). Or you may be working in an Emergency Department where, for reasons of privacy or just Government waiting time targets, all morning after pill requests are directed to Walk in Centres or Pharmacists. Do not make a problem for yourself if by one means or another that problem has been taken out of your path.

5. Know when you cannot win

This applies to the speciality of Obstetrics and Gynaecology in the UK and maybe to one or two others. A career in O&G is, in my opinion, just not possible above Senior House Officer level. There are a number of misconceptions around about why this is the case.

It has nothing to do with discrimination, failure to respect the conscience of Catholics, refusal to perform abortions (there are O&G doctors who do not get involved and become Consultants) or an anti-Catholic ethos. It is actually all to do with service commitment. Quite simply, a Catholic trying to be perfect just cannot do a large part of the day-to-day work involved. It would be like a Consultant Emergency Physician appointing a Jehovah's Witness with a conscientious objection to giving blood transfusions to a training rotation in Emergency Medicine. (Of course, in the O&G case, the work you cannot do is not, like a blood transfusion, in the patient's true best interests.)

The other aspect of "knowing when you cannot win" is to know yourself. If you have a weakness for gambling then the sensible thing to do is to run away from casinos. On the same principle one should choose one's speciality according to one's own strengths and weaknesses.

7. Conclusion

Finally, do not worry. We are still privileged to work in a profession where the vast majority of its members are kind, compassionate and understanding people. I struggle in my own professional life to emulate the standard of patient care that my colleagues achieve; quite simply there are thousands of really good people working in medicine. This means that a person trying to be sincere in his or her beliefs often has a very receptive audience.

Also, there are lots of colleagues around who have "been there and done that" in difficult cases involving cooperation. With this in mind, be prepared to seek advice. The Linacre Centre is the source par excellence in the UK but other sources include the Guild of Catholic Doctors, your Parish Priest or just write to me!

8

General medical practice: the problem of cooperation in evil

Mike Delany

1. Introduction

Few would question that, for the Christian, these are trying times. Most areas of life are tainted by the spirit of a post-Christian culture. Manifestations of this range from sharp practice in business to widespread corruption of the family ideal and increasing sexual licence. Faced with this, we may develop an envy for the cloistered life but, without a religious vocation, might instead seek an existence in the secular world which engages it least – a pseudo-cloister. This may provide blanket protection from temptation and an unsullied feeling, but refusal to engage the world inevitably results in failure to evangelise it and, having buried our talents, we could find ourselves empty-handed when account is finally rendered. The Christian life does involve risk.

The medical world springs readily to mind as representative of modern attitudes to the ultimate value and purpose of life. Pope John Paul II spoke of a "culture of death", and it is clear from statistics alone that the medical profession leads as a proponent of this trend: current WHO figures estimate a global abortion rate in excess of fifty million per year. There are, in addition, numerous other practices which threaten human life, directly or indirectly, from its beginnings as well as in maturity. The question must then be asked whether a practising Christian can survive in the profession and retain the nobility for which medicine was once renowned. Can he or she faithfully observe the principles of the Hippocratic and Judeo-Christian traditions in their entirety *and* remain free to pursue a medical specialisation of his or her choice? I would say that, for a GP, the answer is in the affirmative, but not without emphasising how morally precarious the situation may become. Further, the minefield we need to cross is not merely one of particular moral transgressions but also the rather more ensnaring danger of a disabling scrupulosity. For the greater part of the time, the evil in which we might cooperate presents itself starkly and the means to circumvent it may be obvious; but increasingly complex procedures in the realm of reproductive medicine in particular, coupled with often irregular relationships between the sexes, threaten to catch us unawares. With this in mind, I believe our starting point should be an authentic perception of a deeply personal God, a perfectly loving father who seeks not to outwit us by multiplying and complicating the dilemmas we face but rather, yearns for our sanctification in and through the practice of medicine. Struggle is vital, and surely needs to begin with a concerted effort to properly inform the conscience by familiarisation with authentic Church teaching on morality. Concurrent with this, ongoing ascetical formation with constant recourse to prayer and the sacraments will serve to nurture the intrepidity required and protect us from discouragement when we fall short of perfection.

2. The current situation in general practice

The debate continues as to the wisdom of socialised medicine as we know it in the UK. There does seem to be a consensus within general practice, though, that fifty plus years of the National Health Service (NHS) has inclined many to an over-dependence on and even abuse of medical services which remain free at the point of contact. Recent government initiatives on waiting times and accessibility threaten to compound and exacerbate this trend. For individual GPs the end result is spiralling stress, and it is within this context that a Catholic will incur the additional tension found when confronting society with the teachings of Christ to which it is largely hostile.

For a GP, conflict of interest is inevitable in those areas relating to contraceptive services and reproductive medicine. At a time when most Catholics as well as society in general contracept, an authentically Catholic approach in medicine represents a genuine voice in the wilderness. In light of this it is prudent to approach the medical consultation armed with a set of well-planned strategies which will suffice in the majority of challenging situations likely to arise. There will continue to be uncomfortable moments and embarrassment, but these can be minimised.

3. Gaining acceptance in general practice

As an undergraduate in medicine, I took university life to be an authentic microcosm of the real world. Involved in pro-life campaigning and known to be a Catholic, I experienced frightening skirmishes with radical political groups which openly attacked the Church and its stance on abortion in particular. The prospect of a lifetime spent working against such pressures became daunting, but within days of beginning my first paid job in medicine, it became clear that men and women engaged in the serious business of earning a living simply did not have time to pursue political ideologies in the workplace. What we in fact have to contend with is more a sense of indifference and bemusement on the part of our colleagues. I have yet to see evidence of an orchestrated campaign against Catholic doctors.

In the UK, general practitioners are subcontracted to the NHS and tend to form small business partnerships which mostly emerge as lifelong professional relationships and, it is often said, have to be approached with the caution appropriate to choosing a spouse. The uppermost question for prospective business partners is whether they can work together in reasonable harmony. If we take, as our only agenda, Catholic teaching on abortion, contraception etc. we will inevitably raise hackles at interview rather than our chances of being hired. Having failed even to be employed we find ourselves in no position to further the mission of the Church within medicine.

In my experience, the key to acceptance as a Catholic in general practice lies in presenting ourselves as good and competent doctors through what may initially be a non-confessional approach. By first of all establishing a rapport on common ground, the way can be opened to candid discussion of those areas likely to present moral difficulty for us. Once we feel things to be progressing favourably, it may be time to drop the *Humanae Vitae* "bomb". The initial response is likely to be one of disbelief: the provision of contraceptive services, in particular, is now such an integral part of general practice that it would seem impossible to work in the field without it. The first attack then has to be followed up with a salvo of enticements designed to turn the tables. My own strategy was to explain that a clearly displayed notice would be placed in the practice reception area politely advising patients that I would not be providing contraceptive services. This tends to avert the open conflict which could arise where the Pill, for example, is denied to a patient. I went on to explain that I did not wish to share in the practice profits derived from family planning; I did not expect to carry a lesser workload and would happily see extra general medical patients who would otherwise have been seen by my colleagues now engaged in additional family planning work. These measures do, I believe, have the effect of demonstrating consistency of belief, as well as providing a small financial incentive to prospective business partners.

The above strategy has worked well for me personally. There may have been good fortune involved initially, but after five years in an essentially secular practice, I have been left free to practise as I wish and have not encountered major complaints although, undeniably, some level of background anxiety does persist.

4. Frameworks of medical ethics

In a certain sense, when seeking to practise medicine guided by Catholic principles, we will not clash with any formalised set of opposing principles because, at undergraduate level, medical ethics is taught either badly or not at all. Mostly we encounter a random cocktail of situation ethics not guided by any absolute moral norms. However, where there has been defined study of ethics in the secular realm, it is likely to be based around the four principles formulated by Beauchamp and Childress of Beneficence, Non-Maleficence, Respect for Autonomy and Justice. Their definitions are as follows:

1. Beneficence	The obligation to provide benefits and balance benefits against risk.
2. Non-Maleficence	The obligation to avoid causation of harm.
3. Autonomy	Respect for the decision-making capacity of autonomous persons.
4. Justice	The obligation of fairness in distribution of benefits and risks.

These seem to me to be open to interpretation to some extent. What, for example, does avoidance of harm imply if harm itself is not first defined according to absolute criteria? The advantage of this vagueness is that a free interpretation of Beauchamp and Childress's thinking which identifies with Catholic teaching on morality is quite feasible. From this, I would suggest that two basic guiding principles can be derived:

(i) To act always in the best interests of the patient – in light of Church teaching on morality. This of necessity implies avoidance of harm in Christ's terms.

(ii) To respect the autonomy of the patient – i.e., the freedom to accept or reject treatment and advice offered and ultimately to seek a second opinion from a doctor of his or her choice unobstructed.

5. Key areas of conflict

Because all except immediate emergency services are designed to be accessed initially via GPs in the UK, we find ourselves dealing with many more situations of moral import than do doctors in most other disciplines. Requests for contraception are made direct to GPs, who will also be asked to make referrals to specialists regarding abortion, sterilisation, IVF etc. Additionally, GPs may be expected to continue treatments initiated in the hospital setting but required to be maintained in the community. There are increasing varieties of procedures and medications which are not in accordance with Catholic morality, but I have identified five broad areas of difficulty which can be expected to arise regularly, and challenge a Catholic GP. These are:

1. Abortion
2. Contraception
3. Sterilisation
4. Some infertility investigations and treatments
5. Erectile dysfunction treatments for the unmarried.

5.1. Abortion

Contrary to what might be expected, abortion requests do not constitute the greatest difficulty. In terms of the 1967 Abortion Act, most cases do not fulfil the stated criteria of legitimacy and remain essentially unlawful; we may therefore decline requests on purely legal grounds. The Act seeks to legitimise abortion where two doctors are of the opinion that either:

(a) "The continuance of the pregnancy would involve risk to the life of the pregnant woman or of injury to the physical or mental health of the pregnant woman or any existing children of her family, greater than if the pregnancy were terminated"

OR

(b) "there is a substantial risk that if the child were born it would suffer from such physical or mental abnormalities as to be seriously handicapped."

For us who are obliged to do no harm, we simply cannot, in good conscience, countenance the notion that the killing of an unborn child could do other than harm to all concerned: it could never benefit either the mother or her born children. Scenarios in which there is a direct threat to the life of the pregnant woman are rare, although there may be occasional situations when removing, for example, a diseased, pregnant uterus or a fallopian tube damaged by an ectopic pregnancy constitutes a lifesaving measure. However, history reveals that hard cases make bad law, and in any case, such procedures do not qualify as abortion but have, as an unintended secondary effect, the death of the unborn child.

My approach to the patient requesting abortion or any other illicit procedure, for that matter, is to view the situation as I would any other medical consultation: I have training in medicine alone and can only offer a medical opinion. There are few, if any, circumstances where I am prepared to bow to a patient's demands without first considering the implications for all concerned: only where I conclude that my actions will not constitute moral or physical harm either to myself or the patient and will be in his or her best interests do I proceed. This principle applies as much to prescribing antibiotics as it does to weightier matters. So, I begin by taking a history and performing whatever examination or further investigation is appropriate; I am then in a position to discuss my findings with the patient and propose a course of action. This may produce an opportunity for a change of heart capable of sparing mother and child the abject misery of abortion, but seizing this opportunity requires effort. As already mentioned, these dramas of conscience are often played out against a backdrop of the stress inherent in general practice which, although of little moral import, serves nonetheless to heighten tension. The consultation may very well be one of twenty or more crammed into a morning surgery. Conjuring suffi-cient time to deal effectively with a young woman contemplating her difficult or unsupported future as a mother is often extremely challenging. It may be that a purely operative type of charity is called for when we discover, confronted with real life, that the warm sentiment we experienced at a stirring pro-life rally gives way to the onerous burden of fulfilling profes-sional obligations in far from ideal circumstances. Sufficient time to address the concerns of a reluctant mother-to-be is of paramount importance.

In the limited time available at a first consultation, I begin by outlining what I *am* able to offer: I will do all I can to provide support through this pregnancy and facilitate connection with other services available. Where this is not well received, I allow the patient to direct the consultation. If she persists along the lines of seeking an abortion, I share my experience of treating the aftermath of this procedure. An explanation of the possible physical and highly probable deleterious psychological sequelae is informa-tion to which every patient has a right. As with any surgical procedure, the doctor is obliged to inform fully of the nature of the procedure and the risks entailed. If no change of heart emerges, I invite the patient to discuss the matter with loved ones and return to me as often as she wishes, having first emphasised that, as a doctor, I do not feel abortion to be in her best interests and cannot support her in that choice. Sadly, few are swayed, and most simply ask how they should proceed with obtaining an abortion referral – it is here that delicacy is required if complicity is to be avoided. The first precept of doing no harm has been honoured; the rather thornier issue of respecting autonomy follows. My own response has been to lean heavily on the time-honoured principle that all are entitled to a second opinion from a doctor of their choosing. I do not have an obligation to arrange that second opinion and, in any case, I would be likely to choose a doctor who shared my view, which could be construed as an infringement of autonomy. My approach is to inform the patient of her right to seek a second opinion and leave the rest to her. Invariably there is minor friction and exasperation on her part as I repeat my advice that where and from whom she obtains a further opinion is a matter entirely for the patient. I am frequently asked whether she can see one of my colleagues and I reply that she certainly can but again she chooses. Almost inevitably, this is what does happen: she consults one of my colleagues who will almost certainly comply with her wishes.

It is an uncomfortable feeling to be rubbing shoulders with the evil of abortion, but I am satisfied that I am not complicit in it and grateful that I do at least have some opportunity to attempt averting it. Up to now, I have received no major complaints and those that have arisen were more to do with a clash of personalities than the principle being upheld.

5.2. Contraception

There may have been genuine, if misguided, good intentions behind the liber-alisation of contraceptive services in the 1960's. What was not foreseen by its proponents, however, was widespread sexual promiscuity and social devasta-tion as the family began to disintegrate. Most people born after about 1970 will have been raised on the principle that contraception is a good and sensible thing for all, married or otherwise. To oppose this notion is to incur ridicule or even malice. Whilst the majority will respect a conscientious objection to abortion, few can comprehend an anti-contraceptive mentality as a logical corollary. A steady nerve is required in the realm of contraception and all that follows in its wake – i.e., sterilisation, IVF etc.

As already outlined, in my own practice I have sought to construct a protective mechanism efficient at deflecting contraceptive requests on most occasions; when the system fails, a patient requesting (usually) the Pill will present.

In many cases, simply informing the patient that I am not a family-planning doctor brings the consultation to a swift and mostly amicable conclusion where the patient leaves to seek an appointment with a different doctor. However, some persist or even insist and thereby avail themselves of my medical opinion which, after all, is the only thing I have to offer. Proceeding then through the usual protocol of history, examination and special investigation, I arrive at my conclusion that I do not believe contra-ception to be in this person's best interest. This may provoke an immediate and angry response or, possibly, prepare the way for a discussion of the philosophical principles underpinning Catholic teaching in this area; there may even be an opportunity to introduce the possibility of natural family planning (NFP) as an alternative. Other than this, the consultation evolves as with abortion matters: the patient is advised of my opinion and informed of the right to seek another elsewhere.

Where contraception is concerned, tempers fray more readily than with abortion matters and one tends to feel a greater sense of humiliation and ridicule on the receiving end of the common response. However, complaints are unlikely to be sustainable where autonomy has been observed and the all-important second opinion left unobstructed.

5.3. Sterilisation

Most women of child-bearing age who read my advisory notice regarding contraception will conclude that the umbrella extends to surgical sterilisation but, since the notice is addressed to female patients, men will tend to slip through the net. Interestingly, the man's response, when denied this particular request, is more one of disbelief than anger; he finds himself unable to apprehend the notion that the snipping and tying of a couple of tubes should have such moral significance. But, as ever, I have been approached in my role as a doctor and therefore respond accordingly – history, examination etc. My conclusion, of course, is that vasectomy is not good for men. Once again, there may be an opportunity to explain why, but failing this, I proceed to an outline of what the operation entails, its potential side effects and the (mostly) extreme difficulty of reversal at a later time. Finally, I advise of the right to a second opinion.

5.4. Infertility

Without personal experience of an infertile marriage, I cannot entirely identify with the type of suffering incurred by couples in this situation. Certainly, from my observations as a GP, it appears to be profound. To anticipate children as the fruit of a marital union is natural and logical: when they fail to materialise a sense of failure or of having been cheated may ensue. These sentiments may arise in individuals or couples of any social or religious background but, increasingly, overcoming infertility by any means likely to succeed is viewed as an absolute right. The child has been commodified, and it is this, along with the numerous morally abhorrent methods of achieving pregnancy, which render the field of infertility treatment so perilous for a Catholic doctor.

The key problems are raised by procedures which remove conception from the setting of marital intercourse and those designed to produce multiple embryos, with the inevitable loss of most. A GP will rarely be directly involved in the procedures themselves but will certainly be approached with a view to initial investigation and subsequent referral to a specialist who may engage the couple in morally illicit tests or treatments. A particular difficulty for the GP is the question of obtaining a semen sample. The post-coital test, which did not present moral difficulty, seems to be out of vogue today: most specialists will now recommend masturbation. To the majority, this is a trifling matter but obviously it constitutes a serious moral transgression for a Christian.

When a childless couple or single person presents to me, I will not, in most cases, be in a position to cooperate with infertility treatments. However, my practice is to view the problem in a wider medical context as perhaps a case of primary infertility but also, quite possibly, an indicator of other underlying pathology such as diabetes or even more sinister conditions; and, of course, psychological malaise should not be ignored as a potential precipitant. A thorough history and examination along with urine and blood tests and perhaps scans or X-rays are then perfectly legitimate or even obligatory, but an uncomfortable line has to be drawn where the question of a semen sample is concerned. We might be fortunate enough to live close to a centre willing to undertake the post-coital test but, most likely, we will find it necessary to explain our conscientious objection to the couple or individual – the question is what to do next. Having taken patients part-way through the investigative process, it would seem uncharitable to suddenly wash our hands of the situation. I have not entirely resolved this matter for myself but have the feeling that the most charitable way to proceed is with a referral for further investigation, having first advised both patient and specialist that I am unable to cooperate in certain of the tests or therapies which might be suggested.

Making such referrals is a difficult balance of potential harm and good. On the one hand, I am fairly certain that masturbation will be advised for semen collection, and the overall treatment of the couple is highly unlikely to meet the moral criteria of legitimacy established by the Church. On the other, whilst the couple do not have an absolute right to a child, they have rights regarding investigation and treatment of disease in general; I therefore feel that I have an obligation to obtain some form of specialist help for them. There is also the advantage that, by engaging with the couple, an opportunity to explore NFP methods aimed at optimising conception rates might arise, as well as the chance to discuss adoption.

5.5. Erectile dysfunction

Requests for treatment of erectile dysfunction seem to be more frequent these days, probably because of the greater ease with which people feel they can discuss such intimate matters. The condition has often been the subject of humour but, in reality, is a tragic loss of the integrity of marriage, particularly for young couples. As with infertility, erectile dysfunction may be attributed to a primary failure or some underlying pathology of organic, psychological or mixed origin. Once again, it is a medical problem requiring a medical approach.

Where is the moral significance in this? The answer lies in the variety of unions formed by couples at the present time. Many still marry for life but, with a divorce rate now exceeding one in three and with some subsequent remarriage, it follows that there must be a considerable number of marriages where validity is, at least, questionable. Consider further that cohabitation and civil marriage are commonplace, along with rising numbers of same-sex unions. And what of the single person who has relations with serial partners? The question is to which of these unions is it licit to restore erectile function. The answer is not straightforward but can, I believe, be simplified by considering erectile dysfunction in the separate contexts of a primary problem and one resulting from underlying disease.

Patients are likely to simply present with a request for Viagra or other treatments but, as already emphasised, their condition requires full assessment before treatment can be contemplated. A full medical and psychological history and examination are vital; these, together with blood and urine tests, may very well reveal a cause amenable to a treatment which effectively restores potency – no moral dilemma here: erectile function returns concurrent with health. Whether the individual now chooses to engage in illicit sexual intercourse is not the doctor's concern in terms of cooperation. The doctor has simply fulfilled his or her professional obligation to investigate and treat disease. But what of those cases where a thorough search for conditions, the treatment of which could restore normal erectile capacity, proves fruitless? In these circumstances, the use of, say, Viagra facilitates an erection on demand but does not restore overall health, only a facet of it for a brief period. Since the erect penis has only one function, the doctor may find himself or herself cooperating, if not directly, at least proximately in an act of illicit intercourse. So, the doctor is faced with the task of assessing the validity of marriage among patients.

During the earlier part of my career in general practice, I wrestled with this problem and felt that it might preclude working as a GP for me. However, after several years experience and having sounded various experts, I have, I hope, arrived at a solution which will suffice in moral terms. Firstly, since I have nothing other than medical training, I am not in a position to make a competent judgement on the validity of a given marriage. In a ten-minute consultation, I cannot hope to ascertain what a marriage tribunal might take years to rule on. Further, it may be extremely offensive and damaging to pry too deeply into a couple's marital history. I believe, therefore, that the most good and least harm is achieved by a simple enquiry as to marital status; I accept the answer at face value, proceeding to treat the married and withhold treatment where a couple are unmarried, cohabitating or of the same sex. This again is an area where one feels the burden of personal humiliation, especially when a heightened emotional response ensues. However, recourse to the principle of respect for autonomy and the right to a second medical opinion is usually an effective diffusing tactic.

6. Conclusion

The experience of continuing to practise medicine in an environment where the Hippocratic tradition has been effectively turned on its head has a surreal quality when we are deeply immersed in what is happening but somehow entirely separated from it. It is sobering to consider objectively the true nature of what is going on. For me, this came into sharp focus during my hospital career prior to general practice when I spent time as a junior anaesthetist. I remain indebted to the consultants I worked for who treated me very well and entirely respected my position as a Catholic. When assigned to gynaecology operating sessions I would obviously not anaesthetise for abortions or sterilisations; another doctor would take over, leaving me to wander the corridors or drink coffee whilst, the truth is, a baby was crushed and dismembered. When I returned to anaesthetise the next case, the blood from the abortion might still be drying on the floor. My cooperation in this was zero; in general practice, I believe my level of cooperation also to be either zero or very remote and indirect at worst and then on very few occasions. However, having to work at such physical proximity to the evil being perpetrated remains disturbing. The only alternative I see, though, is not to work as a doctor at all and, as implied in my opening remarks, this would be to abandon ship and forego all hope of restoring nobility to our profession.

9

Cooperation problems in care of suicidal patients

Helen Watt

As a general rule, the lives and health of adults are entrusted to their own care. The authority of healthworkers over adult patients is delegated by the patient.[1] Healthworkers must respect the boundaries of their patients' bodies both by refusing to intervene harmfully – especially where the harm is serious and permanent – and by refusing to intervene without consent except for good reasons.[2] In other words, they must respect both the patient's bodily flourishing and the patient's prime responsibility for that bodily flourishing. That said, a choice of suicide causes such damage to the patient and to others that the threat of suicide dramatically changes the health-worker–patient relationship. This is so even when the suicidal person is thought to be fully competent, such that many choices by that person would have some claim to be respected.

1. Suicidal refusals

Suicide can, of course, be carried out by omission, as well as by an act. A patient who fears the extension of a life which is felt to be both painful and pointless may refuse treatment and/or care with the aim of accelerating death. Those around the patient, such as doctors and nurses, may realise themselves that the patient's life has value – despite the patient's current

---

[1] See e.g. Pius XII, "Address to the First International Congress of Histopathology". *AAS* 44 (1952), 779–89; Pius XII, "Address to Gregor Mendel Genetic Institute". *AAS* 49 (1957), 1027–1033.

[2] This is not to say that a doctor (for example) has no responsibility for trying to persuade a non-suicidal patient to accept treatment which seems clearly indicated. Complicity in wrongful, though non-suicidal, refusals is a real possibility.

feelings – and may be unwilling to facilitate suicide, even unintentionally, by omitting treatment or care. In this paper, I will look at the responsibilities of healthworkers in this situation, and at what counts as "complicity" or wrongful cooperation with the patient's plan. I will look, in particular, at cases where the patient also sees what he or she refuses as too burdensome, though this is not the patient's only reason for refusing the procedure.

Of course, if a procedure *really is* too burdensome – either in itself, or in relation to the benefits it promises – that procedure should not be offered,[3] especially to an unwilling patient. The burdens involved are a individual matter: a procedure which is genuinely too burdensome for one patient, due to his or her particular sensitivities, may not be too burdensome for another. Having said this, the *benefits* of a procedure also vary from patient to patient. Such benefits include social benefits – which would include giving patients who are suicidal and despairing the chance to reacquire a sense of the value of their lives. We should not too quickly give up on a patient's ability to resolve conflicts and be reconciled with life, with other people and, indeed, with God, given time and support.

What I want to focus on initially are cases where procedures are *unreasonably* refused by the patient *both* on the grounds of their perceived burdens and with the aim of ending life. Even taking into account particular sensitivities, the burdens involved do not justify refusal; moreover, the patient is also clearly motivated by the aim of hastening death. There are four possible scenarios of this kind which I would like to explore.

2. Mixed motives

In the first scenario, the patient refusing the procedure is "strongly suicidal". That is, the suicidal motive would suffice to account for the refusal even without the patient's other motive of avoiding the procedure itself. Moreover, the aim of avoiding the procedure is an "underdetermining" motive: were it not for the fact he wants to die – or at least, sees his life as worthless – the patient would not count the procedure's burdens as a reason to refuse it. On the contrary, those burdens would have been accepted had the procedure promised what the patient saw as a life worth supporting. Perhaps the patient sees *any* procedure as involving burdens too great for its benefits if continued life is not seen by the patient as a benefit at all.[4] Though

---

[3] Just as a doctor with a suicidal patient may give pain relief which could shorten life if the pain relief is otherwise warranted, so the doctor may withhold unwarranted treatment, despite the fact that the patient's refusal of that treatment has a suicidal motive.

[4] Alternatively, a suicidal patient may simply not focus on the procedure's burdens – particularly if the procedure is very straightforward or one to which he or she is accustomed.

only the background to a suicidal purpose, the view that life is not worth-while is very closely linked to that purpose.[5] For this reason, it should not be regarded as an independent reason for respecting refusals that are also suicidal.

There are three possible variations on the scenario just outlined. In the second scenario, the patient is also strongly suicidal, but is, in addition, strongly set on avoiding the procedure itself. Either of these motives would alone be sufficient to account for the patient's refusal, though in the event, the patient is refusing on the basis of both combined. In the third scenario, the patient is weakly (or more weakly) suicidal: only in conjunction with the strong motive of avoiding the unwanted procedure does the weaker motive of shortening life come into play. In the fourth scenario, the patient is weakly suicidal, and also weakly motivated by the aim of avoiding the unwanted procedure. Only in combination do the two desires – the desire to die, and to avoid the burdens of the procedure – give rise to intentions, and to subsequent behaviour. Neither the wish to die nor the wish to avoid the minor burdens of treatment or care would suffice on its own,[6] though they suffice in combination to form the intentions which ground the refusal. The two motives are jointly determining, but separately underdetermining. (Perhaps I should say here that in referring to determining motives, I am not denying free will. Rather, I am simply referring to the "strength" or explanatory power in various situations of the motives of someone who may have been fully free to make a different choice.)

It may be objected that my four scenarios are, in fact, unrealistic. Surely those who are truly suicidal, or truly anxious to avoid a certain procedure, will have that and that alone as an explanation of their behaviour? However, it is often the case that we do, or refrain from doing, something with two independent motives, each of which may be over- or under-determining of

---

[5] The view that life is not a benefit does not yet amount to – though it is often accom-panied by – the aim of ending life. However, where it is so accompanied, it should not be seen as giving independent grounds for respecting the patient's refusal. That would mean that any suicidal patient could claim the right to have his or her refusal respected, simply by reference to what is now an integral part of a suicidal plan.

The suicidal person may, of course, see life as a benefit, but nonetheless want to die – for example, so as to benefit other people. However, this is probably not the most common reasoning behind the choice of suicide.

[6] It may be psychologically impossible to intend something one does not sufficiently want in some sense, even if a "sufficient" desire need not lead automatically to a choice that favours that desire. Of course, we often have some control over what we find desirable, and can often choose to recognize the rational appeal of a competing consideration.

our decision when we act. For example, I may decide not to go to Bali both because I dislike Bali and because I find the journey burdensome. In the same way, a patient may recoil both from the burdens of treatment and from what the treatment will achieve: an extension of life. Such recoiling may give rise to mutually reinforcing aims: the aim of avoiding the burdens of treatment, and the aim of hastening death.

The scenario in which one intention is over- and the other intention under-determining also accords with our experience. The fact that one intention is doing more work than the other need not reduce the other to mere foresight of a (welcome) result. Admittedly, the bigger the distance between the strength of the motives – the work they are doing in explaining one's behaviour – the more likely it is that one motive will take over, and the other will cease to be considered. However, a motive which is insufficient to account for our choices by itself may still be a bona fide motive, existing side-by-side with what we otherwise intend. Thus a patient may be strongly suicidal, and less strongly set on avoiding the burdens of treatment (we can imagine that he would accept those burdens if the life which the treatment would extend were even slightly beneficial in his eyes). Alternatively, the patient may be strongly set on avoiding the burdens of a certain procedure, and aiming at his own death only as a secondary intention. Perhaps the patient has a moral objection to suicide, and wrongly believes he is justified in aiming at death providing he is also aiming at avoiding a burdensome procedure. (I am not, of course, making a judgement about the *culpability* of such a person, who may be making what I see as a moral mistake through no fault of his own.)

3. Conclusive motives

How, then, is the health professional to act amid these possible scenarios? I would argue that a weak, undetermining suicidal motive may often be set to one side in responding to refusals of some procedure, in the presence of a much stronger motive of avoiding the procedure itself. Only if the suicidal motive has some visible, outward effect (that is, if it determines the refusal, alone or in conjunction with some other motive) will there be a particularly strong reason to override the refusal. However, in cases where the life-avoiding motive is both weak and inconclusive, doctors and nurses should still make it clear that they themselves are not intending death. "That's not why we're stopping treatment", the doctor might say. "We don't want you to die, we just don't want to give you treatment you feel you can't cope with." (Of course, if the patient has, as we are imagining, an exaggerated view of the treatment's burdens, the doctor should first make a reasonable effort to persuade the patient to accept it.)

How should the doctor or nurse respond if the patient's suicidal motive is sufficient – or at least conclusive – in accounting for his or her refusal? In this case, the healthworker should, prima facie, override the patient's refusal – always assuming the procedure's burdens are not objectively too great. A few simple questions to the patient should throw some light on his or her motives, providing the patient is willing and able to respond. For example, "Is it mostly that you don't like the treatment, or mostly that you want to die?" "Would you still say you didn't want that treatment if you didn't want to die?" There is – at very least – a strong presumption in favour of preventing suicide: a choice particularly harmful to the patient, to those about him or her and to society at large. It is important to give suicidal, and especially strongly suicidal, people the message that others are trying to help them, and will not give up trying simply because they say no. There should be a policy of treating patients with conclusive suicidal motives in their best interests, just as we treat, or should treat, patients who are non-competent in their best interests. (It may, however, be the case that some procedures practically require the compliance of the patient. In what I say here, I am assuming that overriding the refusal will be feasible, bearing in mind the healthworker's other commitments.)

It may be asked why it should be so important to determine if the suicidal motive in the patient is strong and/or conclusive. Morally, there is some significance to the fact that the will to end one's life is strongly held.[7] An intention that is morally wrong does more moral harm to a person the more firmly rooted it is in the person's psyche, such that it would be likely to be retained (at least in the short term) even without a second motive. However, perhaps moral harm *per se* is not the central issue here. Intentions which have visible causal effects[8] (apart from their sheer presence being detected or reported) are arguably more in the public domain – more the business of others – than intentions which do not have such effects. Of course, in the term "visible causal effects" I am including the effects of omissions, where the wrongful intention was significant for subsequent events.

---

[7] It might be argued that a weak suicidal motive does not become stronger in itself for being jointly conclusive with a weak non-suicidal motive. While there is more to the cooperation question (I am arguing) than a moral assessment of the patient's state of mind, there is possibly some moral significance to the fact that the suicidal motive is conclusive, assuming the patient knows this. If the suicidal motive is what "sways the balance", the refusal would seem to represent a stronger commitment to suicide than where the suicidal motive makes no practical difference.

[8] Thus if homicide or suicide is attempted by wildly ineffective causal means (for example, hostile thoughts) this is of less concern to society than when more conventional means are chosen.

4. Legal/professional pressures

What are some other factors that might influence the doctor or nurse's response? Here I will look at various factors which might be morally relevant, whether or not the suicidal patient has a second aim in his or her refusal. The first factor is legal or professional pressure: doctors, for example, may fear repercussions if they fail to comply with suicidal refusals, or pass the patient to a colleague who will do so. What should a doctor do when expected either to respect the patient's wishes – suicidally motivated or otherwise – or pass the patient to a colleague with fewer qualms? What kind of risk of legal or professional penalties should a doctor be prepared to accept? The pro-life doctor may, of course, argue that suicidal refusals and/or cooperation with such refusals are, in fact, unlawful. However, this defence will not be open to doctors in all legislatures: deliberate assistance in suicide by omission may well be legally permitted in the place in which the doctor works.

Positive duties – that is, duties to make (as opposed to avoiding) certain choices – are not normally absolute. It is negative duties, such as the duty not to choose death by act or omission – leaving aside the requirements of justice – which bind absolutely. If a relative pointed a gun at a nurse's head and told her not to feed a suicidal patient, the nurse would surely be entitled to omit the choice to feed. Of course, the penalty, if one exists, for intervening to prevent suicide would normally be much less certain, and much less severe. Moreover, we can imagine particular circumstances which would mean a higher risk of repercussions should be taken by the health professional. It might be argued that a higher risk should be taken in the case of patients who are now incompetent (we can think, for example, of those who have signed advance directives with a suicidal motive). Such patients seem more completely and permanently entrusted to the health-worker's care than do competent patients who are actively seeking to prevent their lives being saved. In view of this, withholding treatment or care from an incompetent patient may be difficult to justify, and may encourage similar neglect of other incapacitated people. This applies particularly to the with-holding of food and fluids, which is particularly likely to be seen by others as deliberate killing of the patient, even if the healthworker does not, in fact, have this aim.

On the other hand, there are factors which could make withholding treat-ment or care from a *currently* suicidal patient difficult to justify. Cooperation in an ongoing – and therefore in a future – suicidal plan seems in itself more serious than cooperation in a plan formed in the past by a patient who is now incompetent. In addition to the ongoing moral harm involved in the patient's current suicidal plan, there is a *benefit* available only to patients who are competent: the benefit of reassessing the value of one's life and/or the burdens of what one is refusing.[9] If this benefit seems at all achievable, again, it is possible that higher legal/professional risks should be taken by the health professional.

5. Referral

Difficult questions are also raised by the issue of referral. The General Medical Council (GMC) allows a doctor who is unhappy with a patient's refusal of life-prolonging treatment – including tube-feeding – to withdraw from that patient's care. However, the GMC also requires that senior doctors in this situation ensure "that arrangements have been made for another suitably qualified colleague to take over their role, so that the patient's care does not suffer".[10] While the GMC does not, on the face of it, require that the doctor referred-to take a different view from the doctor who refers, this may nonetheless be a foreseeable result of referring the patient to a colleague. The colleague may be indifferent to, or even disapproving of, the patient's wish to die, but may nonetheless think him or herself obliged to respect the patient's refusal. May a pro-life doctor refer to such a doctor, in the limited sense of transferring the patient to him or her? I would say yes, at least in some cases: it is neither formal nor very close material cooperation to refer to a doctor one knows will fail to prevent suicide, if one is not referring for that reason, and is under serious pressure to refer. Such an action is more like what a doctor does when going off duty: the doctor passes patients to the care of others without necessarily endorsing how those others will behave. However, if, in withdrawing from a patient's care, one passes the patient oneself to another doctor it is important not to give the impression that the doctor is chosen as someone with different moral views from one's own. On the contrary, one would gladly refer to a

---

[9] One might argue that there was more of an onus on the doctor not to respect a refusal with an "underdetermining" suicidal motive, in that the patient's mind could potentially be changed by addressing the patient's other motive. On the other hand, an "overdetermining" suicidal motive may be more scandalous, in that the issue of burdens may be less to the fore.

[10] General Medical Council, "Withholding and Withdrawing Life-prolonging Treatments: Good Practice in Decision-making", par. 28. Moreover, a recent letter by the head of the GMC standards commission helpfully made the point that deliberately causing death by omission of food and fluids was regarded by the standards commission as unlawful and unethical behaviour (H. Thomas, "GMC guidance on withholding life prolonging treatment". 326 (2003) *BMJ*: 1215). Doctors could perhaps use this statement as a defence for their non-referral to a doctor who will share the patient's aim to hasten death (see also note 14 below). Having said that, it still leaves the problem of referral to someone expected to facilitate that aim by complying with the patient's refusal but without intending death.

pro-life colleague if such a colleague was available. Of course, there will sometimes be an overriding reason not to refer to a non-pro-life colleague: for example, to a doctor who is strongly pro-suicide, rather than simply unprepared to override a suicidal refusal.

6. Active interventions

There is another factor which can influence the doctor's responsibilities. Doctors may rightly be unwilling to cooperate with a strongly suicidal patient if such cooperation involves an active intervention which itself causes harm. For example, the doctor may be unwilling to turn off a respirator at the request of such a patient.[11] In cases where harm is not intended, but will nonetheless occur, there is a special onus on the doctor not to cause harm by an active intervention. While it is not reasonable, in view of competing opportunities to do good, to expect that people always intervene to prevent harm, there is more of a presumption against intervention where this itself does only serious harm, even if the harm is not intended. Assuming there is no other reason for turning off the respirator than the patient's suicidal request, it is, I would argue, wrong for the doctor to accede to this request, even under threat of disciplinary action. Admittedly, such an act is a "prevention of a prevention" – i.e. it merely reverses the effect of a previous intervention to sustain life.[12] In this way, it differs from the sheer initiation of a causal chain leading to death. Nonetheless, in one respect, such an act involves closer complicity in suicide than failing to treat – or even supplying dangerous drugs – in that the act itself is one which leads inexorably to death. While even closer complicity can be envisaged – such as injecting, under threat, a lethal substance into the patient[13] – an active intervention which itself causes death in a strongly suicidal person is something the doctor should avoid, even at the risk of serious repercussions. Again, some forms of active, non-intentional cooperation with a suicidal refusal will be more scandalous than others: more likely to be interpreted as euthanasia or assisted suicide, or at least as agreement with a policy of neglect. An example might be the

---

[11] We can also envisage active interventions which do not themselves cause death but are nonetheless morally problematic – such as arranging for transport to take a suicidal patient home to die.

[12] There is a danger in all these cases, but perhaps especially in those involving an active intervention, of the doctor coming to see him or herself as collaborating "formally" or intentionally with suicide.

[13] I have argued that such an act, while it need not involve the aim to kill, is nonetheless wrong in itself, as a form of mutilation (H. Watt, "Beyond Double Effect: Side-Effects and Bodily Harm", in D. Oderberg and T. Chappell (eds) *Human Values: New Essays on Ethics and Natural Law*. Houndmills: Palgrave MacMillan 2004: 236–251).

removal of a feeding tube from a patient who had made a prior, suicidally-motivated request that this be done.

7. Conclusion

Sadly, such situations are likely to become more common in the future, with the spread of the concept of the "worthless" life, in combination with an exaggerated stress on patient autonomy. In particular, with the passing of the Mental Capacity Act in Britain, there will be many such dilemmas of conscience for doctors, nurses and others.[14] It is unclear whether (for example) the GMC will sufficiently respect conscientious objection, though human rights law on respect for freedom of religion can also be invoked. Health professionals have a special responsibility to protect their patients from harm, and their profession from a growing disregard for human life and health. Courage, prudence and prayerful reflection will certainly be needed, in years to come, by those with suicidal patients in their care.

---

[14] Some protection is, however, offered by e.g. clause 5, section 4 of the Act, which states that someone determining the best interests of an incapacitated person must not be motivated by a desire to bring about death.

10

The Holy See and the Convention on the Rights of the Child: moral problems in negotiation and implementation

Jane Adolphe

1. Introduction

The 1989 Convention on the Rights of the Child (hereafter "the Convention") has been the subject matter of much controversy. At first glance, one might argue that the Convention, negotiated and drafted within the United Nations, has attained almost universal acceptance having been ratified or acceded to by 191 States, with the exception of Somalia and the United States.

Yet, upon deeper reflection, one can see that battle lines have been drawn between those who argue that the Convention drives a wedge between children and their parents, and others who maintain that the Convention finally recognizes children as autonomous beings and merely seeks to strike a balance between the individual rights of children and those of their parents. Through the course of this debate, the Holy See has come under attack from both sides. The former group contends that the Holy See should not have ratified the Convention, while the latter argues that the Holy See in ratifying but entering (what are known in international law as) reservations, failed to treat the child as an autonomous being.

Other considerations, which are rarely highlighted, are those concerning the relationship between the Committee on the Rights of the Child (hereinafter "the Committee"), and the Holy See. When the Holy See ratified the Convention she agreed to submit a report to this monitoring body. She submitted her first report and later appeared before the Committee to answer questions. From a perusal of these documents, it is clear that the Committee treated the Holy See like any other State party, and in so doing either misunderstood or ignored her *sui generis* status in international law, which is integrally tied to her spiritual and moral mission. In particular, the Committee recommended that the Holy See withdraw her reservations, which uphold parental rights and duties and reject contraception and abortion as legitimate means of family planning. In addition it asked her to change her magisterium and internal legal system in a way that would render them more in line with the "spirit of the Convention."

Whatever the polemics surrounding the Convention, it enjoys the distinction of being the only United Nations agreement to have reached near universal acceptance. Its global influence on the consideration of children's rights, therefore, cannot be underestimated, marginalized, or easily reversed.

This presentation is a case study, then, of the participation of the Holy See in the drafting and implementation of the 1989 Convention on the Rights of the Child, with a view to understanding her involvement. To flesh out the issues, the presentation is divided into four parts. Part I discusses the Holy See and the international order with a view to highlighting the Holy See's legal personality within the international system, and her status within the United Nations system. Part II gives a brief overview of the Convention, and its problems. Part III seeks to address three questions: Why did the Holy See participate in the drafting process? Why did she ratify the Convention? Why does she continue to participate in the implementation process? Part IV highlights some important implications and then makes a few concluding remarks.

2. The Holy See and international order

The Holy See is recognized as a subject of international law, or in other words, a member of the international community with rights and duties. This means she contributes to the creation of international law and accepts, adopts, or accedes to those practices, laws, or principles which do not contradict her particular nature and spiritual mission.

The Church, which is neither a State nor an organization, participates as a member of the international community predominately through her governing organ the Holy See, which is itself a juridical subject.[1] In canon

---

[1] It is argued that since her earliest origins, the Catholic Church has been an independent juridical entity having a normative order analogous to that of States but radically different in its ontological and theological constitutive elements which justify its independence and sovereignty. See for example: Ignio Cardinale, *The Holy See and the International Order*. London: Colin Smythe, Gerrards Cross 1976 at 73–82; Robert John Araujo, "The International Personality and Sovereignity of the Holy See." 50 (2001) *Catholic University Law Review*: 291; Jude M. T. Okolo, "The Holy See: A Moral Person." Ph.D. diss., Pontificia Università Urbaniana, Rome 1990 at 51.

law, the Holy See is defined as the Pope or the Pope and the Roman Curia.[2] The Holy See is at the same time the governing authority of Vatican City, which is a neutral and independent territory serving as a base of operations for her spiritual and moral mission.[3] In brief, to understand the complex reality of the Holy See one must come to grips with three entities: the Church, the Holy See and Vatican City.

A related question is whether the Holy See signed and ratified the Convention as (1) an organ of the supreme power of the Catholic Church having a juridical effect in canon law; (2) a sovereign organ of the State of Vatican City having a juridical effect in its legal system; or (3) an organ that combines two distinct realities having effects in both juridical systems? The most coherent perspective is that of the third paradigm. As we will discuss, by reserving on issues pertaining to parental authority and family planning, the Holy See protects the integrity of the deposit of the faith as embodied in the magisterium and provided for in canon law, and by reserving on the question regarding the application of the Convention in Vatican City, she highlights the *sui generis* nature of this small State.

The Holy See, though a unique body on the world scene, has therefore a specific and well-justified role to play in international affairs. Indeed, by reason of the Gospel, she is a perennial voice on the international level in defense of Christian morals, and in particular, human dignity, rights and duties of the human person, and world peace. Her presence at the United Nations and her participation in various discourses concerning these themes are fully in keeping with her nature and divinely ordained mission. Yet to safeguard her independence she does not participate as a member of the United Nations. Rather she is a non-member State of the United Nations having the status of Permanent Observer,[4] with an office in New York since

---

[2] "Nomine Sedis Apostolicae vel Sanctae Sedis in hoc Codice veniunt non solum Romanus Pontifex, sed etiam, nisi ex rei natura vel sermonis contextu aliud appareat, Secretaria Status, Consilium pro publicis Ecclesiae negotiis, aliaque Romanae Curiae Instituta." *Codex iuris canonici,* 1983, c. 361.

[3] Vatican City was set up in 1929 with the Lateran Agreements entered into between the Holy See and the Italian Government. The Agreements are comprised of three treaties: "(1) a political treaty recognizing full sovereignty of the Holy See in the City of the Vatican; (2) a concordat regulating the position of the Catholic Church and religion in the Italian State; and (3) a financial convention by which Italy gave to the Holy See" a sum of money. Cardinale, 103.

[4] For a comprehensive academic treatment of observer status with the United Nations, see: E. Suy, "The Status of Observers in International Organizations," Académie de droit international, *Recueil des Cours,* vol. II (1978): 79–160; Russel A. Jay, *United Nations Observer Status: An Accumulation of Contemporary Developments* (Washington, D.C.: World Association of Lawyers 1976), and R. G. Sybesma-Knol, *The Status of Observers in the United Nations.* Brussels: Vrije Universiteit Brussel Centrum voor de

1964, and in Geneva since 1967.[5] She also cooperates with various specialized bodies and agencies working within the United Nations system.[6]

Through her position as Permanent Observer, the Holy See has made her presence felt at the United Nations. The Pope himself has spoken before the General Assembly on three separate occasions: 1965, 1979 and 1995. On each occasion he stressed the spiritual and moral mission of the Holy See, and emphasized the United Nations' good work before delivering a Christian message involving the correction of various errors.

Pope Paul VI addressed the General Assembly on 4 October 1965 and delivered a message of peace to all humanity. He congratulated the United Nations for establishing a system of solidarity, and stressed its important role when he noted that "it represents the obligatory path of modern civilization and of world peace." He also underlined the Holy See's role at the United Nations as an "expert in humanity," and one qualified to speak on behalf of the human person. In addition, he spoke of the need of modern civilization to return to spiritual principles capable of sustaining, illuminating and animating its development and progress. He also highlighted the spiritual mission of the Holy See and the role its temporal sovereignty plays in promoting this mission.[7]

Studie 1981; see also a brief discussion of the topic by Araujo, 347–353. For treatment of the issue by the United Nations itself see: United Nations General Assembly, *Question of Criteria for the Granting of Observer Status in the General Assembly: Note of the Secretariat* (hereinafter, *Question of Criteria*), Forty-ninth Session, 9 November 1994, Agenda Item 157, A/C.6/49/WG.3/CRP.1; see also "Selected Legal Opinions of the Secretariat of the United Nations and Related Inter-Governmental Organizations," *United Nations Juridical Yearbook 1962* (hereinafter, "Selected Legal Opinions"), 22 August 1962, ST/LEG/8.

[5] United Nations, *Information on the Status of Permanent Observer Mission to the United Nations* (hereinafter, *Information on the Status*). New York: Public Inquiries Unit, October 1992: 2.

[6] The *Annuario Pontificio per l'anno 2003* (Città del Vaticano: Libreria Editrice Italiana 2003, at 1241–1243) includes a list of permanent observers at the following: the Office of the United Nations and Specialized Bodies, at Geneva and Vienna, United Nations Industrial Development Organization (UNIDO); United Nations Food and Agriculture Organization (FAO), United Nations Educational, Scientific and Cultural Organization (UNESCO); Council of Europe; Organization of American States; and World Organization of Tourism.

[7] "He is your brother, and even one of the least among you, representing as you do sovereign States, for he is vested – if it please you so to think of Us – with only a mute and quasi symbolic temporal sovereignty, only so much as is needed to leave him free to exercise his spiritual mission and to assure all those who treat with him that he is independent of every worldly sovereignty. He has no temporal power, no ambition to compete with you. In point of fact, We have nothing to ask for, no question to raise; at most a wish to express and a permission to request: to serve you, within Our competence, disinterestedly, humbly and in love.... Whatever your opinion of the Roman

Fourteen years later, on 2 October 1979, Pope John Paul II addressed the General Assembly and praised and thanked the United Nations for its initiatives promoting peaceful coexistence and cooperation among nations. In particular, His Holiness mentioned the work done in the areas of culture, health, food, work, and the peaceful use of nuclear energy. He also pointed out important issues directly related to world peace: the Middle East crisis, the arms race, and threats against human rights. In this speech, he argued for a better relationship between spiritual and material values, claiming: "The pre-eminence of the values of the spirit defines the proper sense of earthly material goods and the way to use them. This pre-eminence is therefore at the basis of a just peace."[8] On the issue of the Holy See's relationship with the United Nations, Pope John Paul II stated:

> The formal reason for my intervention today is, without any question, the special bond of cooperation that links the Apostolic See with the United Nations organization, as is shown by the presence of the Holy See's permanent observer to this organization. The existence of this bond, which is held in high esteem by the Holy See, rests on the sovereignty with which the Apostolic See has been endowed for many centuries. The territorial extent of that sovereignty is limited to the small state of Vatican City, but the sovereignty itself is warranted by the need of the papacy to exercise its mission in full freedom and to be able to deal with any interlocutor, whether a government or an international organization, without dependence on other sovereignties. Of course the nature and aims of the spiritual mission of the Apostolic See and the Church make their participation in the tasks and activities of the United Nations very different from that of the states, which are communities in the political and temporal sense.[9]

On 5 October 1995, Pope John Paul II spoke again to the General Assembly, emphasizing the rights of nations and respect for differences. He went on to offer authentic definitions of freedom and moral truth, arguing that "utilitarianism, the doctrine which defines morality not in terms of what is good but of what is advantageous, threatens the freedom of

---

Pontiff, you know Our mission: We are the bearer of a message for all mankind" (Araujo, citing Pope Paul VI, Address to the General Assembly of the United Nations Organizations, 4 October 1965, at 315).

[8] Pope John Paul II, Address to the General Assembly of the United Nations Organizations, 2 October 1979. http://papal-library.saint-mike.org/John_PaulII/Addresses/UN1979.html

[9] *Ibid.*

individuals and nations and obstructs the building of a true culture of freedom."[10] In regard to the mission of the Holy See and its relationship with the United Nations, Pope John Paul II stated:

> The Holy See, in virtue of its specifically spiritual mission, which makes it concerned for the integral good of every human being, has supported the ideals and goals of the United Nations Organization from the very beginning. Although their respective purposes and operative approaches are obviously different, the Church and the United Nations constantly find wide areas of cooperation on the basis of their common concern for the human family.[11]

3. The Convention: philosophical and practical problems

3.1. Philosophical issues

Efforts at the international level have developed hand in hand with an increasing reliance on children's rights rhetoric, and a review of the literature reveals that a number of different perspectives on children's rights can be loosely grouped into two major approaches, described as the protectionist and autonomist theories of children's rights.[12] The protectionist theory was the prevalent approach to children's rights during the pre-Convention period; namely in the drafting of the 1924 League of Nations Declaration of the Rights of the Child and 1959 UN Declaration on the Rights of the Child. The autonomist theory, on the other hand, is that which seems to have won out in the drafting and implementation process of the 1989 Convention on the Rights of the Child.

A. Protectionist theory

The protectionist theory of children's rights is characterized by its embrace of traditional conceptions of marriage, the family and parental authority as developed in Western cultures under a Judeo-Christian belief system.

According to this theory, the family is the best environment for the growth and development of children. Parents have a keen interest in seeking the best for their children, and society has a strong interest in ensuring that children are raised to become responsible citizens, cognizant of the common good. Moreover, this theory asserts that it is unrealistic for a child, or any other

---

[10] Pope John Paul II, Address to the General Assembly of the United Nations Organizations, 5 October 1995 (Available online at the Vatican website, <http://www.vatican.va/holy_father/john_paul_ii/speeches/index.htm>, last accessed 7 October 2003).

[11] *Ibid.*

[12] Jane Adolphe, *A Light to the Nations: The Holy See and the Convention on the Rights of the Child.* J. C. D. diss., Pontificia Università della Santa Croce, Rome 2003, 75–106.

member of a family living under the same roof, to expect to enjoy total autonomy at all times – indeed, individuals must choose to act not only in the interests of the family, but also in the interests of the community, or society at large, which people have come to acknowledge and accept that they belong to.

The main justification for the above theory is that children are different from adults due to their immaturity and vulnerability, and therefore require parental protection, education and supervision to ensure they develop in a manner that will allow them to responsibly exercise their autonomy once they become adults. Parental authority is protected and supported by the State, which (1) favors the rights of children within families; (2) relies upon families as children's best and first protectors; and (3) respects family integrity and privacy through minimal interference. Indeed, the State generally intervenes only in exceptional cases when parents have demonstrably failed children (i.e., neglect, abuse or abandonment).

B. Autonomist theory

The autonomous child theory, on the other hand, maintains that families are likely to fail children and that the solution to this problem is to free children from their families and endow them with adult rights (i.e., freedom of expression, freedom of religion, the right of association, and the right to privacy) all of which will be safeguarded largely, if not primarily, by the State, which must, to fulfill this role, actively monitor parents' treatment of their children and participate in educating and providing for them.

This theory is based on the assumption that children should, as far as possible, be free to exercise choice and self-determination in all important areas of their lives, since only the individual is in a position to know his or her own best interests: efforts to judge the interests of others necessarily represent coercion or intolerance – a prelude to favoring certain ideas, thoughts or behaviour over others.

This distorted vision of freedom – "to do what one wants" – has important implications for rearing children. It necessarily follows that children should have the right to choose their own moral, spiritual and religious value systems, and that parental permissiveness should be the fundamental principle for child-rearing.

Before moving on to the discussion of the Convention and how the autonomist theory plays itself out in the Convention, I wish to address two main objections to classification of the literature into these two categories. The first objection is that any reduction of the various perspectives into two main categories – protectionist and autonomist – is an oversimplification of the literature on children's rights. While this is partly true, given the diversity of opinions on the topic of children's rights, one is compelled to make generalizations in order to discuss the issues adequately in the space allotted. Further, the decision to reduce the categories to two, instead of three or even more, is due to the essential underpinnings of each proposed position in comparison with the two theories or categories proposed in this paper. As described above, the autonomist and protectionist theories rest on certain presumptions that are fundamentally inconsistent. Upon a review of the literature, scholarly works are placed in one of the two categories corresponding to the underlying presuppositions the author promotes in his or her own theory. Certainly, some children's rights scholars as well as Convention proponents argue that various academics and the Convention itself have successfully combined elements of the autonomist and protectionist schools into one coherent whole. However, my review of this area of study has not borne this out. While people may often have mixed feelings about a given perspective, arguments made in support of children's rights generally reflect a pattern of thinking that is consistent with one of the two visions. For example, many of the Committee recommendations cited below reveal an autonomous perspective of children's rights because such suggestions undermine parental rights and duties – a key concern in the protectionist approach. This is not to say that a better legal balance cannot be developed that would ensure respect for children's rights as their capacities evolve without undermining the rights and duties of parents. However, to date, this has not been achieved.

The second objection maintains that such an analysis demonstrates a Western bias in its approach to children's rights. In this regard, it is frequently emphasized that the reality of family life differs across the globe. Families in Africa do not meet the same challenges as families in the United States. This is, of course, true. However, the Convention was predominately drafted by Western nations, and as a consequence, a Western vision permeates the Convention and Committee interpretations of the Convention.[13]

Turning again to the autonomist school of thought: how, then, are the philosophy and the Convention related?

The Convention marks a radical shift in thinking about children's rights, moving away from the protectionist approach to children's rights to the autonomist model that attempts to free the child from parental control,

---

[13] In this regard, Cynthia Price Cohen observes: "Finally, as the drafting of the Convention on the Rights of the Child neared completion, there were rumors that, because most of the less developed countries had not participated in the drafting of the Convention, they viewed it as a Northern-Western treaty that failed to reflect their concerns. As a result, there was fear that even if these attitudes did not derail the process completely, they might still prevent the Convention from being widely accepted." (Cynthia Price Cohen, "The Developing Jurisprudence of the Rights of the Child" [hereinafter, "The Developing Jurisprudence"]. 6 (1993) *St. Thomas Law Review*: 85, n. 474).

and through such efforts downgrades the integrity of the family and under-mines parental rights and duties.

The United Nations itself admits this evolution in stating that the Convention "charts new territory"[14] – that it promotes "the right of the child to be an actor in his or her own development, to express opinions and to have them taken into account in the making of decisions relating to his or her life."[15]

The 1989 Convention consists of a lengthy list of rights (54 articles in total), which spring up without any apparent connection to prior declarations embodying international principles on children's issues.[16] The Convention does not just embody recommendations or aspirations but rather creates international legal obligations that are enforced with the assistance of its monitoring body, the Committee on the Rights of the Child. This Committee, originally composed of 10 members, has been expanded to 18 members, and is the single most important mechanism for enforcing the Convention worldwide.

Its primary role is to determine whether State Parties are meeting international standards and, if not, to determine what measures State Parties must take to ensure the standards are met in the future. The Committee considers reports submitted to it by State Parties and makes recommendations, which are not legally binding, but are frequently carried out by State Parties seeking to avoid bad publicity internationally when Committee comments and recommendations are picked up by the media, usually with the assistance and pressure of both non-governmental organizations (NGOs) and inter-governmental organizations (IGOs).

The importance of the NGOs cannot be underestimated. They greatly assist the Committee by also submitting what are referred to as "shadow reports" designed to supplement State reports. These NGO reports frequently provide additional information, correct misstatements or errors in State reports as well as highlighting specific problems. To ensure their findings are not ignored, NGOs request the Committee to participate in the "pre-sessional meeting," a private meeting closed to the media and State delegates, which is held about two months in advance of the hearing of a State's report. At the conclusion of every pre-sessional meeting a list of questions is drafted by the Committee, which is then sent to the State for response. It is within a couple of months of the pre-sessional meeting

---

[14] United Nations, *The Convention on the Rights of the Child: World Campaign for Human Rights* (hereinafter "World Campaign"). New York: United Nations, May 1991.

[15] *Ibid.*

[16] Cynthia Price Cohen, "The Relevance of the Theories of Natural Law and Legal Positivism", in M. Freeman and P. Veerman (eds) *The Ideologies of Children's Rights*. Dordrecht, The Netherlands: Kluwer Academic Publishers 1992.

that State delegates appear before the Committee expected to address the list of questions received.

Just recently, in response to the sexual abuse scandal in the United States, "Catholics for a Free Choice," a pro-choice group led by Frances Kissling, organized a special briefing and produced a report which alleged that the Holy See was in breach of her obligations under the Convention.[17] The Holy See has not yet submitted her second report, which was due in 1999, but when she does she should expect many questions on the topic.

On a more positive note, awareness has increased with respect to international moral problems, and more conservative NGOs have been engaging the process. For example, in regard to Canada's hearing to discuss its Second Report scheduled for 17 September 2003, three NGOs presented their reports at the pre-sessional meeting held on 10 June 2003 in Geneva and two of them promoted the natural family based on marriage. In particular, Focus on the Family argued that Canada was in breach of the Convention for not helping children by promoting and supporting the natural family. In support of their argument they proffered statistics setting out the ills suffered by children raised in alternative families in comparison to those growing up in natural families. The report noted increased rates of depression, poverty, teen pregnancy, teen suicide, teen crime, neglect and abuse.[18] Another NGO,

---

[17] Catholics for a Free Choice, *Clergy Sexual Abuse: Out of the Shadows*, prepared for the Special Session of the General Assembly on Children held in May 2002. See also a second report *The Holy See and the Convention on the Rights of the Child: Shadow Report*, September 2002, submitted to the Committee on the Rights of the Child during the Thirty-first Session, available online at <http://www.cath4choice.org/spotlight.htm>, last accessed 7 October 2003.

[18] See, for example, the scientific literature in Canada: the *Family Health Index* (available at http://www.nffre.org/resreports.php) published by the Canadian-based National Foundation for Family Research and Education, which links various problems (i.e., hyperactivity, teen suicide, and smoking) to the decline in traditional marriage and family (cited in Brad Evenson, "Two-Parent Family Healthiest, Study Finds," *National Post*, 27 November 1998); see also the Canadian government's *National Longitudinal Study of Children and Youth* which considers 23,000 Canadian children, and shows that children of poor single parents or parents living in common law relationships suffer more from behavioral, physical and emotional health problems than other children living in families that earn higher incomes (HRDC Update 1996, n. 294, Part III, Ottawa: Government of Canada, at http://www.hrdc-drhc.gc.ca/sp-ps/arb-dgra/nlscy-elnej/home.shtml., updated every two years); see also the study, *Giving Mom and Dad a Break: Returning Fairness to Families in Canada's Tax and Transfer System*, Commentary No. 117, by K. Boessenkool and J. B. Davies of the Canadian-based C. D. Howe Institute (Toronto, Canada, 1998), which calls for changes in federal income tax policy and the elimination of taxing one-income couples more than two-income earners at the same income level. For a discussion of this study see: Tom Arnold, "Families Need Income Tax Break: Report," *National Post*, 27 November 1998.

REAL Women of Canada, introduced a report arguing that gay adoption contravened Convention provisions due to the physical and moral dangers associated with gay role models and exposure to a gay lifestyle.

3.2. Practical application issues

Turning now to the practical issues, the Convention combined with Committee interpretations transforms traditional relationships between the child, the family, and the State. We can see this transformation in three main areas of the Convention: (1) general principles, (2) civil and political rights for children, and (3) rights and duties of parents.

A review of Convention provisions and Committee reports clearly demonstrates that the Convention is being interpreted by the Committee as granting children adult rights, transferring parental duties to the State, diminishing parental rights and duties, increasing State intervention, calling for a massive welfare State, and empowering the Committee on the Rights of the Child to become the highest world authority on ethics and values in regard to children.

A. General principles

The Committee has concluded that there are four general principles which must aid in the interpretation of the Convention. They are Art. 2 (1) (non-discrimination); Art. 3 (1) (best interests of the child), Art. 6 (2) (survival and development) and Art. 12 (the right to be heard).[19]

In so concluding, the Committee implicitly rejects the principle that preambular provisions should inform the interpretation of the Convention, and thus avoids preambular references to the family and the right to life, which is a point I will return to later.

(a) First general principle: Article 2: Non-discrimination

With respect to the non-discrimination principle set out in Art. 2 (1), the Committee on the Rights of the Child has pinpointed two basic forms: age-based and gender-based discrimination.

According to Art. 2 (1), "State Parties shall respect and ensure the rights set forth in the present Convention to each child within their jurisdiction without discrimination of any kind." While in principle this sounds fair,

---

[19] See, for example, the principles expressly enumerated by the Committee on the Rights of the Child, "Concluding Observations of the Committee on the Rights of the Child: Paraguay," Seventh Session, 24/10/94, CRC/C/15/Add. 27, para. 7 wherein Paraguay is criticized for not fully taking into account the provisions of the Convention, "including its general principles, as reflected in its articles 2, 3, 6, and 12."

the provision opens the door to attacks on age-based discriminations that have traditionally been employed to protect children in some countries. For example, commenting on the report submitted by El Salvador, the Committee challenges limits on the exercise of children's rights according to age-based categories:

> [T]here is a need to consider seriously questions relating to the legal definition of the child, in particular the minimum age for marriage, employment, military service and testimony before a court. It appears that these provisions do not sufficiently take into consideration the principles of the best interest of the child and non-discrimination.[20]

In its examination of initial state reports, the Committee has frequently found what it refers to as "gender discrimination."[21] It is important to note that the term "gender" may mean different things to different people. For example, many who participate within the UN system, especially those who work at the local level, may understand the term to mean simply "relating to the male and female sex". For example, in countries like Africa it is a known fact that girls do not, as a general rule, receive the same level of education as boys and so references to "gender discrimination" or initiatives designed specifically for the "girl child" may seem reasonable.

What the Committee means by "gender," however, may differ greatly, for the word has come to represent a particular understanding of human sexuality that places a gap between man's physical and psychic/emotional characteristics. In contemporary usage, the term "gender" denotes that "one's biological sex is a natural given" but that all other sex-related differences between men and women, such as masculinity, femininity, manhood, womanhood, motherhood, fatherhood, and heterosexuality are culturally constructed "gender roles," and therefore artificial and arbitrary.[22]

---

[20] Committee on the Rights of the Child, "Concluding Observations: El Salvador," Fourth Session, 18/10/93, CRC/C/15/Add. 9, par. 10.

[21] Rachel Hodgkin and Peter Newell, *Implementation Handbook for the Convention on the Rights of the Child*. New York: UNICEF 1998, 23–24.

[22] The term has been defined as follows: "Gender is a concept that refers to a system of roles and relationships between women and men that are determined not by biology but the social, political and economic context. One's biological sex is a natural given: gender is constructed... gender can be seen as the process by which individuals... are born into biological categories of... women and men through the acquisition of locally defined attributes of masculinity and femininity" (United Nations International Research and Training Institute for the Advancement of Women [hereinafter, "INSTRAW"], *Gender Concepts in Development Planning: Basic Approach* [Santo Domingo, 1995, Instraw/SER.B/50, available at INSTRAW website: <http://www.un-instraw.org/en/resources/publications.html#a7> 16/08/02]). See also

This approach to human sexuality is clearly a borrowing from radical feminism where the word "gender" has become "the focus of the feminist revolution."[23] From a gender perspective, motherhood, a vocation necessarily unique to women, is frequently undermined by this kind of thinking, since the goal of statistical equality between men and women in the work force, women's autonomy, and access to political power can never be met "if even a significant percentage of women choose mothering as their primary vocation."[24]

Radical feminist ideology, in fact, permeates thinking on children's issues, especially that concerning the "girl child." For example, in preparing for the Fourth World Conference on Women: Action for Equality, Development and Peace, held in Beijing, China in 1995 (hereinafter, "the Beijing Conference"), the Committee on the Rights of the Child held a General Discussion on the "girl child," and later submitted its report to the Beijing Conference. The report addressed concerns of inequality and discrimination based on gender discrimination arising from "harmful traditions and prejudices

---

the critique of gender definition by Dale O'Leary, *The Gender Agenda: Defining Equality* (LaFayette, Louisiana: Vital Issues Press 1997), 120: O'Leary discusses the development of the term in feminist literature and its employment within the context of UN conferences, i.e., the Cairo and Beijing Conferences. For a similar analysis within the scope of the Beijing Conference, see Martha L. de Casco, Michael Cook, Catherine Dalzell *et al.*, *Empowering Women: Critical Views on the Beijing Conference* (Crows Nest, New South Wales, Australia: Little Hills Press 1995). For a brief overview of feminist thought, see Rosemarie Tong, *Feminist Thought: A Comprehensive Introduction* (San Francisco: Westview Press 1989); and for an overview of feminist thought in the field of human rights, see Rebecca J. Cook (ed), *Human Rights of Women: National and International Perspectives*. Philadelphia: University of Pennsylvania Press 1994.

[23] O'Leary, 120; see also de Casco *et al.*

[24] O'Leary, 120–121. This deconstruction of motherhood is a recurring theme in the INSTRAW booklet, where the following quote, from Maureen Macintosh, appears: "[N]othing in the fact that women bear children implies that they exclusively should care for them throughout childhood…" (INSTRAW, 18). The booklet continues: "The fact of sexual difference is used to arbitrarily limit women's autonomy, economic activities and access to political power" (INSTRAW, 19). To eradicate the problem, INSTRAW advocates increasing "[w]omen's access to political and economic power," and the development of a "broad view of human reproduction activities," including abortion and contraceptive services, thus articulating the connection between production and reproduction (INSTRAW, 21–22). O'Leary's review of feminist literature reveals that any woman who aspires to mothering is seen as a threat to other women who have not been so "socially conditioned to want the wrong things" (O'Leary, 124). For a review of some of the feminist literature see Rebecca J. Cook (ed), *Toward a Feminist Theory of the State*. Philadelphia: University of Pennsylvania Press 1994.

160

against women."[25] This criticism has chilling connotations, since these "harmful traditions and prejudices against women" could very well refer to any education of children within families about traditional roles, for example, that of fatherhood or motherhood.

Such has already been the case: in its "Concluding Observations" to the report submitted by Jamaica, the Committee notes that the traditional attitudes, beliefs, or customs supporting and promoting differentiation of roles carried out between men and women are conducive to "the persistence of gender stereotypes and the existing role distribution between boys and girls,... which might affect very young girls."[26] Similarly, as publicists Rachel Hodgkin and Peter Newell of the *Implementation Handbook for the Convention on the Rights of the Child* observe, the Committee has been greatly concerned about the girl child; that is, "the way roles [are] traditionally distributed within the family," especially "in rural or remote areas under the strong influence of community and religious leaders."[27]

(b) Second general principle: Art. 3 (1): Best interests of the child

Article 3 (1) makes the best interests of the child "a primary consideration" in "all actions concerning children." The concept of "the best interests of the child" is also specifically mentioned in other articles pertaining to the separation of children from parents (art. 9 [1]); parental responsibilities (art. 18); deprivation of family environment (art. 20); adoption (art. 21); restriction of liberty (art. 37 [c]); and criminal matters involving juveniles (art. 40 [2][b][iii]).

The Committee has elevated the "best interests of the child" to a general principle of the Convention, and exhorts State Parties to incorporate it into plans, policies, and workings of parliaments and governments both nationally and locally, and to include it in considerations with respect to budgeting,

---

[25] This report stated: "In fact, girls are simply human beings who should be seen as individuals and not just as daughters, sisters, wives or mothers, and who should fully enjoy the fundamental rights inherent to their human dignity.... Within the larger movement for the realization of women's rights, history had clearly shown that it was essential to focus on the girl child in order to break down the cycle of harmful traditions and prejudices against women..." (Hodgkin, Newell, 29, quoting from the Committee on the Rights of the Child, "General Discussion Report on the Girl Child," Report on the Eighth Session, January 1995, CRC/C/38).

[26] Committee on the Rights of the Child, "Concluding Observations: Jamaica," Eighth Session, 15/02/95, CRC/C/15/Add. 32, par. 11.

[27] Hodgkin, Newell, 29, quoting from the Committee on the Rights of the Child, "General Discussion Report on the Girl Child," in preparation for the Fourth World Conference on Women: Action for Equality, Development and Peace, held at Beijing, China in September 1995.

allocation of resources, and assessments of child impact. For example, in examining the Paraguay Report, the Committee stated that it wished "to emphasize the importance of the provisions of article 3 of the Convention, relating to the best interests of the child, in guiding deliberations and decisions on policy, including with regard to the allocation of human and economic resources for the implementation of the rights guaranteed under the Convention."[28] In short, no significant action in society or by individuals or institutions should be undertaken without due consideration as to whether or not it will serve children's best interests.

The wording of article 3 (1) is extremely broad, so as to embrace a full range of activities affecting children, including State-initiated actions as well as those of private bodies and families. For example, in considering the Bulgarian Report, the Committee stated that it had concerns about "the insufficient consideration of the principle of the best interests of the child in tackling situations of detention, institutionalization, and abandonment of children, as well as in relation to the right of the child to testify in court."[29]

Stephen Toope, Law Professor at McGill University, emphasizes what art. 3 (1) will mean for parents: "the overall thrust of the Convention is to declare that best interests of children may not be what parents think they are . . . provisions concerning privacy (Art. 16), freedom of expression (Art. 13), and freedom of thought, conscience and religion (Art. 14) . . . undercut any notion that the parent may dictate what is 'best' for the child."[30] Indeed, this subjective and value-laden standard means that decision makers informed by their own moral, religious, and political beliefs and opinions about children, the family and child-rearing can shape families through application of the standard. And in the liberal culture in which we live this often translates into the promotion of contraception and abortion services for children.[31]

(c) Third general principle: Art. 6: Right to survival and development
Pursuant to article 6 (1), "State Parties recognize that every child has the inherent right to life," and (article 6 (2)), they "shall ensure to the maximum extent possible the survival and development of the child."

---

[28] Committee on the Rights of the Child, "Concluding Observations: Paraguay," Seventh Session, 24/10/94, CRC/C/15, par. 9.

[29] Committee on the Rights of the Child, "Concluding Observations: Bulgaria," Fourteenth Session, 24/01/97, CRC/C/15/Add. 66, par. 12.

[30] Stephen J. Toope, "The Convention on the Rights of the Child: Implications for Canada," in *Children's Rights: A Comparative Perspective*, at 48.

[31] See for example the discussion about the promotion of "reproductive health needs for adolescents" in Robert J. Araujo, "Sovereignty, Human Rights, and Self-determination: The Meaning of International Law." 24 (2001) *Fordham Int'l L.J.*: 1477.

The notion of "survival and development" rather than "right to life" or "the right to life, survival and development" is the fundamental principle behind this article. Authors Hodgkin and Newell assert that "[t]he concept of 'survival and development' to the maximum extent possible is crucial to the implementation of the whole Convention."[32] Similarly, the group of NGOs calling themselves the International Save the Children Alliance[33] designates "survival and development" as a general principle along with discrimination, best interests, and participation.[34]

The focus on the right to "survival and development" is indeed curious: if life itself is not protected, then all other rights are irrelevant. On the other hand, one may argue that the right to survival includes the right to life. But why not be clear? Why is there no specific mention of the right to life? In response, focusing on the "survival and development" phraseology is presumably an attempt to avoid the controversy surrounding the right to life issue. In this regard, Hodgkin and Newell make the following comment:

> Contentious ethical issues arise in relation to the right to life, which the Committee has not as yet tackled – for example the responsibility to sustain significantly disabled children at birth and to sustain the life of very premature babies.... As medical technology advances, these issues of rights may become more complex and pose a greater number of ethical dilemmas and possible conflicts between the rights of the child and the mother.[35]

(i) Article 6 (1): Right to life

Article 6 (1) and preambular paragraph 9 both raise the abortion question. The Preamble quotes from the 1959 Declaration of the Rights of the Child that "the child, by reason of his physical and mental immaturity, needs special safeguards and care, including appropriate legal protection, before

---

[32] *Ibid.*, 85.

[33] Save the Children was founded in London in 1919. Today there is an organization called the International Save the Children Alliance made up of about 29 member organizations. The Alliance's work is devoted to the rights of the child as enshrined in the Convention on the Rights of the Child. It has been very active in providing information about the reporting and implementation process to NGOs. See, for example, "Who We Are," 2000, Save the Children website: <http://www.savethchildren.net/stc/publicsite/editor/readnew.asp?id=138> (2000).

[34] International Save the Children Alliance, *Integrating Work on the Convention on the Rights of the Child into Policy and Practice*, 1998, CRIN website: <http://www.crin.ch/crc/integr.htm> (2000).

[35] Hodgkin, Newell, 88–89.

as well as after birth." Delegations that supported the inclusion of the paragraph "argued that their national legislation contained provisions protecting the rights of the unborn child from the time of conception."[36] Those that opposed argued that its inclusion would preclude the possibility of State Parties legalizing abortion, thereby violating "the right to make decisions concerning one's body and health."[37] They also opposed the idea of using the preambular provision to assist in interpreting article 1, which defines the term "child" to mean that the life of a child begins at conception: "Every human being below the age of eighteen years unless, under the law applicable to the child, majority is attained earlier."

The debate was resolved by a compromise that left the decision to State Parties about when "childhood" begins – conception, birth, or somewhere in between.[38] This was achieved by including the preambular provision "before as well as after birth," but tempering its legal effect with the following statement in the *travaux préparatoires*: "In adopting the preambular paragraph, the Working Group does not intend to prejudice the interpretation of Article 1 or any other provision of the Convention of State Parties."[39]

The Committee's position on abortion is far from consistent. On the one hand, it has condemned the use of abortion as being destructive to family culture. For example, in considering the Report submitted by the Russian Federation, the Committee expressed its concern for "the breakdown of family culture as regards abandoned children, *abortion* [emphasis added], the divorce rate, the number of adoptions, the number of children born out of wedlock, [etc.] . . . ."[40] Yet, in other cases, the Committee promotes the provision of sex education and health services to children and adults which include the dissemination of material and services on various methods of contraception, including abortifacients and "safe" abortions. The Committee stated that "to reduce the practice of abortion, greater efforts should be made to provide family education . . . to disseminate widely knowledge about modern methods of family planning,"[41] which include, however,

---

[36] David Johnson, "Rights of the Child and Cultural and Regional Pluralism," in Michael Freeman and Philip Veerman (eds) *The Ideologies of Children's Rights*. Dordrecht, The Netherlands: Kluwer Academic Publishers, 108.

[37] *Ibid.*, 108–109.

[38] Hodgkin, Newell, 1.

[39] David Johnson, 109.

[40] Committee on the Rights of the Child, "Concluding Observations: Russian Federation," Third Session, 18/02/93, CRC/C/15/Add. 4, par. 10.

[41] Committee on the Rights of the Child, "Concluding Observations: Romania," Fifth Session, 07/02/94, CRC/C/15/Add. 16, par. 15.

those methods promoted by UNFPA programs for adolescent sexual and reproductive health: "the pill, IUD, injectable, implant, female barrier method, spermicide or condom – or voluntary sterilization,"[42] new forms of male contraception,[43] and safe abortions.[44]

Further, the Committee has criticized governments for not providing abortions to alleviate the problems of teenage pregnancy and clandestine abortions. For example, during the review of the Nicaraguan Report, Committee member Mrs. Karp, promoting broader access to abortion services, criticized Penal Code provisions that limited abortion to therapeutic grounds alone.[45]

Hodgkin and Newell observe that the Committee in the future may be tackling difficult ethical and spiritual issues relating to "the responsibility to sustain significantly disabled children at birth and to sustain the life of very premature babies."[46] If it were to embark upon this analysis, one should expect the same inconsistent treatment of the issues.

(ii) Article 6 (2): Right to survival and development

Article 6 (2) provides that State Parties "shall ensure to the maximum extent possible the survival and development of the child." In the *General Guidelines Regarding the Form and Contents of Periodic Reports*, published by the Committee, paragraph 40 promotes massive State intervention when State Parties are asked:

> [to] describe specific measures... to create an environment
> conducive to ensuring to the maximum extent possible the
> survival and development of the child, including physical, mental,
> spiritual, moral, psychological and social development, in a

---

[42] UNFPA, *Hope and Realities: Closing the Gap between Women's Aspirations and their Reproductive Experiences* (New York, NY: UNDPI 1998), 5.

[43] UNFPA, *Population Issues Briefing Kit 1998* (New York, NY: UNDPI 1998), 6.

[44] *Ibid.*, 4. It is noteworthy that the term "safe abortion" in practical terms implies that "for abortion to be safe it must be legal" (O'Leary, 60).

[45] According to the summary records, Mrs. Karp noted that "under the Penal Code abortion was prohibited except for 'therapeutic reasons.'" If the mother was under age or had been the victim of rape, could those be considered legitimate therapeutic grounds for an abortion? Were abortion services available for under-age girls who had been the victims of sexual abuse and, if so, were they free? She suggested that however sensitive the religious and moral issues involved in that area, and despite the fact that abortion was not in itself a good form of family planning, consideration needed to be given to changing some of the prevailing social attitudes to abortion (Committee on the Rights of the Child, "Summary Record of the 212th Meeting: Nicaragua," Ninth Session, 29/05/95, CRC/C/SR.212, par. 22).

[46] Hodgkin, Newell, 88.

manner compatible with human dignity, and to prepare the child for an individual life in a free society.[47]

That "parents... have the primary responsibility for the upbringing and development of the child" (art. 18) seems merely cosmetic, lost in the myriad of articles requiring extensive State action, including: art. 24 (right to the highest attainable standard of health); art. 27 (right to a standard of living); art. 29 (compulsory State education); and art. 31 (right to rest and leisure).

(d) The fourth principle: Article 12: Right to be heard

Article 12 (1) provides that a "child who is capable of forming his or her views has the right to express those views freely in all matters affecting the child, the views of the child being given due weight in accordance with the age and maturity of the child."

According to Hodgkin and Newell, art. 12 underlines that children are "active subject[s] of rights... [and] individuals with fundamental human rights, and views and feelings of their own,"[48] which essentially means there is "no area of traditional parental or adult authority – the home or school for example – in which children's views have no place."[49] Michael Freeman has described this article as the "linchpin of the Convention,"[50] because it recognizes the child as a "full human being, with integrity and personality and with the ability to participate fully in society."[51] In other words, this notion has become a general principle under the Convention because it clearly seeks to establish children as autonomous beings having the ability to participate fully in society, independently from the family, and with the assistance of the State.

The Committee has stressed the need to reflect article 12 in the legislation of nation States. For example, in consideration of the Report submitted by the United Kingdom, the Committee suggested that the State develop

---

[47] *Reporting Guidelines to Governments: General Guidelines Regarding the Form and Contents of Periodic Reports To Be Submitted by State Parties under Articles 44, Paragraph 1(b), of the Convention* (hereinafter, "*General Guidelines*"), adopted by the Committee on the Rights of the Child at its 343rd meeting, Thirteenth Session, 11/10/96 (cf. Hodgkin, Newell, appendix, 604–618).

[48] Hodgkin, Newell, 145.

[49] Ibid., 149.

[50] Michael Freeman, "Whither Children: Protection, Participation, Autonomy?" 22 (1993–1994) *Manitoba Law Journal*: 307, 319, n. 8.

[51] *Ibid.*

mechanisms to ensure that children are granted full participation rights within the family and community life.[52]

In brief, what this necessarily means is the creation of a bureaucracy readily available to provide these services or entitlements, and corresponding tax increases in order to pay for them. This, in turn, means further State intervention into families and, in some cases, further conflict when children are legally represented during divorce proceedings over the protests of those parents who may desire to protect their children from the stresses associated with the legal process.

B. Civil and political rights

The general principle set out in art. 12; namely, the right to participate or the right to be heard, is integrally connected with the other autonomous child rights provided for in the Convention. The right to express one's own views is restated and further developed in art. 13 (the right to seek, receive, and impart information and ideas of all kinds), art. 14 (freedom of thought, conscience, and religion), and art. 15 (freedom of association).

While arts. 13 to 15 potentially have very broad applications (i.e., allowing children to decide with whom they socialize, study or worship, including individuals determined to cause them harm in some way), they also interfere with parents' rights to exercise discretion over their children's education and socialization, especially on matters relating to ethics and religion.

(a) Article 13: Freedom of expression

Article 13 guarantees children "the right to freedom of expression; this right shall include freedom to seek, receive and impart information and ideas of all kinds, regardless of frontiers."[53] The only acceptable limitations are those set

---

[52] The Committee suggested that "greater priority be given to incorporating the general principles of the Convention, especially the provisions of its article 3, relating to the best interests of the child, and article 12, concerning the child's right to make their views known and to have these views given due weight, in the legislative and administrative measures and in policies undertaken to implement the rights of the child. It is suggested that the State Party consider the possibility of establishing further mechanisms to facilitate the participation of children in decisions affecting them, including within the family and the community" (Committee on the Rights of the Child, "Concluding Observations: United Kingdom of Great Britain and Northern Ireland," Eighth Session, 15/02/95, CRC/C/15/Add. 34, par. 27).

[53] It is noteworthy that article 13 of the Convention is closely linked with article 17, which addresses the role of the mass media and the importance of every child having "access to information and material from a diversity of national and international sources especially those aimed at the promotion of his or her social, spiritual and moral well-being, physical and mental health." In regard to "access to information" no mention is made of parental guidance. Yet, for many parents, the article immediately

out in art. 13 (2) which are: "provided by law and are necessary: (a) For respect of the rights or reputations of others; or (b) For the protection of national security or of public order (*ordre public*), or of public health or morals." There is no restriction mentioning parental rights or familial integrity, and States are encouraged to give the limiting provision a very restrictive interpretation. For example, in examining Indonesia's Report, the Committee expressed its concerns about authorities giving "a wide interpretation to limitations for 'lawful purposes' of the exercise of these rights to freedom of religion, expression and assembly which may prevent the full enjoyment of such rights."[54]

In other words, according to art. 13 (2), the State has sole authority for determining appropriate limits on a child's "right to information" and "freedom of expression."

(b) Article 14: Freedom of thought, conscience, and religion

Under art. 14 of the Convention, children have "the right to freedom of thought, conscience and religion," subject to two limitations. Firstly, according to art. 14 (2), parents and legal guardians are "to provide direction to the child in the exercise of his or her right in a manner consistent with the evolving capacities of the child." Secondly, pursuant to art. 14 (3), "Freedom to manifest one's religion or beliefs may be subject only to such limitations as are prescribed by law, and are necessary to protect public safety, order, health or morals or the fundamental freedoms of others."

The limitations set out in art. 14 (3) will be interpreted restrictively. For example, the Committee examining China's Report stated: "The Committee wishes to emphasize that the implementation of the child's rights to freedom of thought, conscience and religion should be ensured in the light of the holistic approach of the Convention and that limitations on the exercise of this right can only be placed in conformity with para. 3 of art. 14 of the Convention."[55]

---

raises a number of questions, such as: Who is to determine what constitutes spiritual, moral or physical well-being, and which sources of material are most likely to promote it? Ought the material to include information relating to sex, contraception, or abortion, even for very young children? What about pornography or realistic, but potentially upsetting, portrayals of violence? What about information on the therapeutic benefits of marijuana? Does the article prohibit parental supervision of their children's television viewing or of their use of the Internet?

54 Committee on the Rights of the Child, "Concluding Observations: Indonesia," Seventh Session, 24/10/94, CRC/C/15/Add. 25, par. 13.
55 Committee on the Rights of the Child, "Concluding Observations: China," Twelfth Session, 07/06/96, CRC/C/15/Add. 56, par. 17.

Parents are only permitted to provide "direction" to the child on matters of conscience or religion, and that direction must be given in "a manner consistent with the evolving capacities of the child." Article 14 (2) significantly diminishes the rights and duties of parents in comparison with those expressed in the 1966 Covenant on Civil and Political Rights which recognized "the liberty of parents and, when applicable, legal guardians to ensure the religious and moral education of their children in conformity with their own convictions" (art. 18). Article 14, in effect, leaves children entirely free to follow their consciences in matters of thought and religion. This has some potentially seriously consequences for children and others, should no religious beliefs, values or ethics be learned at all, or should parents be prohibited from preventing their child from joining a dangerous religious sect or a satanic cult or from associating with those who are already members of such organisations.

Hodgkin and Newell argue that the wording of art. 14 and the Convention's general principles "certainly do not support the concept of children automatically following their parents' religion until the age of 18;" however, should a child choose to follow the parents' religion, "article 8 (preservation of identity), article 20 (preservation of religion when deprived of family environment), and article 30 (right to practice religion in community with members of the child's group) support children's right to acquire their parents' religion."[56]

According to Hodgkin and Newell, the Algerian interpretative declaration which "stipulates that a child's education is to take place in accordance with the religion of its father" is incompatible with art. 14.[57] Indeed, in reviewing the report submitted by Algeria, the Committee argued that Algeria was in breach of the Convention and recommended that the report be withdrawn.[58] They also note that "The Committee has as yet made little comment on the effective implementation of art. 14," but maintain "It is apparent from a range of declarations and reservations that in some States the right of the child to freedom of religion conflicts with tradition and, in some cases, with legislation. Few States appear to have reflected the child's rights in domestic legislation, and in many, it is parents who determine the child's religion."[59]

When conflicts arise between parents and children, the practical reality of Convention provisions assures that "neither parent should have 'authority'

---

[56] Hodgkin, Newell, 180.
[57] *Ibid.*, 181, citing Committee on the Rights of the Child, "Concluding Observations: Algeria," Fifteenth Session, 18/06/97, CRC/C/2 Rev. 5, 10.
[58] "Concluding Observations: Algeria," Fifteenth Session, CRC/C/15 Add. 76, pars. 11, 28.
[59] Hodgkin, Newell, 177.

over such matters. Where there is disagreement and the matter goes to court, the matter should be decided on the basis of the child's right under art. 14, with the child's views taken seriously according to his or her age and maturity."[60]

(c) Article 15: Freedom of association

Article 15 (1) recognizes "the rights of the child to freedom of association and to peaceful assembly," subject only to the restrictions laid down in art. 15 (2), namely, "those imposed in conformity with the law and which are necessary in a democratic society in the interests of national security or public safety, public order (*ordre publique*), public health or morals or the protection of the rights and freedoms of others."

Here again, no reference is made to the parental right to guide and educate a child on how he or she may best exercise this freedom. Only the State is to decide the limits on the exercise of such a right. Again, the possibility exists that a movement to see the Convention implemented in a particularly literal fashion raises the possibility that parents may be prevented from taking action to protect their children from harm. If a parent seeks, for instance, to prohibit his child from associating with youth offenders, drug users, heavy drinkers, gang members, criminals, pimps, members of religious cults and so forth, a question arises whether, under the terms of the Convention, parents could be accused of infringing a child's freedom of association.

Moreover, the Committee urges children to employ individualistic rights rhetoric to advance claims. For example, the Committee, reviewing Jordan's Report, stated: "The active participation of children should be encouraged. Similarly, efforts should be undertaken to develop new channels, including membership of associations, through which children may make their views known and have them taken into account."[61]

Furthermore, the Committee encourages children's involvement in political activities. In considering the Belarus Report, the Committee wondered whether the law which prohibited children from engaging in political activities until age eighteen infringed art. 13 of the Convention.[62]

In sum, from what we have hereto described, it is not unfair to ask whether the Convention, in its zeal to provide for the child's autonomy, is at the same time depriving the child of adult guidance, education, and protection that

---

[60] *Ibid.*, 181.

[61] Committee on the Rights of the Child, "Concluding Observations: Jordan," Sixth Session, 25/04/94, CRC/C/15/Add. 21, par. 24.

[62] Committee on the Rights of the Child, "Summary Record of the 125th Meeting: Belarus," Fifth Session, 26/01/94, CRC/C/SR.125, par. 13.

may, in the long run, better serve the child's best interests than unfettered freedom. Let us now consider the effects of the Convention on parental authority and family integrity.

C. Rights and duties of parents

It is difficult to see how the above provisions can be reconciled with references to the family. The preamble of a Convention is, in theory, supposed to set out the values and principles that will inform interpretation of provisions. With respect to the Convention, the Committee has delineated a set of general principles that have little or no bearing on preambular provisions.

Paragraph 5 of the preamble recognizes the family as "the fundamental group of society and the natural environment for the growth and well-being of all its members and particularly children," and states that the family "should be afforded the necessary protection and assistance so that it can fully assume its responsibilities." Preambular para. 6 stresses the need for a child to "grow up in a family environment, in an atmosphere of happiness, love and understanding."

In the body of the Convention, there is reference to leaving and entering any country for purposes of family reunification (art. 10); and the consequences for children deprived of their family environment (art. 20).

With respect to parental authority, there are numerous articles that refer to parents and their importance to children's well-being, such as the right to know and be cared for by parents (art. 7); maintenance of personal relations and direct contact with parents upon separation (art. 9); and parental responsibilities and assistance by the State (art. 18).

Yet the formal acknowledgments of the importance of the family and parents in the preamble and some other articles are largely offset by the manner in which the Convention requires children to rely on the State to enforce their rights against parents, the State in effect taking on responsibility for children's well-being or for their protection – a role that traditionally has fallen on parents. In this regard, one need only consider the array of government-provided services or entitlements, such as art. 18 (day care), art. 26 (social assurance for all children) and art. 27 (an "adequate standard of living"). Further, as previously mentioned, Art. 3 calls on the State to ensure that parents are "acting in the best interests of the child;" and Art. 5 limits parents to carrying out their rights and duties "in a manner consistent with the evolving capacities of the child," and in a way that only directs and guides them "in the exercise by the child of the rights recognized" in the Convention.

The incongruity between the Preamble, on the one hand, and some of the Convention Articles along with Committee interpretations of them, on the other hand, sheds light on why the Convention is "schizophrenic" in its approach to parents and the family. In the words of J. W. Mohr:

> There is a curious form of schizophrenia here, a split and dissociated mind, not recognized because it is assumed to be normal, which tells us on the one side that the family is the place of all evil and on the other that it is the source of our deepest needs and expectations.[63]

3. The Holy See and the Convention

Having set out a few of the key problems associated with the Convention, let us turn to a discussion as to why the Holy See participated in drafting the Convention, what effect, if any, she had, and what problems have arisen in the Convention's implementation.

3.1. *Why did the Holy See assist in drafting?*

Firstly, the Holy See has a serious and profound interest in the care and defence of children. Such activities are shown to derive from the nature of the Church and her divinely ordained mission. However, perhaps more importantly, a review of the drafting process reveals how the Holy See acted as a light to the nations when she intervened on a number of occasions to correct error. She was able to positively influence the flow of some important discussions. The *travaux préparatoires* for the Convention reveal that the Holy See intervened on topics such as the right to life. The Holy See spoke about the necessity of adequate health care and an adequate standard of living, the right to education, and the importance of religious formation. The Holy See also expressed concern regarding the influence of the mass media on children, and concern for the best means by which the young can profit from rest and leisure, and be protected from exploitation, trafficking, and armed conflict. Moreover, the Holy See pushed to ensure the recognition of a child's "moral and spiritual" development and the rights and duties of parents in ensuring this formation. Finally, the Holy See contributed to discussions aimed at the practical application of the Convention's work: the

---

[63] Mohr made these comments not in relation to the Convention but rather in regard to the revolution in Canadian family law that embraced an increase in children's autonomy and parental responsibility almost to breaking point. J. W. Mohr, "The Future of the Family, the Law and the State," in B. Landau (ed) *Children's Rights in the Practice of Family Law*, 366–378, at 366.

formation of the Committee, the procedures for State reports, and the methods to be employed.[64]

Perhaps the Holy See's greatest contribution was in regard to the drafting of paragraph 9 of the Preamble where, as previously stated, she pushed for the inclusion of the following phrase: "the child, by reason of his physical and mental immaturity, needs special safeguards and care, including appropriate legal protection, *before as well as after birth.*"

3.2. Why did the Holy See ratify?

There are numerous Convention provisions which are not disputed. Paragraph 5 of the Preamble, for example, recognizes the family as "the fundamental group of society and the natural environment for the growth and well-being of all its members and particularly children," and states that the family "should be afforded the necessary protection and assistance so that it can fully assume its responsibilities."

Preambular paragraph 6 stresses the need for a child to "grow up in a family environment, in an atmosphere of happiness, love and understanding." In the body of the Convention, there is reference to leaving and entering any country for purposes of family reunification (art. 10), and mention of the consequences for children deprived of their family environment (art. 20). With respect to parental authority, there are numerous articles that refer to parents and their importance to children's well-being, such as the right to know and be cared for by parents (art. 7); maintenance of personal relations and direct contact with parents upon separation (art. 9); and parental responsibilities and assistance by the State (art. 18).

Further, there are provisions that protect children from various dangers, and others that offer special assistance in special circumstances. Such provisions include those relating to illicit transfer (art. 11); the disabled (art. 23); refugees (art. 22); illicit drugs (art. 33), unlawful sexual activity (art. 34); abduction (art. 35); armed conflict (art. 38); and criminal procedure (art. 40).

Lastly, the Convention's attention to the poor, uneducated and sick child evident in Arts. 30, 28, 29, 24, where this does not relate to abortion or contraception "services" and/or usurpation of parental rights/duties is also a positive step.

However, the Holy See could not concur entirely with the Convention, and so, while showing that she was in accord with the majority of the Convention provisions when she ratified the Convention in 1990, she invoked article 51 of the Convention to attach three reservations. A reservation is a unilateral

---

[64] See Sharon Detrick (ed), *The United Nations Convention on the Rights of the Child: A Guide to the 'Travaux Préparatoires.'* Dordrecht, The Netherlands: Martinus Nijhoff 1992 (Distributed in U.S. by Kluwer Academic Publishers).

statement, generally entered at the time of ratification, which "purports to exclude or to modify the legal effect of certain provisions of the treaty in their application to that State,"[65] and it is based on the concept that "no State is bound in international law without its consent to the treaty."[66]

Through her reservations, the Holy See objected to the content of the Convention where such content diverged from the magisterium of the Church as supported and protected in her internal legal system. The Holy See excluded and modified the legal effect of Convention provisions within her jurisdiction, stating in particular that she would:

1. interpret the phrase "family planning education and services" in article 24 (2) to mean only those methods of family planning which she considers morally acceptable; that is, the natural methods of family planning;
2. interpret the Convention in a way which safeguards the primary and inalienable rights of parents, in so far as these rights concern education (arts. 13 and 28), religion (art. 14), association with others (art. 15) and privacy (art. 16); and
3. apply the Convention taking into consideration the particular nature of the Vatican City State.[67]

The first two reservations go to the heart of the controversy in which the Holy See has historically been engaged. With these two reservations, the autonomous view of the child as an isolated, independent chooser on important matters such as religion, freedom of association, privacy, education and human sexuality, is rejected outright. In this way, the Holy See remains a light to Christians and the world at large in regard to the authentic dignity of the child.[68]

---

[65] The term "reservations" has been defined in the three Vienna Conventions: Vienna Convention on the Law of Treaties (1969), Convention on Succession of States in respect to Treaties (1978), and Convention on the Law of Treaties between States and International Organizations or between International Organizations (1986). The 1978 and 1986 definitions of reservation are modeled on the 1969 Convention and "adapted to the particular object" of these Conventions (*Third Report on Reservations to Treaties by Alain Pellet, Special Rapporteur*, 1998. International Law Commission 50th Session, 5 May 1998, A/CN.4/491/Add. 1, 10).

[66] *Second Report on Reservations to Treaties by Alain Pellet, Special Rapporteur*, 1996. International Law Commission 48th Session, 21 May 1996, A/CN.4/477/Add. 1, 18.

[67] Committee on the Rights of the Child, *Reservations, Declarations, and Objections Relating to the Convention on the Rights of the Child: Note by the Secretary General*, 12 March 1998, CRC/C/2/Rev. 7, 24; see also CRC/C/2/Rev. 6, 20.

[68] It is noteworthy that the average person may be unaware of the Holy See's reservations because copies of the Convention on the Rights of the Child are rarely sold in stores with the reservations attached, and discussions of the Convention, on the plethora of websites devoted to children's rights, may not allude to the existence of reservations *per se*.

The third reservation addresses the possible application of the Convention in the State of Vatican City, since there is always the possibility for children to reside in Vatican City and, indeed, a few do.[69]

The Holy See also entered an important declaration that addresses the right to life issue: "The Holy See remains confident that the ninth pre-ambular paragraph will serve as the perspective through which the rest of the Convention will be interpreted."[70] One cannot underestimate the importance of this declaration since the preambular paragraph, were it to be employed as an aid in interpreting Convention provisions, would protect the right to life which is at issue in article 1 (the definition of the child) and article 6 (the right to life).

3.3. Why does the Holy See assist in implementation?

What becomes less clear is the continued role of the Holy See in the process when: (1) pursuant to Convention provisions she is required to submit herself to the temporal authority of the Committee on the Rights of the Child; at a time when (2) since her ratification of the Convention in 1990, a discernible trend is noted in the Committee's interpretation of the Convention which clearly advocates an autonomous child philosophy of children's rights.

In regard to the Holy See's reporting obligations, pursuant to article 44, she must submit reports outlining her progress in implementing the Convention and then appear before the Committee to discuss these reports. The Holy See submitted the *Initial Report* in 1994,[71] which, due to her *sui generis* nature, did not conform strictly to Committee guidelines. Instead of treating various thematic issues related to Convention provisions, her report was divided into the following three sections: affirmation of the rights of the child in the teachings of the Holy See; activity of the Holy See on behalf of children; and activities of the Pontifical Council for the Family for the protection of the rights of the child.

According to the Summary Records of the Meetings of the Committee on the Rights of the Child held on 14 November 1995, the delegation of

---

[69] According to a discussion during the week of 15 July 2002 with Mons. Giorgio Corbellini, Vice Segretario Generale and Capo Ufficio of the Ufficio Legale of the Segreteria Generale of the State of Vatican City, there were about ten children living in Vatican City at that time.

[70] Committee on the Rights of the Child, *Reservations, Declarations, and Objections Relating to the Convention on the Rights of the Child: Note by the Secretary General*, 12/03/98, CRC/C/2/Rev. 7, 24; see also CRC/C/2/Rev. 6, 19–20.

[71] Committee on the Rights of the Child, *Initial Report of the Holy See*, CRC/C/3/Add. 27.

the Holy See appeared before the Committee at the *Palais des Nations* in Geneva for approximately two three-hour sessions.[72]

During this meeting, the Committee focused on the nature of the Holy See as an organ of the Roman Catholic Church. It vigorously questioned the Holy See regarding her commitment to promote and disseminate the Convention with respect to the content of her doctrine and in regard to her educational programmes, activities and institutions, as well as on the problem of sexual abuse and "gender" and religious discrimination directed at Catholic children.

Yet the Committee had only a few questions relating to the State of Vatican City. This is surprising since there is no prohibition on children living in Vatican City. In fact, children have lived there in the past and a few are living there today: a fact that could have opened the door to a barrage of questions relating to civil rights and freedoms, availability of schools, adequate health care, and the availability of contraception and abortion education and services.

The Committee ultimately concluded:

1. The Holy See should "consider reviewing its reservations to the Convention with a view to withdrawing them;"
2. "In view of the moral influence wielded by the Holy See and the national Catholic Churches, the Committee recommends that efforts for the promotion and protection of the rights provided for in the Convention be pursued and strengthened," and that the Convention be widely disseminated and translated into various languages;
3. The Holy See should see that the Convention is included in school curricula, and that adequate training and education of professionals and voluntary workers be carried out in accordance with the principles of the Convention, and that teaching methods be adopted which reflect the "spirit and philosophy of the Convention;"
4. The Holy See should clarify the relationship between article 5 (parental rights and duties) and article 12 (the child's right to be heard). In this regard the Committee "wishes to recall its view that the rights and prerogatives of the parents may not undermine the rights of the child as recognized by the Convention;"
5. The Holy See should take into account when conducting all of its activities, "the spirit of the Convention and principles set forth therein,

---

[72] Committee on the Rights of the Child, "Summary Record of the 256th Meeting" (hereinafter, "Tenth Session"), Tenth Session, 14/10/95, CRC/C/SR.256.

in particular the principles of non-discrimination, of the best interests of the child and of respect for the views of the child."[73]

4. Implications and conclusions

Without a doubt, the Holy See's participation in the Convention has implications for the whole of humanity, with special relevance to her doctrine, internal legal system, and the laws of the Vatican City State. The Roman Catholic Church, like any other religious community, represents a social group having its own proper identity characterized by the sharing in a well-defined system of beliefs or articles of faith. Modification of the content of belief implies an alteration of the Church's identity, and every external influence destined to precipitate such change is against the Church's fundamental right to freedom of religion as articulated and protected in a plethora of international instruments.

Certainly, her participation in the drafting stage was of great benefit, and by ratifying the Convention she demonstrated her support for the good contained in it, and through her reservations and declarations, she put the world on notice as to its grave errors. Yet certain concerns exist with respect to her participation in the implementation process. Clearly, the Committee has a view of the Convention that differs from that of the Holy See. Further, one of the Committee's main tasks is to ensure that State Parties, including the Holy See, withdraw reservations and implement the entire Convention in internal legal systems, complete with its new philosophy for children.[74] Moreover, the Committee does not understand, or does not want to accept, the very special and complex nature and purpose of the Holy See. And the limited time period allotted for discussion with the Committee does not seem sufficient for the Holy See to give full and complete answers to the Committee's questions nor to clear up grave misunderstandings.

Certainly there are protections in place for the Holy See. After all, she acts as the light of Christ, with all the graces that flow from this reality. In addition, there are rules of international law. The Holy See ratified the Convention with reservations, which are permissible under art. 51 of the Convention. Furthermore, Committee recommendations are not legally

---

[73] Committee on the Rights of the Child, "Concluding Observations: Holy See," Tenth Session, 27/11/95, CRC/C/15/Add. 46, pars. 10–14.

[74] See, for example, the Committee's *General Guidelines*, par. 13, wherein State Parties are asked to "indicate the status of the Convention in domestic law . . . [its] recognition in the Constitution or other national legislation . . . the possibility for the provisions of the Convention to be directly invoked before the courts and applied by national authorities."

binding, and any State party, even the Holy See, may argue that she falls within art. 41 of the Convention, which provides: "Nothing in the present Convention shall affect any provisions which are more conducive to the realization of the rights of the child, and which may be contained in the law of a State Party." Moreover, the Holy See's failure to submit the second and third reports confirms that not much can be done should a state fail to report in a timely manner. Finally, it is always open to the Holy See, like other State parties, to work behind the scenes to reason with Committee members of good will, and to exercise her influence to effect changes in Committee membership. This paper merely suggests that there be further reflection and study on the manner by which the Holy See actually partici-pates in the implementation process.

In closing, the Holy See is in a delicate position when, after signing and ratifying a Convention, she subjects herself to the scrutiny of a monitoring body like the Committee on the Rights of the Child, which essentially works as a political tribunal. Despite her reservations, the Holy See should expect continued pressure to bring her doctrine, as protected and promoted in canon law, in line with Convention provisions and principles, not to mention greater scrutiny with respect to the laws of the State of Vatican City. This is a sobering fact that should engage the interest of all Catholics, and of all men and women of faith. How the Church understands herself is not always the way she is perceived by others. The implications of the Committee's misapprehension, then, are serious, as are the challenges to what the Holy See teaches, lives, and holds out to the world as the light of salvation.

11

Problems of principle in voting for unjust legislation

Colin Harte

1. Introduction

The particular "problem of principle" considered in this paper is the one raised by Pope John Paul II in the third paragraph of number 73 of his encyclical letter *Evangelium Vitae* (*EV* 73.3):

> A particular problem of conscience can arise in cases where a legislative vote would be decisive for the passage of a more restrictive law, aimed at limiting the number of authorised abortions, in place of a more permissive law already passed or ready to be voted on.[1]

When *Evangelium Vitae* was published it was widely held that the Pope was teaching that legislators could actually vote for a law "limiting the number of authorized abortions, in place of a more permissive law already passed or ready to be voted on." The teaching of *EV* 73.3 is not, however, the part above, describing the "problem of conscience," but the Pope's resolution of that problem, which follows a few sentences later:

> ... when it is not possible to overturn or completely abrogate a pro-abortion law, an elected official, whose absolute personal opposition to procured abortion was well known, could licitly support proposals aimed at *limiting the harm* done by such a law ...[2]

What sorts of legislative proposals, aimed at limiting the harm, does the Pope have in mind? Are all proposals acceptable? Are any ruled out? My contention is that many proposals that restrict abortion are unjust – in

---

[1] John Paul II, Encyclical letter *Evangelium Vitae* (1995), n. 73.3.
[2] *Ibid.*

fact, intrinsically unjust – and that this poses an ethical problem for those who wish to vote for such proposals. Moreover, immediately before addressing the question of how to respond to abortion laws John Paul II stated in a short paragraph that it is never licit to vote for an intrinsically unjust law:

> In the case of an intrinsically unjust law, such as a law permitting abortion or euthanasia, it is therefore never licit to obey it or to "take part in a propaganda campaign in favour of such a law, or vote for it."[3]

This short paragraph, *EV* 73.2, immediately precedes the Pope's consideration of the "problem of conscience" in *EV* 73.3, and it is clearly the background according to which that "problem of conscience" must be understood. Accordingly, the Pope is necessarily teaching that the proposals he has in mind to "limit the harm" of an abortion law must be just: it is never licit to vote for legislation restricting abortion that is unjust.[4]

In response to an article of mine countering some of the arguments that have been proposed to justify votes for restrictive legislation,[5] Professor William May commented:

> Harte maintains that "he [Pope John Paul II] has not taught... that a legislator may vote to enact (unjust) restrictive abortion legislation...." I know of no one who has defended the view that John Paul II taught that a legislator may enact "unjust" restrictive abortion legislation. Those who disagree with Harte maintain, however, that he has taught that "legislators... may vote for restrictive abortion legislation."[6]

Contrary to May's assertion, the Pope has taught nowhere that "legislators... may vote for restrictive abortion legislation."[7] May's remarks are, however,

---

[3] *Evangelium Vitae*, n. 73.2

[4] See Harte, "Challenging a Consensus: Why *Evangelium Vitae* Does Not Permit Legislators to Vote for 'Imperfect Legislation,'" in L. Gormally (ed) *Culture of Life – Culture of Death*. London: The Linacre Centre 2002: 322–342.

[5] See Harte, "Inconsistent Papal Approaches towards Problems of Conscience?" 2.1 (2002) *National Catholic Bioethics Quarterly*: 99–122.

[6] W. E. May, "*Evangelium vitae* 73 and the Problem of the Lesser Evil." 2.4 (2002) *National Catholic Bioethics Quarterly*: 577–579, at 577.

[7] Professor May helpfully commented upon an early draft of this paper and expressed an objection to what I have written here, citing the sentences from *EV* 73 that I have already quoted above, and then saying: "This clearly supports my interpretation I think." As will be seen from those sentences, the Pope does not say: "legislators... may vote for restrictive abortion legislation," and May's view is, as he stated, merely an "interpretation." My paper "Challenging a Consensus..." gives a very different interpretation, and one cannot reasonably say that *EV* 73 supports something "clearly" when it is open to contradictory interpretations.

noteworthy, for not only does he say that he knows no one who has defended the view that John Paul II taught that a legislator may enact *unjust* restrictive legislation, but he implies that no one would or could defend the view that the Pope might have taught that a legislator can enact *unjust* restrictive legislation.

May gives two examples of the sort of restrictive legislation he believes pro-life legislators could vote for. The first is Poland's 1993 legislation which (i) repealed the Conditions for the Permissibility of the Termination of Pregnancy Act 1956 under which abortions had been extensively permitted, and (ii) made it a criminal offence to abort an unborn child except in certain specified instances, notably if the continuation of the pregnancy constituted a serious threat to the life or health of the mother, if the pregnancy resulted from a criminal act (i.e. rape), or if the unborn child would be born with a serious and permanent disability.[8] The second example, which May clearly believes to be equivalent to voting for the 1993 Polish legislation, is one which has been proposed by Professor John Finnis, who says: "in a state in which abortion is legally permitted up to (say) 24 weeks gestation, it is not necessarily unjust for a legislator to support a proposal to enact a bill of the form 'Abortion is permissible up to 16 weeks'."[9] In another text, Finnis argues that legislators can vote for restrictive legislation, using the same sort of illustration: "Say: the existing law or the threatened alternative bill says abortion is lawful up to 24 weeks, while the law or bill for which the Catholic legislator is voting says abortion is lawful up to 16 weeks."[10] If John Paul II has not and could not have taught that legislators can vote for "unjust" restrictive legislation (a point on which William May and I appear to be agreed) then it must be clearly established whether the restrictive legislation is, in fact, just or unjust.

---

[8] "Ustawa z dnia 7 stycznia 1993 r. o planowaniu rodzniy, ochronie połdu ludzkiego i warunkach dopuszczalności przerywania ciaży" [The family planning, protection of the human conceptus, and the conditions for the permissibility of termination of pregnancy Act, 7 January 1993], in *Dziennik Wstaw Rzeczypostpolitej Polskiej* 17 (Warszawa, 1 March 1993): 429–431.

[9] J. Finnis, "Unjust Laws in a Democratic Society: Some Philosophical and Theological Reflections". 71.4 (1996) *Notre Dame Law Review*: 595–604, at 601. This paper was also produced in Italian as "Le Leggi Ingiuste in una Società Democratica: Considerazioni Filosofiche," in J. Joblin and R. Tremblay (eds) *I Cattolici e la Società Pluralista: Il Caso delle 'Leggi Imperfette'*. Bologna: Edizione Studio Domenicano 1996: 99–114. May produces (at p. 578 of his paper, *op. cit.*) the Italian text and his own translation. I have reproduced Finnis' own English text and not May's (equivalent, but slightly different) translation from the Italian.

[10] J. Finnis, "The Catholic Church and Public Policy Debates in Western Liberal Societies: The Basis and Limits of Intellectual Engagement," in L. Gormally (ed) *Issues for a Catholic Bioethic*. London: The Linacre Centre 1999: 261–273, at 268–269.

The title I have been given for this paper refers to the problem of principle in "voting *for* unjust legislation." The focus is specific. The problem of principle is not that which concerns voting for *just* legislation which, in spite of its enactment, leaves in place other unjust legislation. I am not saying that voting for this sort of just legislation is unproblematic (as I shall explain), but it is not the "problem of principle" that this paper is addressing. More specifically, voting "*for*" unjust legislation means voting *to enact* it (and not earlier procedural votes). In other words, we are looking at the vote by which the lawmaker – whether it be an individual with sole law-making authority, or a legislator in a parliament, or a citizen entitled to vote in a legally binding popular referendum, or the head of state whose consent would also be required – expresses his or her will that a specific proposal (the bill for a law) be enacted as law.

Given that Poland's 1993 law and a bill to reduce abortions from 24 to 16 weeks have been cited as illustrations of "restrictive" legislation that legislators can vote for, it is helpful to keep in mind such proposals when discussing what is at issue in this paper. A possible difficulty is that, when considering these as concrete proposals, the reader may feel that he or she does not have sufficient background knowledge of the Polish situation to fully understand what is at issue. Another difficulty is that, in presenting his example of reducing abortions from 24 weeks to 16 weeks by means of the bill "Abortion is permissible up to 16 weeks," John Finnis displays an uncharacteristic inattention to detail. Of course, Finnis is presenting a simple illustration and this is unobjectionable. However, it is not clear what, precisely, Finnis has in mind, because no bill to amend the law from 24 weeks would be presented in the way he proposes. It could specify either: "In Act X [permitting abortions to 24 weeks] replace '24' with '16'," (a bill which means "Amend Act X so that abortion is permitted up to 16 weeks, not 24 weeks"); or "Act X [permitting abortions to 24 weeks] is repealed. Abortion is permissible up to 16 weeks and prohibited after 16 weeks." To overcome these difficulties, and to enable the reader to consider what precisely is at issue, I shall rely neither on the Polish law, nor on Finnis' illustration, but shall consider (not dissimilar) hypothetical attempts to restrict abortion in two imaginary countries, which I shall call Noland and Tyrannia. I shall also compare attempts to restrict abortion in these two countries with the opportunities present in a third imaginary country, Littalia, which has a codified system of law, like some European countries, but unlike the UK and Noland and Tyrannia.

2. The proposals to be considered

Just as John Finnis illustrated his point by means of the simplified proposal "Abortion is permissible up to 16 weeks" I shall also present simplified proposals. They deal mainly with the substantive parts of abortion laws – the permissions, tolerations or prohibitions of abortion in certain instances – and do not generally include other secondary matters, such as regulations about funding, specifications about who can perform abortions and where, and any conditions, such as a requirement for counselling, that in some places may be found within abortion laws. When the proposals mention that abortion is "prohibited," this means that those who violate the prohibition will be subject to the criminal law and subject to a just penalty on conviction.

In the following discussion I shall use the term X2 to refer to the proposal (the bill) being considered for enactment, Y2 to refer to the enacted bill (the Act), and Z2 to refer to the country's abortion law in its totality after the enactment of the bill. The content of X2 and Y2 is always identical; the distinction is merely whether or not the proposal has been enacted as law. The Act and the country's abortion law prior to the introduction of a bill will be denoted by Y1 and Z1 respectively. If the whole of a country's abortion law is contained in a single Act (Y1 or Y2), then Y1 = Z1 and Y2 = Z2.

2.1. Noland

The specific hypothetical situation in Noland is that for nearly 40 years abortion has been extensively permitted, virtually throughout the whole of pregnancy. There are about 200,000 abortions each year. The Nolish "abortion law" (i.e. all the relevant permissions and regulations about abortion = Z1) is contained entirely within two Abortion Acts, P and Q. If these two Acts are repealed and replaced by a law prohibiting all abortions, abortion will be totally illegal in Noland. After much public debate and campaigning by groups with different views about abortion, the following bill, "Proposal A", is subject to a vote for enactment in the Nolish parliament:

Proposal A
Abortion Acts P and Q are repealed. Every human being has the right to life from the moment of conception. Whoever assists in an abortion will be punished, on conviction, according to the range of punishments established for the crime of homicide. It shall not be unlawful or a punishable offence if a doctor aborts a non-viable unborn child in a registered health care institution if: (a) the pregnancy is deemed to constitute a serious danger to the life of the mother; (b) the doctor has reasonable grounds to believe that the pregnancy occurred after rape; or (c) prenatal tests indicate a serious and irreversible foetal disability.

Proposal A represents the bill (X2), the enacted bill (Y2) and the whole abortion law of Noland if the bill is enacted (Z2). If Proposal A is enacted it is anticipated that there will be less than 1,000 legal abortions each year.

2.2. Tyrannia

The specific hypothetical situation in Tyrannia is that the country's abortion law is expressed entirely in a single Abortion Act R: "Abortion is permitted up to 24 weeks and prohibited after 24 weeks." This Act has been in force for over 20 years, and there are about 200,000 abortions each year. Here $Y1 = Z1$.

In Tyrannia, there have been mixed attitudes towards abortion which have, in part, been influenced by anti-semitism. Trying to prohibit all abortions in Tyrannia seems impossible largely because many anti-semitic legislators will not prohibit abortion of Jewish babies: they want to keep the Jewish population as low as possible. At the same time there has been general unease about aborting as late as 24 weeks, unless the baby was Jewish. After much debate and discussion, the legislature has decided to vote on alternative proposals: Proposals B and C. Proposal C will be considered only if Proposal B is not accepted:

Proposal B
Abortion Act R is repealed. Abortion is permitted up to 24 weeks if and only if one or both of the parents of the foetus is Jewish. All other abortions before 24 weeks, and all abortions after 24 weeks, are prohibited.

Proposal B represents the bill (X2), the enacted bill (Y2) and the whole abortion law of Tyrannia if the bill is enacted (Z2). If Proposal B is enacted it is anticipated that there would be about 3,000 legal abortions each year.

Proposal C
Abortion Act R is repealed. Abortion is permitted up to 16 weeks and prohibited after 16 weeks.

Proposal C represents the bill (X2), the enacted bill (Y2) and the whole abortion law of Tyrannia if the bill is enacted (Z2). If Proposal C is enacted it is anticipated that there would be about 170,000 legal abortions each year.

2.3. Littalia

As in Noland, Littalia's abortion law was not enacted in a single Act. In contrast to Noland, however, Littalia's laws are codified, and the country's abortion law – all the permissions, prohibitions and regulations relevant to abortion – is itemized in separate articles of law from number 90 in the code. Littalia's abortion law (Z1), as found in the code, is as follows:

Art. 90: Abortion is prohibited except where it is specifically permitted.

Art. 91: Abortion is permitted up to 16 weeks on request.

Art. 92: Abortion is permitted up to 24 weeks if two doctors agree that it would benefit the health of the pregnant woman.

Art. 93: Abortion is permitted up to 30 weeks if tests indicate the likelihood of foetal disability.

Art. 94: Abortion is permitted at any time if pregnancy is reasonably believed to have occurred after rape.

Art. 95: Abortion is permitted at any time if performed to save the life of the pregnant woman.

Art. 96: Abortion is permitted up to 24 weeks if one or both parents of the foetus is Jewish.

Art. 97: Medical personnel have a right not to be involved in any way with abortions.

Art. 98: Taxes and other public funds cannot be used to pay for abortions.

Under Littalia's abortion law (Z1), abortion is widely permitted and there are about 200,000 abortions each year. For the purposes of our discussion we will consider five different proposals that could be considered for enactment, each proposal being considered with respect to the abortion law, Z1, as presented above.

Proposal D
In the code, repeal articles 91, 92, and 96.

Proposal D represents the Bill (X2) and the Act (Y2) but it does not represent the country's abortion law (Z2) if the proposal is enacted. Z2 will be the articles of law not repealed by Proposal D (thus the articles permitting abortion in cases of disability, rape, and threat to the mother's life are not repealed). The repeal of the articles of law mentioned in Proposal D would mean that about 199,000 of the 200,000 abortions taking place each year would no longer be permitted.

Proposal E
In the code, repeal articles 91–95.

Proposal E represents the Bill (X2) and the Act (Y2) but it does not represent the country's abortion law (Z2) if the proposal is enacted. Z2 will be the articles of law not repealed by Proposal E (thus the article permitting Jewish babies to be aborted is not repealed). The repeal of the articles of law mentioned in Proposal E would mean that about 197,000 of the 200,000 abortions taking place each year would no longer be permitted.

Proposal F
In the code, repeal articles 92–96.

Proposal F represents the Bill (X2) and the Act (Y2) but it does not represent the country's abortion law (Z2) if the proposal is enacted. Z2 will be the articles of law not repealed by Proposal F (thus the article permitting abortions up to 16 weeks is not repealed). The repeal of the articles of law mentioned in Proposal F would mean that about 30,000 of the 200,000 abortions taking place each year would no longer be permitted.[11]

Proposal G
In the code, amend article 91, replacing '16' by '8.'

Proposal G represents the Bill (X2) and the Act (Y2) but it does not represent the country's abortion law if the proposal is enacted. Z2 will be the articles of law not repealed by Proposal G, as well as article 91, as amended, specifying: "Abortion is permitted up to 8 weeks on request." The juridical "meaning" of Proposal G is: "Amend article 91 of the code, so that abortion is permitted on request up to 8 weeks, not 16 weeks." Article 91 is the article of law under which most abortions are permitted. The amendment of Article 91 by Proposal G would mean that about 100,000 of the 200,000 abortions taking place each year would no longer be permitted.

Proposal H
It is prohibited (i) for a pregnant woman to take an abortion-inducing drug (such as mifeprex/RU486) and (ii) for a doctor or any other person to prescribe or distribute such a drug to a pregnant woman.

Proposal H represents the Bill (X2) and the Act (Y2) but it does not represent the country's abortion law if the proposal is enacted. Z2 will include all the articles of law included in the previous law (Z1), as well as this new law, which may be codified as two articles, say:

Art. 99:   It is prohibited for a pregnant woman to take an abortion-inducing drug (such as mifeprex/RU486).

---

[11] In a concrete situation it is likely that this sort of proposal, like Proposal C in Tyrannia, would only slightly reduce the number of abortions. Those abortions that previously took place under articles 92–96 could still take place, at least up to 16 weeks, under article 91. And if women could no longer abort under any circumstances after 16 weeks it is likely that they would make greater efforts to abort earlier.

Art. 100: It is prohibited for a doctor or any other person to prescribe or distribute an abortion-inducing drug (such as mifeprex/RU486) to a pregnant woman.

Let us assume that this law is being passed before mifeprex/RU486 has been licensed for distribution. In itself, the new law does not permit or tolerate any abortions, nor will it stop any abortions currently taking place. However, it is believed that the advent of drug-induced abortions will make abortions cheaper and that some women will have abortions who otherwise might not have. It could also be the case that abortion is regarded as a less serious matter if it does not require surgical intervention. In short, pro-life legislators may have good reasons to want to prohibit drug-induced abortions.

Which of the eight proposals could morally upright legislators justly vote for? Because the "problem of principle" arises when faced with intrinsically unjust legislation which it is never licit to vote for (cf. *EV* 73.2), we must first identify which, if any, of the Proposals A–H are intrinsically unjust. Some general remarks about abortion legislation are called for.

3. Abortion legislation

3.1. "Permitting" and "tolerating" abortion in law

Bearing in mind the teaching of *EV* 73.2, quoted above, which mentions that "a law permitting abortion" is "an intrinsically unjust law" for which one cannot licitly vote, it would seem self-evident that legislators could not vote licitly for Proposals B and C because they specifically "permit" abortion. Although Proposal G does not mention "permission" in itself, it is meaningless unless it is understood in the context of the article to which it refers. Understood with respect to Article 91, Proposal G must be understood as ratifying and continuing some (though not all) of the permission that was previously included in article 91: Proposal G *permits* abortion on request up to 8 weeks. Unlike Proposals, B, C and G, Proposal A does not specifically "permit" abortion. It does not say abortion is "lawful", but that it is "not unlawful" and "not . . . a punishable offence." Is this, therefore, not intrinsically unjust?

At this point further attention should be given to the question of "permitting" and "tolerating" actions in law. Human law is not always required to prohibit that which is prohibited by the natural moral law. It is not required, then, that legislators pass laws prohibiting adultery or pre-marital sex, even though the moral law prohibits these actions. But this does not mean that legislators can "permit" these actions – that is, "authorize" them or make them "lawful." As St Thomas Aquinas teaches,

> The human will can, by common agreement, make a thing to be
> just provided that it be not, of itself, contrary to natural justice,
> and it is in such matters that positive right has its place.... If,
> however, a thing is, of itself, contrary to natural right the human
> will cannot make it just, for instance, by decreeing that it is lawful
> to steal or to commit adultery. Hence it is written: "Woe to them
> that make wicked laws" (Isaiah 10:1).[12]

Aquinas is not saying that human law must prohibit adultery, even though
it cannot be "permitted," i.e., made lawful. It is legitimate to legally "tolerate"
adultery by repealing a law that made it a criminal offence or by refraining
from the passing of a law prohibiting it. Such "toleration" is distinct from
"permission." Perhaps the point can be better understood by considering
what is commonly regarded as "Age of Consent" legislation. Many countries,
like the UK, have legislation prohibiting sexual intercourse with a minor, the
age being set at 14, 16, 18 or whatever. The legislation does not normally say
that those older than the specified age are *permitted* or *authorized* or *have a
right to* engage in sexual activity (with others who have also reached the
specified age). It simply says that once they reach the specified age *they are
not committing a criminal offence*. To this extent the law can be said neither
to permit, nor to prohibit, but rather *to tolerate* – not to impede – immoral
sexual activity of those who are no longer minors.[13] This is legitimate. To
specifically permit such activity, however, is not legitimate, and any such
law permitting it would be a "wicked law": in every instance it would be
unjust.

Whilst noting that human law is not required to prohibit all immoral
actions, Aquinas indicates that some immoral actions can be neither
permitted nor tolerated but must be prohibited:

> Human laws do not forbid all vices from which the virtuous
> abstain, but only the more grievous vices from which it is possible
> for the majority to abstain; and chiefly those that are to the hurt of
> others, without the prohibition of which human society could not
> be maintained: thus human law prohibits murder, theft, and
> suchlike.[14]

---

[12] St Thomas Aquinas, *Summa Theologiae* (*ST*) II-II, q. 57, a. 2, ad 2.

[13] Pius XII speaks of toleration as the principle of "*non impedire*" in his Discourse to the Fifth Convention of Italian Catholic Jurists, 6 December 1953, published in *The Catholic Mind* (April 1954): 244–251, at 247. Janet E. Smith has used the same term to signify toleration in *Humanae Vitae: A Generation Later*. Washington DC: Catholic University of America Press 1991: 93.

[14] *ST* I-II, q. 96, a. 2.

The first action which Aquinas says must be prohibited – that is, can be neither permitted nor tolerated – is murder, i.e. all murders. This prohibition derives from the natural law.[15] A law that fails to prohibit the murder of some people – e.g. if it were to specify that "It is prohibited to murder those aged between the ages of 3 and 70" – does not prohibit murder, but only *some* murders. A law of this form would tolerate murder of those aged younger than 3 and older than 70. This sort of law is unacceptable, given that human law, derived from the natural moral law, requires that all murders must be prohibited.[16]

---

[15] See R. P. George, "Natural Law and Positive Law," in R. P. George (ed) *The Autonomy of Law*. Oxford: Clarendon Press 1996: 321–334, at 328.

[16] Legislation illustrated by the proposition "It is prohibited to murder those aged between the ages of 3 and 70" entails that if someone is tried and found guilty for the crime of murdering someone between the ages of 3 and 70, then they will be punished. Punishment is associated with any sort of "prohibiting" law. Even though the law does not "permit" or "authorize" anyone to kill those aged below 3 or over 70, nevertheless the law's toleration of such offences against their lives would be shown by the fact that anyone killing a two year old would not be arrested or tried or convicted, because no criminal offence would have been committed. If human law must prohibit murder – that is, all murders – then the introduction of the ages of 3 and 70 in the context of a "murder law" is arbitrary, and insofar as the ages are introduced in such a way as to deny the due protection of the law to some people that is being afforded to others, it is unjust. The "murder law" itself is unjust, and this sort of law is, in itself, always unjust, i.e. it is intrinsically unjust.

Now, let us suppose that in a country there is a murder law of the form: "It is prohibited to murder those aged between the ages of 3 and 70." Morally upright legislators, acknowledging this to be an unjust law, might want to prohibit all murders, but realise there is not a parliamentary majority for this. They discover that it is impossible to protect those younger than 3, but think they can persuade enough fellow legislators to extend the murder prohibition for those aged over 70. At this point we see that the use of simple propositions to illustrate laws is not always adequate for discussing the finer points of the question of changing unjust laws. However, the sort of law to be introduced would normally be one which independently of the previous law, which would continue to remain in force, protected those aged over 70 (e.g. a proposal of the form "It is prohibited to murder those aged 70 or more"), or one which would essentially replace the previous law (e.g. a proposal "It is prohibited to murder those aged 3 years or more"). Supporting the change in the law poses a problem, however, because just as the original law "It is prohibited to murder those aged between 3 and 70" is in itself unjust – because it unjustly tolerates some murders – similarly the two proposals to prohibit murder for those over 70 are each *in themselves* unjust. Even though they would prohibit some murders, both proposals can be regarded *in themselves* as tolerating other murders. The legislative proposals themselves are intrinsically unjust; by failing to provide the protection of the law to some people, in a legislative context in which such protection is required, the proposals can be seen to be a violation of the natural law which requires the prohibition of murder.

In *Evangelium Vitae* John Paul II notes that the whole tradition of the Church has supported "the doctrine on the necessary *conformity of civil law with the moral law*."[17]

> This is the clear teaching of Saint Thomas Aquinas, who writes that "human law is law inasmuch as it is in conformity with right reason and thus derives from the eternal law. But when a law is contrary to reason, it is called an unjust law; but in this case it ceases to be a law and becomes instead an act of violence."[a] And again: "Every law made by man can be called a law insofar as it derives from the natural law. But if it is somehow opposed to the natural law, then it is not really a law but rather a corruption of the law."[b][18]

Immediately after this John Paul II says:

> Now the first and most immediate application of this teaching [of the conformity of the civil law with the natural moral law] concerns a human law which disregards the fundamental right and source of all other rights which is the right to life, a right belonging to every individual.[19]

The relevant point is not whether the law specifically permits or authorizes abortion, but whether it fails in any way to protect the right to life, and this is something which occurs not only with laws that permit or authorize abortion, but also with those that make it compulsory and command it, as well as those that tolerate it. A law tolerating immoral actions like adultery or pre-marital sex can be regarded as being in conformity with the moral law, but a law tolerating abortion or any other offence against the life of a person contradicts the natural law, and accordingly must be judged, as Aquinas observed, to be "contrary to reason" or "unjust."[20] The UK's

---

[17] *EV* 72.1. Emphasis in original text.

[a] Footnote reference in the text to *ST* I-II, q. 93, a. 3, ad 2.

[b] Footnote reference in the text to *ST* I-II, q. 95, a. 2.

[18] *EV* 72.1.

[19] *EV* 72.2.

[20] The account I have presented (in line with the teaching of Aquinas and the Church's whole tradition) of human law's capacity to tolerate some immoral actions, whilst always being obliged to prohibit offences against life, seems also to be accepted by John Finnis. See his *Aquinas: Moral, Political and Legal Theory* (Oxford: Oxford University Press 1998), 222–228. For an account of how human law's defence of life is required by natural law see W. Waldstein, "Natural Law and the Defence of Life in *Evangelium Vitae*," in J. Vial Correa and E. Sgreccia (eds) *Evangelium Vitae: Five Years of Confrontation with the Society* [Proceedings of the Sixth Annual Assembly of the Pontifical Academy for Life, 11–14 February 2000]. Vatican City: Libreria Editrice Vaticana 2001, 223–242.

Abortion Act 1967, rightly condemned as being intrinsically unjust, is one which does not "permit" but, rather, "tolerates" abortion: women do not have a "right" to abortion; the law specifies, rather, that it is not a criminal offence to abort if certain conditions have been met. Proposal A, if enacted, would similarly be a law that "tolerates" abortion, although it would tolerate fewer abortions than the UK 1967 Act. Though it does not "permit" abortion it is still intrinsically unjust.[21]

3.2. A matter of law

Voting for legislation is, of course, a matter of law, and we must clearly understand some fundamentals about law: *what is law?* St Thomas Aquinas defines it as "nothing else than an ordinance of reason (*rationis ordinatio*) for the common good, made by him who has care of the community, and promulgated;"[22] law is "nothing else but a dictate of practical reason (*dictamen practicae rationis*) emanating from the ruler who governs a perfect community."[23] Certainly, one can propose and prefer more elaborate

---

[21] Proposal A in Noland corresponds with the 1993 legislation passed in Poland. In an unpublished address "Learning from the Polish Experience," delivered to the annual conference of the UK Society for the Protection of Unborn Children, 13 September 1997 (at which I was present), Dr Kazimierz Janiak, Vice-President of Solidarity, attempted to justify pro-life legislators' support for the Polish law on the grounds that it did not specifically say that abortions were "legal" (i.e. permitted) in the instances I have already mentioned; rather, the law did not criminalize them. As I have argued, the "toleration" of some abortions renders the law intrinsically unjust no less than does their "permission". Dr Janiak implicitly acknowledged the permitting-tolerating distinction, even though he was wrong to believe that the distinction affects the moral judgment about voting for abortion laws. However, the distinction does not appear to be widely acknowledged. For example, the pro-life President of the Polish Senate, Alicja Grzeskowiak, speaks of the 1993 legislation as having *legalized* ("legalizzato") some abortions. She does not suggest that the Polish legislators were justified in supporting the 1993 law on the grounds that they were merely "tolerating" abortions. Rather she regards it as a *compromise* ("il compromesso") which she claims is permitted by the teaching of *Evangelium Vitae* 73. See Alicja Grzeskowiak, "Difesa della famiglia e della vita nell'Est dell'Europa." 3.3 (1998) *Familia et Vita*: 66–81, at 75–76.

[22] *ST* I-II, q. 90, a. 4.

[23] *ST* I-II, q. 91, a. 1.

definitions,[24] but the "essence" of law always focuses on its being a dictate or ordinance of reason.

Another way of saying that law must be a dictate or ordinance of reason is to say that it must be "just,"[25] and justness – being in accordance with reason – can be regarded as the essence of law.[26] Some laws such as those commanding, permitting or tolerating murder, abortion, or destructive embryo experimentation can, and indeed must always, be judged to be unjust because the primary function of human law is to protect human life itself.[27] They are in themselves unjust: they are *intrinsically unjust*. A consideration of the circumstances or the intentions of legislators voting for a law cannot make just a law that is intrinsically unjust. Other laws – for example, specifying that 80% of one's income should be taken in tax, that young adults must receive full-time education until they are 20, or that cars cannot burn petrol with lead in it – are not intrinsically unjust. Whether such laws are, in fact, just or unjust depends on a consideration of the circumstances and the anticipated consequences of their enactment. Even if it can be judged that at a particular time it would be unjust to enact any of these measures, the measure cannot be regarded as *intrinsically* unjust, because at another place or at another time the measure could be judged to be just.

Aquinas observes that "laws framed by men are either just or unjust."[28] A definite judgment about their justness or unjustness can and must be made. More specifically laws can be identified as: (a) just, or (b) unjust in view of the circumstances, or (c) unjust in themselves irrespective of the

---

[24] For example John Finnis uses the term law "to refer primarily to rules made, in accordance with regulative legal rules, by a determinate and effective authority (itself identified and, standardly, constituted as an institution by legal rules) for a 'complete' community, and buttressed by sanctions in accordance with the rule-guided stipulations of adjudicative institutions, this ensemble of rules and institutions being directed to reasonably resolving any of the community's co-ordination problems (and to ratifying, tolerating, regulating, or overriding co-ordination solutions from any other institutions or sources of norms) for the common good by features of specificity, minimization of arbitrariness, and maintenance of a quality of reciprocity between the subjects of the law both amongst themselves and in their relations with the lawful authorities." See his *Natural Law and Natural Rights* (Oxford: Clarendon Press 1980), 276–277. This definition of law seems to me to be entirely consistent with, though more elaborately expressed than, Aquinas' definition.

[25] *ST* I-II, q. 95, a. 3.

[26] See Edward J. Damich, "The Essence of Law According to Thomas Aquinas." 30 (1985) *American Journal of Jurisprudence*: 79–96.

[27] "Therefore, in order that man might have peace and virtue, it was necessary for laws to be framed," *ST* I-II, q. 95, a. 1.

[28] *ST* I-II, q. 96, a. 4.

circumstances, i.e. intrinsically unjust.[29] When voting to enact legislation on abortion it is insufficient simply to regard the legislation as "favourable to the pro-life cause" or, as is commonly the case nowadays, as "imperfect"[30] or "imperfectly just."[31] Voting to enact legislation on abortion is in the first place a matter of law, and it must be established whether the bill being considered for enactment as law is just or unjust.

3.3. *Focusing on the matter of a legislative enactment*

An "abortion law" in its entirety (Z1 or Z2, as described above) has a single identity as a "law," and is subject to a judgment of being either just *or* intrinsically unjust. Such a law can also consist of separate propositions of law, which, considered separately, are also subject to a judgment of being just or intrinsically unjust. Thus, Littalia's abortion law as a whole (Z1) is intrinsically unjust, but each of its articles is also "law," some of which (Articles 90–96) are intrinsically unjust, while others (Articles 97–98) are just.

The justness or intrinsic unjustness of a proposal is not determined simply by looking at the "end state" of the country's abortion law (Z2) if the proposal is enacted. Let us compare Proposals C and F, introduced in Tyrannia and Littalia respectively. The end result (Z2) of voting for the proposals in each country would be the same: the abortion law would

---

[29] *Ibid.* Although Aquinas does not refer specifically to a category of "intrinsically unjust" laws, he identifies two categories of unjust law. His category of laws that are unjust "through being opposed to the divine good" corresponds with what I label intrinsically unjust laws. His category of laws that are unjust "by being contrary to human good" corresponds with those judged to be unjust at a particular time or place, i.e. on account of extrinsic factors. John Finnis would also appear to accept the distinction between intrinsically and extrinsically unjust laws when he refers to "unjust positive laws – and above all, a law whose injustice is not merely a matter of improper motivations or procedural improprieties, but intrinsic...." See his "Natural Law – Positive Law," in *'Evangelium Vitae' and Law* [Acta Symposii Internationalis in Civitate Vaticana Celebrati, 23–24 Maii 1996]. Vatican City: Libreria Editrice Vaticana 1997, 199–209, at 209.

[30] The term has become so acceptable that the Congregation for the Doctrine of the Faith (CDF) used it in the title of a symposium it organized: "Catholics and Pluralist Society – the Case of 'Imperfect Laws'," Rome, 9–12 November 1994. The proceedings were published in Italian: Joseph Joblin and Réal Tremblay, *op. cit.* The former Secretary of the CDF, Archbishop Tarcisio Bertone SDB, argued that legislators could vote for "imperfect" laws in some circumstances; see "Catholics and Pluralist Society: 'Imperfect laws' and the Responsibility of Legislators," in Juan de Dios Vial Correa and Elio Sgreccia, *op. cit.*, 206–222.

[31] See, for example, Robert P. George, "The Gospel of Life: A Symposium." 56 (October 1995) *First Things*: 32–38, viewed at http://www.firstthings.com/ftissues/ft9510/articles/symposium.html.

permit abortion up to 16 weeks. But proposals C and F are radically different. With Proposal C, legislators in Tyrannia would be voting to enact a law permitting abortion up to 16 weeks, and this law (Act) would also be the country's abortion law. With Proposal F, legislators in Littalia would be voting to repeal a series of laws (articles 92–96) that had been previously enacted; they would not be voting *for* any other articles, including article 91 permitting abortion up to 16 weeks.

If a law permitting abortion is intrinsically unjust, then Proposal C cannot be anything other than intrinsically unjust. A proposal *to repeal* intrinsically unjust law can never, however, be intrinsically unjust, and it is not the sort of law that it is never licit to vote for. Voting for Proposal F does not, therefore, involve the same "problem of principle" encountered in voting for Proposal C. Whether or not legislators should vote for it – or the similar proposals of repeal, D and E, – depends on other considerations that I shall discuss later on.

Each of the proposals A, B and C refers to a bill (X2) which when enacted (Y2) will be the country's entire abortion law (Z2). Given that any law which violates the right to life by permitting or tolerating abortion must be judged to be intrinsically unjust, it will be clear that, if Proposals A or B or C are enacted, Noland and Tyrannia have an intrinsically unjust abortion law (Z2). And if the country's law (Z2) is intrinsically unjust, so is the Act (Y2) which is, precisely, the country's law. And the bill (X2) is therefore also intrinsically unjust. It is not possible to claim, without abandoning reason, that a vote for any one of the Proposals A or B or C is not a vote for an intrinsically unjust law.

Proposal G differs insofar as it does not determine Littalia's entire abortion law, but it is still the enactment of "law" and its juridical meaning is that of permitting abortion up to 8 weeks. Whether or not the proposal is just does not depend on the circumstances of whether it is increasing permission from, say, 6 weeks or reducing permission from, say, 16 weeks. The view that the justness of this sort of proposal depends on the context or circumstances fails, fundamentally, to take into account what is meant by the concept of an *intrinsically* unjust law.

If Proposal H is enacted, the country's abortion law (Z2) is still intrinsically unjust. Unlike Proposals A, B and C, where X2 = Y2 = Z2, a vote for Proposal H (X2/Y2) is not a vote for the whole abortion law (Z2). The relevant question is whether X2/Y2 is just or intrinsically unjust. Given that it is solely prohibitive and in no way can be said to tolerate or permit anything unjust, the proposal is not intrinsically unjust. Depending on the circumstances and the consequences legislators could regard it as a just and desirable law, and vote to enact it. Their direct vote is for the proposal (X2/Y2) and not for Z2.

The discussion of these proposals reveals the need to be properly focused as to what, precisely, is subject to the vote of enactment. Law cannot simply be regarded as an amorphous entity, and the discussion highlights, in particular, an awareness of the different "levels" of law, together with the need to respect the integrity of individual laws which are part of what is also, more broadly, "the law."

4. Judging the justness or unjustness of law

The main oversight of John Finnis, William May and others who believe legislators can vote for restrictive measures like the 1993 Polish law, or for proposals permitting abortion up to 16 weeks instead of 24 weeks, would appear to be their failure to identify whether the specific proposal under consideration is just or intrinsically unjust. Thus May says with respect to voting for the Polish law:

> I believe that a proper analysis of the law, given that it was intended to *replace* a very liberal law permitting abortion on demand, would hold that it could be right and indeed obligatory for a legislator, whose personal opposition to abortion is well known and who has exhausted every attempt to proscribe all abortion, could vote for the law endorsed by pro-life people [sic]. The *object* morally specifying his vote would not be to *permit abortion* but on the contrary to *extend the protection of the law to the lives of unborn children whose lives are not protected under the existing legislation, which this legislation is* intended to replace.[32]

With these sentences May gives his reasons for thinking that pro-life legislators could have voted for the Polish law, but where is the "proper analysis of the law" that May suggests is being offered? There is none.[33] John Finnis presents a similar view:

> In a state in which abortion is legally permitted up to (say) 24 weeks gestation, it is not necessarily unjust for a legislator to support a proposal to enact a bill of the form "Abortion is permissible up to 16 weeks." For it is possible to support such a proposal precisely as a proposal to extend legal protection to the life of unborn children after the 16th week.[34]

---

[32] May, "*Evangelium Vitae* 73 and the Problem of the Lesser Evil," 578. Emphasis in original text.

[33] For my reply to William May, see Colin Harte "*Evangelium vitae* 73 and Intrinsically Unjust Laws." 3.2 (2003) *National Catholic Bioethics Quarterly*: 241–243.

[34] Finnis, "Unjust Laws in a Democratic Society," 601.

Finnis says "it is not necessarily unjust" for a legislator to vote for the bill restricting abortion to 16 weeks, but (like May with respect to the Polish situation) he does not say whether the specific proposal is just or intrinsically unjust. If it is never licit to vote for intrinsically unjust legislation, then one must establish first of all whether the legislation that is the subject of a vote for enactment is, in fact, intrinsically unjust, and it is because an analysis of Proposals A, B, C and G reveals them to be intrinsically unjust that I (following the Pope's teaching at *EV* 73.2) maintain that a legislator cannot licitly vote for them. Unless John Finnis disagrees, in principle, with John Paul II's teaching that it is never licit to vote for intrinsically unjust laws, then his support for restrictive legislation would appear to be based on a faulty judgment as to what is, in fact, intrinsically unjust. The intrinsic unjustness of Proposals A, B, C and G is self-evident, and I think that, prior to defending his argument to justify voting for such proposals, John Finnis should address the primary and fundamental question of whether he regards them to be just or intrinsically unjust.

In the hypothetical situations of Noland, Tyrannia and Littalia, all the relevant details have been presented to enable the reader to judge whether or not the proposals are intrinsically unjust. I trust that in his reply to this paper, John Finnis will clarify (a) whether he judges Proposals A, B, C and G – understood precisely as they have been presented – to be just or intrinsically unjust, and (b) whether, in his view, a legislator could or could not justly vote for them.

5. Some problems with John Finnis' argument

Apart from failing to judge the justness or intrinsic unjustness of specific proposals to restrict abortion, there are particular flaws in John Finnis' argument to support votes to enact them.

5.1. Intentions and side-effects

The first flaw arises from Finnis' general theory of what is involved in legislative votes. I refer, in particular, to his apparent belief that a legislator supports only the part(s) of a bill that he or she "chooses" to support and that other parts, though included in the bill, are not part of his or her "choice" when voting and can be regarded as unintended side-effects of the legislator's chosen act. As an illustration of what is meant by this, let us consider a bill that will authorize funding for three things: a school, a hospital and a leisure complex. Some legislators object that funding for the leisure complex has been included, as this means the school and hospital will get less money. They believe it is unjust to fund a leisure complex when the money allocated for it could be better spent on the school and hospital. How, then, should they vote at the final stage of deciding whether to enact the bill as law? According to Finnis' analysis – as he acknowledged when I checked with him – the legislators could vote for the bill, on the grounds that they were intending to support only the parts authorizing funds for the hospital and school, the authorization of funds for the leisure complex included in the bill not being part of their intention, but accepted as a side-effect.

I agree that legislators who object to funding the leisure complex could vote for the bill, but this has nothing to do with a consideration of the legislators' intentions and acceptance of side-effects. Each legislator voting for the bill would be voting to enact as law the bill in its entirety – the bill *as a whole* is the subject matter of the vote for enactment – and he or she would be giving as much support to funding the leisure complex as to funding the school and hospital. If a legislator believes funding for the leisure complex is unjust, is this then an unjust law? I would say no. In itself, it is not unjust to fund a leisure complex (that is, we are not considering something that is intrinsically unjust) though a legislator may think it is unjust considering the circumstances. The circumstance that the school and hospital could make better use of the money may lead some legislators to the view that authorizing funds for the leisure complex is unjust. But a further consideration of the circumstances includes the awareness that unless the bill is passed funding will be withheld not only from the leisure complex but also from the hospital and school. Taking this into account the bill, as a whole, can be regarded as reasonable, i.e. just, and legislators who continue to object to the funding included for the leisure complex could vote for the bill – vote to enact all that it contains – as a legitimate compromise on what is properly speaking a "political" matter. This would be a legitimate political compromise, and indeed in such *political* matters not only is it ethical to compromise, but it can be unethical not to compromise.[35]

Suppose, however, that the bill authorized funding not for a leisure complex but for an abortion clinic. This involves support for abortion and, being a violation of the protection that the law must give to the unborn, it is intrinsically unjust. The unjustness of the bill in this instance is not determined by a consideration of the circumstances, but is intrinsic, and the bill as a whole, if it allows funding for the abortion clinic, is necessarily unjust – intrinsically unjust. According to John Finnis' analysis, it could be justified for pro-life legislators to vote for this bill on the grounds

---

[35] As Cardinal Ratzinger notes "It is not refusal to compromise but compromise that in *political* things is the true morality" (my emphasis). See his *Church, Ecumenism, and Politics* (Slough: St Paul Publications 1988), 149.

that they were intending to support only the proposals authorizing funding for the school and hospital, the funding of the abortion clinic being, in Finnis' view, a side-effect of the pro-life legislator's act.[36] I reject this view as a falsification of what is involved in legislative voting, and maintain that legislators could not vote ethically for its enactment because this would entail, according to a proper analysis of what is being done, not a political compromise but a *moral* compromise. The right to life is a condition *prior to politics*; it is the moral foundation of politics.[37] Voting for legislation which violates the right to life – by obligating, permitting, tolerating or in any way supporting (e.g., by funding) actions against the life of any unborn child – cannot be regarded as a political matter. It is fundamentally a *moral* matter, on which compromise is unethical.[38]

Most legislation in the UK and other parliaments deals with matters that are properly understood to be "political" (described by Aquinas as *ius civile*), and not with matters such as offences against life which violate the "moral" foundations of a society (described by Aquinas as *ius gentium*).[39] When dealing with "political" matters, legislators making decisions in accordance with Finnis' theory of intentions and side-effects would come to the same conclusions as legislators who, acknowledging the legislation not to be intrinsically unjust, vote in accordance with a correct understanding of

---

[36] This illustration corresponds with Finnis' statement in "Unjust Laws in a Democratic Society," at 603: "Reflection on the case of paying one's taxes can assist in showing also that a legislator may support an omnibus budget bill for the financing of the whole or a large and mixed part of public expenditure, and may give this support without intending or cooperating formally in any wrongful act, even when the bill contains some clauses authorizing gravely immoral expenditures. The decent legislator should do what he reasonably can to amend the budget by eliminating the immoral expenditures, and to make public his rejection and denunciation of the immoral expenditures. But in a final vote, where his options have narrowed to supporting or (in effect) opposing the whole Budget, support for the general bill can be intended only to fund good causes and merely accept as a side-effect (material cooperation) the use of public money for funding immoral activities."

[37] See Martin Rhonheimer, "Fundamental Rights, Moral Law, and the Legal Defense of Life in a Constitutional Democracy." 43 (1998) *American Journal of Jurisprudence*: 135–183, at 176.

[38] "When political activity comes up against moral principles that do not admit of exception, compromise or derogation, the Catholic commitment becomes more evident and laden with responsibility. In the face of *fundamental and inalienable ethical demands*, Christians must recognize that what is at stake is the essence of the moral law, which concerns the integral good of the human person. This is the case with laws concerning *abortion* and *euthanasia* . . . . Such laws must defend the basic right to life from conception to natural death" (emphasis in original text). Congregation for the Doctrine of the Faith, *On the Participation of Catholics in Political life* (2002), n. 4.

[39] *ST* I-II, q. 95, a. 4.

political compromise. The fundamental flaw in Finnis' theory is revealed when he applies it to intrinsically unjust legislation like Proposal A. If Finnis' theory were correct, legislators could vote for Proposal A on the basis that they were intending to enact only the part of the bill which would prohibit abortions, with the part of the bill tolerating abortions not being included in what they were "choosing," but simply accepted as a "side-effect." If, however, legislators cannot vote licitly for Proposal A because it is intrinsically unjust, Finnis' general theory of lawmaking must be flawed.

5.2. Acts and side-effects

John Finnis' reference to "side-effects" shows that he is confusing the acts of legislators, and the acts (or Acts) of a Legislature, with the effects of their acts/Acts. What exactly is the Act of a Parliament (or other Legislature)? The term "Act" has a two-fold meaning. It is a noun, i.e. the Act is the formal record of what is tolerated, permitted, commanded, prohibited, etc. It is also a verb, i.e. the Act is that which the Legislature *does*; the act of the Legislature is "to permit" or "to tolerate" or "to prohibit," etc.

Consider a bill for a law specifying: "All teenagers must attend a one hour skate-boarding instruction class each Saturday; skateboarding is prohibited on Sundays." A legislature enacting this law is, in fact, passing two laws – *doing* two things; performing two "acts": (i) mandating attendance at a one hour skate-boarding class each Saturday, and (ii) prohibiting skate-boarding on Sundays. A legislature may decide to enact this law because skateboarding is a typical teen activity which is causing problems: say, many teens are having accidents because they don't skateboard safely, and they are causing inconvenience and nuisance to others by skateboarding in public places; in order for other citizens to have some peace on Sundays it has been decided to prohibit skateboarding on this one day of the week.

The act (or Act) of the legislature consists of the two acts of mandating and prohibiting, mentioned above. The direct effects of these acts are that teenagers will attend the Saturday class (or they will be punished if they fail to attend), and that they will not skateboard on Sundays (or they will be punished if they do). One might anticipate broader effects: if the teenagers learn well from their classes, they may have fewer accidents themselves and cause fewer accidents to others; they may become generally more considerate towards the non-skateboarding public, and they may become more proficient at skateboarding. With respect to the prohibition of skateboarding on Sundays the effects may be that the public is more contented because it is not troubled by the skateboarders, and that teenagers become better members of society (maybe they will go to Church and clean the family car) because they are not indulging in their skateboarding passion.

That, at least, could be what legislators hope and intend when voting to enact the legislation. The reality could be different. The legislation could, amongst other things, help to shape a sullen teen culture, which, because its favourite pasttime is being thwarted, develops anti-authoritarian attitudes. Instead of becoming better members of society on Sundays, the skateboard-less teenagers might indulge in other pursuits to overcome the boredom, such as taking drugs, alcohol, etc., etc. Even if some legislators foresee the possibility of this happening in some places as a consequence of voting for the legislation, they could vote to enact it, if they believe that the legislation would generally contribute to the common good. The negative consequences could be accepted as unintended side-effects.

What I have described is a proper understanding of the side-effects of voting for legislation. According to John Finnis' theory, however, if some legislators favoured the instruction classes but not Sunday's skateboarding prohibition, they could vote for the legislation "intending" to support only the instruction classes, and accepting Sunday's prohibition as an unintended "side-effect." It seems as though Finnis regards a bill as something that is acted upon, *by means of which* an Act is effected, and that if an Act has two "effects" (e.g. if it permits two things), then a legislator could vote for the bill intending one "effect" and not the other. Such a view distorts the reality of what is involved in voting for a bill. A bill is a draft law. A law (Act) is not enacted *by means of* a bill; rather, a law is enacted *by means of the legislators' support (i.e. vote) for that bill* to be enacted as law. Voting for all the permissions, etc. contained in a bill – i.e., voting for the enactment of the entire content of a bill – is what legislators *are doing*.

Whether lawmaking power is invested solely in a single person (say, a King), or in several hundred members of a legislature, or in the entire citizenship voting in referenda, those with that lawmaking power are "making law." Voting to enact "Abortion is permissible up to 16 weeks and prohibited after 16 weeks," or "All teenagers must attend a one hour skate-boarding instruction class each Saturday; skateboarding is prohibited on Sundays," is the *personal act of each lawmaker*, irrespective of whether one is the King with sole lawmaking power or the most lowly citizen voting in a referendum. If law is made by a legislature or by citizens voting in a referendum, the actual enactment of the bill will depend on the agreement of other lawmakers. In view of this it is, perhaps, more precise to speak of a law-maker's vote as being an expression of "willing the enactment," with the understanding that if the lawmaker is part of the relevant "majority" group, the vote expressive of "willing the enactment" also constitutes a "vote of enactment." Each lawmaker's act of voting represents what is willed and hence what is chosen. Legislators voting for Proposals A, B, C and G are willing and choosing to enact precisely what is contained within those proposals. The will of the legislature in enacting legislation is indistinguishable from the will of the legislator voting for the enactment. What the legislature "does" (in willing that certain permissions, tolerations, prohibitions, etc. be enacted as law) is indistinguishable from what an individual legislator "does" (in willing that the proposal with those very permissions, tolerations, prohibitions, etc., be enacted). Voting for the whole of the proposal which is presented as the matter of the vote is *the act of each legislator* just as the enactment of the whole of the proposal is *the act of the legislature*. John Finnis is wrongly regarding as a "side-effect" what is, in fact, an "act."

5.3. Voting "to permit, precisely to permit" abortion

As noted, John Finnis maintains that pro-life legislators can justly restrict abortion from 24 weeks to 16 weeks by voting for a law "Abortion is *permissible* up to 16 weeks." He avoids making any judgment as to whether this is an intrinsically unjust law (the sort of law for which *EV* 73.2 says it is "never licit" to vote) and, instead, engages in a redefinition of the sort of vote that is never licit, claiming that: "the always illicit vote is for a law *as permitting*, precisely *to* permit, abortion."[40] According to Finnis, a pro-life legislator could vote for "the new law which does in fact permit abortion up to 16 weeks,"[41] because, as he explains: "Even though it is a vote for a law which does permit abortion, it is chosen by this legislator as a vote for a law which restricts abortion."[42]

In his redefinition of "the always illicit vote," Finnis distorts the teaching that some legislation cannot be supported because it is, objectively, in and of itself, always unacceptable, i.e. intrinsically unjust. He presents his own version of "the always illicit vote," a version which appears to hold that the licitness of voting for legislation depends upon the context and one's reasons for doing so. Thus, the licitness of voting for the proposal "Abortion is permissible up to 16 weeks" would appear to depend on the circumstances and the legislator's orientation towards the bill. If the legislator is pro-life and supporting the bill for a law "which does in fact permit abortion up to 16 weeks"[43] in order to prohibit the abortions after 16 weeks, and not "precisely" to permit those before 16 weeks, then the vote would (according to Finnis) be licit. But if the legislator is not pro-life, and is supporting the

---

[40] Finnis, "The Catholic Church and Public Policy Debates . . . ," 268 (emphasis in original text).
[41] *Ibid.*, 269.
[42] *Ibid.*
[43] *Ibid.*

proposal in order to prohibit abortions after 16 weeks (the point at which the legislator thinks abortions should no longer be allowed) *and also* "precisely" to permit abortions up to 16 weeks (as the law specifies), then the vote would be "always illicit."

Those legislators who are not pro-life, whose votes for restrictive legislation like the "16 week" law are "always illicit," must be "doing evil." This raises some difficult questions and serious moral problems for pro-life legislators who might be inclined (as experience in the UK and elsewhere indicates) to introduce a bill for a "16 week" law. According to Finnis' analysis the pro-life legislators would not be doing evil in supporting a "16 week" law. But can they and pro-life campaigners ask and, as is often the case, exert pressure upon other legislators – whose votes would be illict and evil, but without which the bill would probably have no chance of being enacted – to vote for it too?

5.4. *Formal and material cooperation*

John Finnis also claims that the principles of formal and material coopera- tion in evil apply to the question of voting for restrictive legislation. Formal cooperation in evil is, of course, never morally permissible.[44] Some forms of material cooperation (e.g. remote) are permissible; others (e.g. proximate) are not.[45] The relevant principles have been well articulated, not least by other contributors to this volume, and Finnis refers to them as relevant to his argument that a legislator can vote for restrictive legislation of the form "Abortion is permissible up to 16 weeks."[46]

If voting for restrictive legislation were to constitute permissible material cooperation in evil, then the voting legislator would be performing a good action which contributes to the evil action of another person. It is *the evil*

---

[44] The teaching of *EV* 74 is included in footnote 46 below.

[45] "The traditional teaching on material cooperation, with its appropriate distinctions between necessary and freely given cooperation, proximate and remote cooperation, remains valid, to be applied very prudently when the case demands it." Congregation for the Doctrine of the Faith, *Haec sacra congregatio* [On sterilization in Catholic hospitals] (1975), n. 3.

[46] Finnis includes two footnotes in the text of "Unjust Laws in a Democratic Society," 601. At footnote 14 he quotes from *EV* 74: "Indeed, from the moral standpoint, it is never licit to cooperate formally in evil. Such cooperation occurs when an action, either by its very nature or by the form it takes in a concrete situation, can be defined as a direct participation in an act against innocent human life or a sharing in the immoral intention of the person committing it. This cooperation can never be justified ...." At footnote 15 Finnis writes: "'Material cooperation' with action X is any cooperation (participation, assistance, etc.) which does not constitute formal cooperation as defined in the text at note 14 above."

action of the other person in which the legislator would be said to be "cooperating."[47] In which evil action, then, performed by which other person, is the legislator cooperating when voting for restrictive legislation? Some have claimed that voting for restrictive legislation is permissible cooperation in abortion itself, one's cooperation being in the woman's act of undergoing the abortion or the abortionist's act of performing it.[48] To decide whether it was indeed permissible material cooperation *in abortion* one would still have to analyse the act of voting for the legislation to determine whether the "cooperation" was a good act, and therefore permissible. However, this is not the sort of cooperation John Finnis has in mind. He speaks of "cooperation" not in the abortion, but in *the enactment of legislation*. In one text he says that "a legislator's support for the bill ["Abortion is permissible up to 16 weeks"] is also material cooperation in something unjust, namely the legislative act of continuing the existing unjust legal permission of abortion *up to* the 16th week...."[49] Elsewhere Finnis speaks of "the legislator's non-formal but obviously real material cooperation in enacting the new law which does in fact permit abortion up to 16 weeks."[50]

If this does involve the principle of material cooperation in evil, then the act in which the pro-life legislator is cooperating must, necessarily, be evil. The act which Finnis identifies as evil is precisely that of "enacting the new law which does in fact permit abortion up to 16 weeks." Who, then, is enacting the new law? In the UK, law is enacted, properly speaking, by the Queen and the whole of Parliament,[51] though, within the Parliament, only those who *vote for the law* can be said to have performed the personal action that constitutes "enacting" the law (or, as I described it in section

---

[47] This is consistent with Germain Grisez's illustrations of permissible material cooperation in evil: e.g. the actions of a grocer providing food to someone who acts gluttonously, of a postman delivering mail which contains pornographic material, or of a tax payer whose government is engaged in unethical activities. See his *The Way of the Lord Jesus: Volume 3, Difficult Moral Questions* (Quincy, Ill.: Franciscan Herald Press 1997), 871. In each instance the action of the "cooperator" is good but it is abused by another to perform an evil act.

[48] For example, Bishop John Myers of Peoria, Illinois, says that a legislator who votes for legislation "permitting some abortions in order to prevent the enactment of legislation permitting even more" is engaged in an acceptable form of "material cooperation in abortion." See his pastoral statement, "The Obligations of Catholics and the Rights of Unborn Children," in *Origins* 20/4 (14 June 1990): 65–72, at 70.

[49] Finnis, "Unjust Laws in a Democratic Society," 203.

[50] Finnis, "The Catholic Church and Public Policy Debates...," 269.

[51] Each Act of the UK Parliament is an enactment *by* the monarch *and by* the Parliament, as is specified on each Act: "Be It Enacted *by* the Queen's most Excellent Majesty, *by* and with the consent of the Lords Spiritual and Temporal, and Commons, in this present Parliament assembled, and *by* the authority of the same, as follows:...."

5.2, the act expressive of "willing the enactment" of the law). Legislators who vote against the enactment of a law, or who (with good reason) abstain from voting, are not morally responsible for the law's enactment, and have not, in a personal sense, "enacted" the law.

If the evil in which pro-life legislators voting for the "16 week" law are said to be "cooperating materially" is that of "enacting the new law...", then it would appear that Finnis is saying one of two things, neither of which is plausible. The first possibility is that Finnis is saying that pro-life legislators, who are themselves voting for the "16 week" law, are "materially cooperating in the evil of their own action." The concept of material cooperation requires that the evil, to which the cooperation refers, be that of another person, so this option is hardly plausible; and if the evil refers to a pro-life legislator's own action, then his or her action must itself *be evil*, and therefore impermissible.

The second possibility is that Finnis is making a distinction between the acts of pro-life legislators who *are not* voting (as he suggests) "to permit, precisely to permit, abortion," and other legislators who *are* voting "to permit, precisely to permit, abortion." As described in the previous section, Finnis appears to believe that though they are voting for the same legislation, at the same time, and within the same context, for some legislators the action is evil, and for others the action is good. Is Finnis saying, then, that pro-life legislators voting to enact the "16 week" law are doing good, but that they are cooperating materially in the evil act of the other (not pro-life) legislators who are also voting for the same law? If he is, and if the "cooperation" is material, one must still ask if it fulfils the conditions of being *permissible* material cooperation. For example, is the "cooperation" proximate or remote? A possible answer to this question is that the actions of pro-life and other legislators are so proximate that, even if the "cooperation" of pro-life legislators is material (and not formal), nevertheless it cannot be regarded as *permissible* material cooperation. A more pertinent question, however, is: in what way does the action of one legislator contribute to the action of any other legislator voting for the legislation? Certainly, the actual enactment of legislation is a collective act; it depends on a majority of legislators showing, by their votes, that they will the enactment and, in this sense, enacting law is a "collaborative" task. In common discourse "collaboration" and "cooperation" may be interchangeable nouns, but "collaboration" (as used in ordinary discourse) should not be confused with the precise meaning of "cooperation" as applied to the formal or material assistance given to another person's evil acts. All legislators voting for a bill are performing entirely separate, individual acts which are in no way dependent upon the actions of other legislators voting for the same bill. Legislators are engaged in a collective, "collaborative" activity insofar as the actual enactment of legislation depends upon a calculation of the numbers who expressed, by voting, their will that the bill be enacted. It is, however, false to say that one legislator's act of voting for a law contributes to the performance of another legislator's act of voting for the same law, and that voting for a proposal like "Abortion is permissible up to 16 weeks" can in any way be regarded as the sort of "cooperation" matter that Finnis suggests.[52]

6. Problems of principle and other considerations

Proposals A, B, C, and G permit or tolerate abortion, and are accordingly the sort of intrinsically unjust proposals that it is never licit to vote for. If Proposals A or B or C were enacted, the abortion law in Noland and Tyrannia would be similar to the abortion law in Littalia if, respectively, Proposals D or E or F were enacted. One notes, not only that these latter proposals (as well as Proposal H) are not intrinsically unjust, but that voting for them simply does not require the introduction of the sorts of arguments cited as justifying votes for Proposals A or B or C or G. The sort of analysis undertaken by John Finnis to justify voting for measures like Proposals A or B or C or G – involving considerations of cooperation in evil, intentions and side-effects, and voting "to permit, precisely to permit" abortion – does not apply to votes for Proposals like D or E or F or H. This is because the latter proposals neither tolerate nor permit abortion and are not intrinsically unjust.

Voting for Proposals A, B, C or G is problematic because it requires the violation of the principle that it is never licit to vote for an intrinsically unjust law. While this problem does not apply when voting for Proposals, D, E, F or H, other considerations would have to be taken into account before voting for any of these proposals in a concrete situation.

Although a proposal to repeal intrinsically unjust law, such as Proposal F, is not intrinsically unjust, its justness in a concrete situation depends on the circumstances and the consequences of the proposal's enactment. A welcome consequence of voting for Proposal F is that several thousand unborn children would not be aborted; another consequence is that the overall abortion law (Z2) would have been shaped so that abortion is permitted

---

[52] An appropriate illustration of possible permissible material cooperation in the enactment of an unjust law would refer not to someone actually voting for the law, but to the actions of someone like a secretary working for a legislative drafting committee creating the law. This illustration is given by William May in "Unjust Laws and Catholic Citizens: Opposition, Cooperation and Toleration," *Homiletic and Pastoral Review* (November 1995): 7–14, at 12.

solely up to 16 weeks "on request." Legislators voting for Proposal F would not be responsible for the law permitting abortion up to 16 weeks, but the goodness of their action in supporting Proposal F cannot avoid a consideration of the consequences. Might legislators be giving the impression that abortion was objectionable only if it occurred later in pregnancy, and that earlier abortions were less, if at all, objectionable? The relevant considerations are more evident when considering Proposals E or D. Is the shaping of the law by Proposal E, i.e., the law being shaped so that abortion would be permitted solely if the unborn child had at least one Jewish parent, something that a morally upright legislator would regard as justified? Unlike legislators voting for Proposal B (in Tyrannia), those voting for Proposal E (in Littalia) cannot be charged with voting *to permit* the abortion of Jewish babies; the shaping of the law in such a prejudicial way is, nevertheless, a serious matter. Similarly, unlike legislators voting for Proposal A (in Noland), those voting for Proposal D (in Littalia) cannot be charged with voting *to permit* (or *to tolerate*) abortion if the unborn child has been conceived after rape, or is disabled, etc.; the shaping of the law in such a prejudicial way is, nevertheless, a serious matter. In the abstract one cannot say that a pro-life legislator *should* vote for Proposals D, E, F or H that are not intrinsically unjust. If pro-life legislators were to judge that proposals like these could be justly supported, a minimum requirement would be that their absolute opposition to all abortions be publicly known so that any misunderstanding about the reasons for their votes will be avoided.

In the previous paragraph I focused solely on the question of *voting for* (i.e. voting to enact) legislation that is not intrinsically unjust and which has a restrictive effect on abortion. If careful consideration needs to be exercised when judging whether to vote for it, even more careful consideration is required before *embarking on a public campaign* for it, especially as campaigns for legislation may take several months if not years. Given the radical unjustness of Littalia's abortion law (Z1), a campaign specifically for Proposals D, E, or F is an inadequate response to the intrinsic unjustness of the whole law. Legislators, and their pro-life supporters, must remain focused on the need to repeal the whole of the unjust law, not simply parts of it. This is particularly so, when the unborn children who will not benefit from proposals to partially repeal an abortion law will normally be those who can be regarded as particularly threatened and vulnerable; like those in the proposals I suggested who are younger, conceived after rape, disabled or Jewish. A danger of campaigning "for" Proposals D, E or F is that this would tend, inevitably, to involve the public presentation of reasons for prohibiting particular abortions, the implication being that these reasons do not apply for the prohibition of those abortions not affected by the particular proposal. Similarly, although proposal H (to prohibit abortion-inducing drugs) is not intrinsically unjust, a campaign to enact it requires a prudence which avoids any suggestion that other abortions are more acceptable.[53]

Since the publication of *Evangelium Vitae* in 1995, the precise meaning of the teaching of *EV* 73 has been disputed. In a previous paper I argued that the "proposals" for which legislators can vote, as taught by *EV* 73.3, to "limit the harm" of an (intrinsically unjust) abortion law, are necessarily *just* proposals.[54] Not only is it counter-intuitive to believe that the Pope could have taught that legislators may vote for *unjust* legislation, but it is flatly contradicted by the teaching of the one-sentence paragraph preceding *EV* 73.3, that *it is never licit to vote for an intrinsically unjust law* (*EV* 73.2). A correct identification of specific proposals as being just or intrinsically unjust is required for a correct understanding of what is taught in *EV* 73.3, and I have presented Proposals A–H, above, in order to highlight some of the relevant considerations. Anyone wanting to justify voting for Proposals A, B, C or G has two options. The first is to acknowledge that the proposals are intrinsically unjust, and to argue that voting for them is justified. The second is to deny that they are intrinsically unjust. The first option requires

---

[53] The sort of error to be avoided is the one made in an article by (Lord) David Alton, "Fight this Dangerous Plan for Do-It-Yourself Abortions," *The Universe* 27 July 2003. Encouraging Catholics to oppose plans to allow RU486 to be taken by women who would then abort at home, he says: "If abortion does have to take place, then surely all stages of the abortion should be conducted in an approved medical environment where medical assistance will be on hand immediately if required?" David Alton's long-standing commitment to the pro-life cause is unquestioned, but this sort of argument, used as a means of furthering the pro-life cause, in fact undermines attempts to prohibit all abortions. Alton's argument may help to prohibit RU486 home-abortions, but it also assists the argument of those who support the continued legal availability of abortions, who maintain that if abortion is prohibited illegal abortions will take place and it is better that "abortion should be conducted in an approved medical environment where medical assistance will be on hand."

[54] See my paper "Challenging a Consensus: Why *Evangelium Vitae* Does Not Permit Legislators to Vote for 'Imperfect Legislation,'" *op. cit.* In that paper I addressed the opportunities to change abortion legislation in legislatures like the UK Parliament, and, given the need to identify just ways of changing the law, I focused particularly on the opportunity to restrict abortion by what I labelled the "secondary" aspects of abortion legislation: matters dealing with funding, the rights of doctors etc. I noted that "codified systems present different opportunities" (pp. 328–329) and it seems appropriate to address those opportunities – notably, the opportunities to repeal unjust law – in this paper. The opportunities to repeal unjust law in the imaginary country Littalia correspond with the opportunities in some European countries with a codified system of law, such as Italy. The opportunities present in such countries should not be confused with the more limited opportunities in other countries.

that the teaching of *EV* 73.2 be overlooked if not rejected, and the second involves an obviously incorrect factual judgment. I trust, however, that those who disagree with the argument in this paper, and who believe legislators could rightly vote for Proposals A, B, C or G, are able and willing to express clearly whether they judge each of these proposals to be just or intrinsically unjust.

12

Restricting legalised abortion is not intrinsically unjust

John Finnis

Summary. The form and wording of an enactment must be distinguished from its legal meaning and effect – i.e. from the propositions of law which the enactment *makes* legally valid. An enactment's legal context determines the legal meaning and effect of its form and wording. It is therefore possible, and rationally necessary, to conclude that not all enactments which declare or textually imply that some abortions are permitted (but others prohibited) are permissive laws within the meaning of the true principle that permissive abortion laws are intrinsically unjust and may never be voted for. A provision in an enactment is permissive, in that sense, only if it has the legal meaning and effect of *reducing* the state's legal protection of the unborn.

1. Permissive abortion laws are unjust and never to be voted for

> In the case of an intrinsically unjust law, such as a law permitting abortion or euthanasia, it is therefore never licit to obey it, or to "take part in a propaganda campaign in favour of such a law, or vote for it".

This sentence, the whole of the second paragraph of section 73 of the encyclical *Evangelium Vitae* (1995), is the foundation of my reflections on the question in issue: Is it ever permissible[1] to vote for a proposal to restrict

---

[1] The question thus is whether such a vote is *intrinsically* wrong. Even if the answer to that question is that such a vote is not intrinsically wrong (i.e. that it is permissible, or can be licit), there is in all actual cases the further question whether it is right in all the circumstances to cast such a vote. The answer to that further, always relevant question is given by moral norms – especially of fairness, commitment, and role-responsibility – which are situation-relative in a way that norms about *intrinsic* wrongness are not.

a state's legal permission of abortion if that proposal at the same time leaves in force some elements of that state's existing legal permission? Must such a proposed bill/statute be regarded as itself enacting an intrinsically unjust law?[2]

There are two things to notice at the outset about *EV* 73.2. The first is the tight parallel it draws between the question of obedience to a permissive abortion law and the question of voting for it: "it is... never licit to obey it or... vote for it". Suppose that a law is *restrictive*, that is, is partly permissive and partly prohibitive.[3] It expressly or tacitly permits some abortions[4]

---

[2] "Intrinsically unjust" replaces the term "intrinsically immoral" [Italian: "una legge intrinsecamente immorale", Latin: "intrinsece inhonesta"] predicated of such laws in the Declaration on Procured Abortion made by the Congregation for the Doctrine of the Faith in November 1974, sec. 22. As predicated of a kind of law, neither term is traditional, and the notion gives rise to certain problems. As is said in the encyclicals *Veritatis Splendor* (1993), secs. 67, 80–2, and *Evangelium Vitae* (1995), sec. 75, acts *intrinsece inhonestae* are those kinds of acts which are picked out in the exceptionless *negative* moral norms of Christian teaching about the content of the natural moral law. The obligation to legally prohibit murder or abortion is the content, however, not of a negative moral norm, but an affirmative or positive one, prescribing that a certain kind of act (in this case, legislation or its equivalent) be done. And as Aquinas teaches constantly, affirmative obligations are always situation-relative (*non ad semper obligant*): see J. Finnis, *Aquinas: Moral, Political and Legal Theory.* Oxford: Oxford University Press 1998: 164. Moreover, justice and injustice are predicated of laws only by an analogy of attribution, for justice is "the steady and undeflected will [*of a person*] to give to others what they are entitled to". These facts create serious strains in extending the traditional and sound idea of intrinsically immoral acts to categories of *laws* and to the positive obligation to make laws about murder and abortion. But I shall ignore those problems in this paper, though they cannot be overlooked in real life. More positively, I would suggest that the newly articulated category, properly understood, picks out three types of law: those that permit the violation of a fundamental human right (e.g. abortion), laws which establish a public policy violating such a right (e.g. licensing and funding human embryo production and/or experimentation), and laws which institutionalise an intrinsically evil type of act (e.g. ratifying "homosexual marriage").

[3] Such a law could also be called "incompletely restrictive" or "incompletely prohibitive". I shall use "restrictive" to mean "incompletely prohibitive". I shall use "prohibitive" and "prohibition" to include both complete and incomplete prohibition, and let the context make clear whether the prohibition I am referring to is complete or incomplete. So: restrictive laws are prohibitive, but only incompletely prohibitive. In virtually all instances, I use "restrictive" as shorthand for "prohibitive but less prohibitive than reason (justice) requires".

[4] By "abortion(s)" throughout this paper I shall mean all and only those terminations of pregnancy which, because they *intend* the death of the unborn baby, or *intend* the cessation of its development, are intrinsically wrong and have been judged wrong by the Christian tradition and Catholic magisterium down to today. So the term as I use it does not include those kinds of termination of pregnancy (some or all of which may be conventionally described as types of "therapeutic abortion") that cause the

but prohibits others. It ought, of course, to prohibit all abortions. So we might be tempted to say: this whole law is simply intrinsically unjust. But the temptation should be resisted. For if the whole law is simply unjust, then it "is never licit to obey it", and so no police officer or judge could rightly obey the law's directive to prevent and punish the abortions it prohibits. *EV* 73.2 cannot have meant that. So, instead of saying that the restrictive law, taken as a whole, is permissive and therefore simply unjust, one should say that this restrictive law is unjust *insofar as* it is permissive but is just (and fit to be obeyed) *insofar as* it is prohibitive.

The point can be put more precisely. What is commonly and acceptably called a "law restricting abortion" must actually comprise two (or more) distinct *propositions of law* – indeed, two (or more) *laws* in a strict sense of the word. One is a proposition of law that certain abortions are prohibited. The other – which may be articulated in the same statute or judgment, or may be implied in the constitution, or in the general legal principle that what is not prohibited is permitted – is the proposition of law that other abortions are permitted. Only by keeping in mind this kind of distinction can we make sense of *EV* 73.2's reference to obedience. And since that reference is in strict parallel to its reference to voting, it follows that *EV* 73.2 – even before we reach 73.3 – opens up the possibility and indeed the necessity of distinguishing, and dealing separately with, (i) rules or elements or propositions of a state's law which permit abortion (and are therefore intrinsically[5] unjust) and (ii) rules, elements, or propositions of the state's law which prohibit abortion, and therefore can rightly (and should) be obeyed *and can rightly be voted for*.

The second thing to notice about *EV* 73.2 is that its reference to voting is by way of a quotation. It is from the Declaration on Procured Abortion made by the Congregation for the Doctrine of the Faith [CDF] in November 1974. *EV* 73.2 is deliberately recalling what the Holy See taught in 1974. When

---

death of the child only as a side-effect (some of which may, however, be unjust albeit not instances of *intrinsece malum*). The terms "termination of pregnancy" and "abortion" in state legislation may in many cases not be so precise, and if used without explicit qualifications or exceptions would entail the legal condemnation of actions which Christian tradition and sound moral analysis would not condemn. This is a serious problem for Catholic and other pro-life efforts at restrictive reform, and needs much more attention than it received in *Evangelium Vitae* and other such documents. In this paper I take for granted that *all abortions should be legally prohibited*, even though this proposition is not true if "abortion" is understood in a different sense, perhaps closer to legal and everyday usage. This paper is not the right context for going deeper into this important practical and theoretical issue.

[5] See fn. 4 above.

the Pope goes on in the Encyclical's next sentences, *EV* 73.3, to take up a "particular problem of conscience", he is alluding to a kind of problem that arose constantly, and was extensively debated among faithful Catholics, during the two decades between the Declaration and the Encyclical. By making a key part of *EV* 73.2 a quotation, the Pope is indicating that in 73.3 he intends to pass judgment on a matter that for two decades had been causing disputes among Catholics (and other pro-life people), had been left unsettled by the 1974 Declaration, and had occasioned statements by and on behalf of bishops, episcopal conferences, and officials of the Holy See itself.

A few main examples from those two decades. First, and closest to the Holy See, an example from Italy in 1981–2, recently recalled by Fr Angelo Luño in his commentary on the whole issue of *EV* 73, in the Holy See's *L'Osservatore Romano*:

> On 28 March 1980, the Italian Radical Party began collecting signatures for a referendum in favour of the modification of Law 194/78 in order to make it more completely and openly favourable to abortion. Faced with the prospect of having to choose between the existing law 194/78 and one which would be worse, the Italian Pro-Life Movement began collecting signatures for two referenda: one giving maximum protection to human life by eliminating every possibility for abortion, except in the case of conflict with the life of the mother, and another which represented the minimal position: it condemned abortion in general terms, but allowed legal abortion in two cases: grave threat to the life of the mother and verified pathologies which constitute a grave risk to her physical health. As expected, on 4 February 1981, the Constitutional Court of Italy declared that the minimum referendum of the Pro-Life Movement was admissible, but the one giving maximum protection was not, since it contradicted an earlier decision of the Court of 18 February 1975 (n. 27).
>
> The question of conscience then arose regarding whether someone who was absolutely opposed to abortion could vote in favour of the minimal referendum as drafted by the Pro-Life Movement. The Italian Conference of Bishops offered an important clarification on 11 February 1981: "The referendum proposed by the Pro-Life Movement is morally acceptable and binding for the consciences of Christians since it seeks, by *overturning some elements in the current abortion law, to restrict, as much as possible, its extent and to reduce its negative effects. It does*

not follow, however, that the remaining elements in the civil law in favour of abortion may be seen as morally licit and may be followed."[6]

Given the relationships between the Bishop of Rome and the Italian Conference of Bishops, it is no surprise that this statement is echoed[7] in *EV* 73.3's response by the Pope to the "problem of conscience" of which the Italian issue of early 1981 was one kind of instance.

Another kind of instance arose later in 1981, when Senator Hatch proposed an amendment to the United States Constitution to overturn the virtually complete legal permission of abortion created by Supreme Court decisions in 1972.[8] The proposal embodied in the Hatch amendment would expressly empower each state in the United States to "restrict and prohibit" abortion, that is, to choose whether to permit it completely, prohibit it completely, *or to restrict it* (i.e. prohibit it *incompletely*).[9] Hitherto the National Conference of Catholic Bishops had supported proposed amendments which would have created a nationwide legal right to life for the unborn, and now, on 18 November 1981, the US Catholic [Bishops'] Conference also fully endorsed the Hatch amendment. At the same time, they communicated to the CDF the doubt expressed by some Catholics about the moral permissibility of this endorsement and of the proposed amendment itself. In reply, the President of the Congregation, Cardinal Ratzinger, wrote in May 1982, implicitly accepting the moral permissibility of the amendment and its endorsement by the US Bishops:

---

[6] A. R. Luño, "Evangelium vitae 73: The Catholic lawmaker and the problem of a seriously unjust law". *L'Osservatore Romano* English ed. 18 September 2002: 3–5 at 3 (emphasis added). This article closely parallels the 2000/2001 article by Archbishop Bertone cited by Harte in sec. 3.2.

[7] *EV* 73.3 echoes even more closely the weighty editorial in *La Civiltà Cattolica* no. 3136, 21 February 1981: 313 at 318–324, which quotes the statement of the Bishops' Conference in the course of arguing that the referendum creates a "grave problema di coscienza per coloro che respingono l'aborto per principio, quindi senza eccezioni [serious problem of conscience for all who reject abortion in principle and therefore without exception]", and that the correct answer to the problem is that voting Yes, to rescue those babies who can be rescued, is not only morally acceptable but is also (esp. p. 321) *doveroso* – the word used in the authoritative Italian text of *EV* 73.3 – which the context makes quite clear means "a matter of duty" (not merely "proper", as in the English of 73.3, but "un devoir" as in the French). The editorial employs with vigour the dynamic and comparative analysis later used in 73.3.

[8] Human Life Federalism Amendment, S[enate] J[oint] Resolution 110.

[9] Congress would also have been empowered to restrict or prohibit abortion nationally, and by the terms of the amendment a state's law would have prevailed over Congress's only if it were "more restrictive than" Congress's.

according to the principles of Catholic morality, an action can be considered licit whose *object and proximate effect consist in limiting an evil* insofar as possible. Thus, when one intervenes in a situation judged evil in order to correct it for the better, and when the action is not evil in itself, such an action should be considered not as the voluntary acceptance of the lesser evil but rather *as* the effective *improvement of the existing situation*, even though one remains aware that not all evil present is able to be eliminated for the moment.[10]

Clearly the CDF did not regard the action of enacting a law authorising states currently disabled from restricting abortion to *restrict* it as the enactment of an intrinsically unjust law or as an action "evil in itself". But Cardinal Ratzinger would have been bound to judge such an enactment unjust and the enacting of it evil if it is true that a law restricting abortion – that is, incompletely and inadequately prohibiting it – is by its nature necessarily simply unjust.

In 1989 the Bishops' Conferences of Great Britain published a statement by the Catholic Bishops' [of England, Wales, Scotland and Ireland] Joint Committee on Bio-Ethical Issues, addressed to the question "How far may I support a bill which *inadequately* protects human rights or other important aspects of the common good", taking, "for simplicity", the example of abortion. The statement declared that a legislator faced with "a law or a bill for weakening restraints on abortion" could never vote for it on the ground that killing an unborn child or stopping its development is sometimes needed, or on tactical grounds such as to preserve one's career even for the sake of doing "greater good in the future". But in a society where securing for the unborn the equal protection of the law is or seems practically impossible for the foreseeable future,

> Catholics may support and vote for a bill or other proposal which would *strengthen the law's protection* for the unborn, even when the bill fails to extend such protection to the full extent that justice truly requires. ... Catholics who are publicly lending their support to such imperfect legislation should not disguise their view that all procuring abortion is unacceptable.[11]

---

[10] Quoted by Mgr R. G. Peters, *Catholic Twin Circle*, 17 September 1989: 14 (emphases added).

[11] "Imperfect Laws: Some Guidelines". 19 (1989) *Briefing* (Bishops' Conferences of Great Britain): 298–300 at 299, para. 6 (emphasis added). Publication was in July 1989, well over three months after the document was forwarded to the Holy See.

Thus the statement treated as decisive the same criterion as the Italian Bishops and Cardinal Ratzinger: Does the amending proposal, bill, or law *change* the existing law by making it *more restrictive*? In the next paragraph this criterion was restated: "a measure of protection which is less than complete but which is greater than that accorded by today's unjust law" and is judged to have "a better prospect of being enacted and brought into force" than any proposal to extend to the unborn what they are entitled to – "fully equal protection" by the law. And this broad and common-sense criterion, stateable in many different but equivalent forms of words, was to be the criterion adopted by the Pope in *EV* 73.3.

The British/Irish statement of 1989 was warmly endorsed by Cardinal O'Connor, then chairman of the Committee on Pro-Life Activities of the National Conference of Catholic Bishops, in a statement he published in his archdiocesan paper on 14 June 1990, prominently reprinted in *Origins* on 28 June. In this statement, later included along with the British/Irish statement in the small CDF dossier distributed during the run-up to the CDF conference preparatory to *EV* 73.3, the Cardinal offered his own version of the dynamic and comparative explanation later found in *EV* 73.3:

> The conflict over imperfect law has definitely been divisive to the pro-life movement. It seems to me that our goal must always be to advance protection for the unborn child to the maximum degree possible. It certainly seems to me, however, that in cases in which perfect legislation is clearly impossible, it is morally acceptable to support a pro-life bill, however reluctantly, that contains exceptions if the following conditions prevail:
>
> (A) There is *no other feasible bill restricting* existing permissive abortion laws *to a greater degree* than the proposed bill.
>
> (B) The proposed bill is *more restrictive than existing law*, that is, the bill *does not weaken the current law's restraints* on abortion. And,
>
> (C) The proposed bill does not negate the responsibility [*scil.* possibility] of future, *more restrictive* laws.
>
> In addition, it would have to be made clear that we do not believe that a bill which contains exceptions is ideal and that we would continue to urge future legislation which would *more fully* protect human life.[12]

---

[12] Cardinal John O'Connor, "Abortion: Questions and Answers". 20/7 (1990) *Origins* (emphases added).

In November 1992 the Irish bishops themselves had to confront the very immediate and politically fraught problem of conscience which had arisen since in March 1992 a Supreme Court judgment had made abortion legal in what the bishops termed "a potentially wide range of circumstances". The Irish government and legislature, in response to that judgment, were promoting amendments to the Constitution. In the opinion of the bishops the principal amendment, while it "would improve the constitutional protection of the unborn as this now stands in the light of the Supreme Court judgment", would "give constitutional support to a principle which is morally false and unjust . . . that it can be legitimate to deliberately destroy a human life." They then outlined "two contrary conclusions" which "can be drawn by people, all of whom are equally opposed to abortion". Some consider themselves bound to vote NO, "whatever the legal and political consequences". But others

> who view abortion with total abhorrence see the Amendment as a means of *curtailing* the worst features of the Supreme Court judgment. They have no confidence that any more satisfactory opportunity of doing so will be presented to them. They do not see a YES vote as bringing about the introduction of abortion. *Abortion, with potentially wide availability, has already been introduced by the Supreme Court judgment.* They consider that the passing of the Amendment would substantially mitigate that totally unacceptable legal position. Their desire is to *improve the situation as best they can,* but they do not intend to endorse the flaws in the Amendment. They believe that they are *restoring, insofar as is open to them* at present, the constitutional guarantee of the right to life of the unborn child.[13]

The Bishops' Conference then gave its "considered opinion that from a moral point of view both of these stances are tenable insofar as each is intended to reflect a total abhorrence of abortion and the determination to make that abhorrence clear."

At just the same time, the bishops and people of Poland had to make their judgments about the justice of a law introducing very extensive prohibitions of abortion but leaving intact the existing permission of abortion in a small number of cases specified by excepting from the new law's prohibitions certain cases involving serious threats to the health or life of the mother, rape, or serious and permanent disability of the child. This legislation was adopted early in 1993. But before the end of 1992, the Congregation for

---

[13] "The Referenda: Statement by the Irish Bishops' Conference", 5 November 1992, para. 10 (emphasis added).

the Doctrine of the Faith[14] began direct preparations for a conference to be focussed entirely on the question what judgment might properly and officially be made, at an ecclesiastical level transcending the national, on "the delicate problem of the collaboration of Catholics with imperfect laws (for example, laws which permit abortion in certain cases, but are *more restrictive* compared with existing laws)."[15] This conference was held in the Vatican in early October 1994, and all the participants were invited to reflect on a sheet of paper articulating (in less than 150 words of Italian) a "possible official position on the problem of imperfect laws". What was articulated on that sheet of paper is what now, reordered and partially reworded but in substance identical, is to be found as *EV* 73.3, which reads:

> [73.3] A particular problem of conscience can arise in cases where a legislative vote would be decisive for the passage of a more restrictive law, aimed at [*volta cioè a*] limiting the number of authorized abortions, in place of a more permissive law already passed or ready to be voted on. Such cases are not infrequent. It is a fact that while in some parts of the world there continue to be campaigns to introduce laws favouring abortion, often supported by powerful international organizations, in other nations – particularly those which have already experienced the bitter fruits of such permissive legislation – there are growing signs of a rethinking in this matter. In a case like the one just mentioned, when it is not possible to overturn or completely abrogate a pro-abortion law, an elected official, whose absolute personal opposition to procured abortion was well known, could licitly support [*suffragari*][16] proposals aimed at [*velint*] *limiting the harm* done by such a law and at lessening its negative consequences at the level of general opinion and public morality. This does not in fact represent an illicit cooperation with an unjust law, but rather a legitimate and proper attempt to limit its evil aspects.

---

[14] Doubtless acting within the framework of the preparations for the encyclical *Evangelium Vitae* which were launched by the special consistory of cardinals summoned by the Pope on 4–7 April 1991 and the papal letter to the episcopate *"De Evangelio vitae"* dated 19 May 1991 (see *EV* 5).

[15] From the President of the Congregation's invitation of 1 July 1993 to the conference (emphasis added).

[16] This word picks up the Latin *suffragiis sustinere* used to translate "vote for" in *EV* 73.2. Note, incidentally, that Colin Harte's statements, in writings cited in his present paper, that the Italian is a translation of the Latin are the converse of reality. The Latin is official and normative, but it is a translation of a document conceived from beginning to end (and in all probability approved and signed off by the Pope) in Italian; the Italian version thus has an authority not shared by translations (such as the English).

2. The meaning and logic of *EV* 73.3

In each of the five national situations I have mentioned, the bishops or the Holy See itself, in indicating or plainly affirming that Catholics may rightly vote "for" a bill that will leave the state's laws inadequately restrictive of abortions and thus unjust, adopted one and the same line of analysis: Casting such a vote is permissible because, and only because, the new statute which the passing of the bill will enact will itself *make* the state's law *more restrictive.* These ecclesiastical authorities and sources of guidance look at what will be the *immediate legal effect* of the bill or referendum and resultant new statute upon the state's laws. If that juridical effect is in itself simply prohibitive, the bill or referendum proposal is, they imply, just. Voting for it can be an act of justice, they imply, because the legislative proposal, and the amend*ing* law enacted if the bill is passed, is a just one – and it will be just because the difference it makes to the state's whole law regarding abortion is just.[17] The new statute's *juridical* meaning and effect is simply prohibitive. The statute *does* nothing but prohibit abortions. (Of course, the state's laws, even as amended, will remain unjust because incompletely prohibitive (= partly permissive).) The analysis, in every case, is *dynamic.* That is, it consists in looking to see what *change* is made by the bill or new statute. And the analysis is *comparative.* That is, it compares the statute about to be made, and the state's law as altered by the new statute, with the existing law. If the change made by the new statute is restrictive, the fact that it does not prohibit everything that might and should be prohibited does not entail that the partial prohibition – the new restriction(s) created by the bill/statute – is an unjust act: the amending statute so enacted should not be regarded as an intrinsically unjust Act or, in itself, an unjust law.[18]

In all these cases, this kind of analysis met with incomprehension and/or outright opposition from a (relatively small) number of Catholics or other pro-lifers who reasoned that any bill or new statute which leaves some abortions permitted is intrinsically (i.e. by its nature) – whatever the good intentions and difficult circumstances of any who vote for it – an unjust proposal or law, and therefore incapable of being justly supported or voted

---

[17] As always, this is an over-simplification. "Just", here as almost everywhere in this paper, means "not intrinsically unjust". In reality, a law is not truly just unless it is not only not intrinsically unjust but also does not violate any of the situation-relative moral norms bearing upon the relation between persons which is under consideration. (See also fn. 1 above.) This is another complexity which I usually ignore in order not to clutter up the discussion.

[18] Of course, a vote for it *can* be described as a vote for an unjust law – a vote, that is, for the state's law remaining unjustly permissive after its amendment. But that description is too broad and undiscriminating to be a proper basis for an analysis of the justice or injustice of voting for the amending bill/statute.

for. From 1974 these Catholics and others could point to the CDF's *Declaration on Procured Abortion* sec. 22:

> man can never obey a law which is in itself (*intrinsece*) immoral, and such is the case of a law which would *admit in principle the liceity of abortion*. Nor can he take part in a propaganda campaign in favor of such a law, *or vote for it*.

These objectors could and did object that any bill or new statute which selects for prohibition some but not all classes of abortions is either tacitly or explicitly – but in either case objectionably – "admitting in principle the liceity of abortion" by failing to simply repeal the existing laws' permission(s). A vote for such a proposal is therefore ruled out, according to the objectors, by the *Declaration* sec. 22.

The episcopal and other ecclesiastical interventions I have sketched above all reject this interpretation of the *Declaration* and this denial of the justice of such amending bills and new laws and of voting for them. *Evangelium Vitae* 73.3 is manifestly intended to ratify what I have called the *dynamic* and *comparative* analysis of an amending bill or law. Phrase after phrase keeps that analysis in the foreground. Proposals of the kind in question are acceptable insofar as they propose "a *more restrictive* law, *aimed* at *limiting* the number of authorized abortions, *in place of* a more permissive law." Acceptable proposals are "*aimed* at *limiting* the harm done by" the state's permissive, pro-abortion law. They represent "a legitimate and proper *attempt* to *limit* [the] evil aspects" of the law they (only partially) supplant. The attempt to enact a new law that will have such an (incomplete) effect can be legitimate and proper provided that "it is not possible to overturn or *completely abrogate* [the] pro-abortion law" whose place the new law will *incompletely* take. In such cases, therefore, so 73.3 plainly teaches, voting for such a bill or new law need not be regarded – and indeed, provided the intentions and circumstances indicated in 73.3 are present, *should* not be regarded – as an instance of the kind of act declared by 73.2 to be always impermissible: voting for a permissive and therefore intrinsically unjust law. Regarded dynamically, in what they juridically *do* – immediately, as a matter of law – such proposals and the bills and new laws (statutes) giving effect to them are, precisely speaking, not permissive but prohibitive. That is how 73.3 and 73.2 must be understood if they are to be regarded as consistent with each other, as they can and therefore must be. It is an understanding that treats them as consistent also with the straightforward dynamic and comparative analysis used by responsible episcopal teachers and pastors in all the cases I have mentioned (and others). It is utterly fanciful to think that the Pope would have left sec. 73 of his encyclical bare of any hint of a correction of that analysis (and its practical conclusion) if he had thought that such analyses, and the many acts of Catholic legislators done in reliance upon them – extending most recently to his own much loved homeland, under the guidance of Catholic statesmen very well known to him – were actually misguided attempts to justify the unjustifiable, the seriously immoral act of voting for a bill or law unjust by its very nature.

3. The relevant criteria for assessing a restrictive statute's intrinsic justice

Readings of sec. 73.2/3 of that unusual kind were, however, proposed by a few objectors, among them Colin Harte. Ignoring the sequence of episcopal responses to legislative events or proposals between 1974 and 1995, and ignoring equally entirely the Holy See's long tradition of teaching by answering *questions* whose terms are carefully devised or refined by the answerer so as to define the answer's meaning and purport, Harte argued that one can sensibly regard the last sentence of 73.3 (the answer) as being separate from the first sentence of 73.3 (the question), in much the same way (said Harte) as a teacher's answer "If you use a calculator you'll get the answer" is separate from the child's question "Does $2 + 2 = 5$?"! On the basis of this inapt analogy, he confidently brushed aside the first sentence of sec. 73.3, with its reference to a "vote ... for the passage of a *more restrictive* law, *aimed* at *limiting* the number of authorised abortions, *in place of* a more permissive law...." Having thus largely removed from his view[19] the dynamic, comparative analysis that unites the Pope's teaching with the teaching and practice of various episcopates through the 1980s and early 1990s, Harte felt able to claim that *EV* 73's teaching is entirely non-dynamic and non-comparative. If *either* the amending bill/statute[20] *or* the amended law

---

[19] In fact the dynamic and comparative analysis is still clearly present in the "answer" sentence, which says that the answer applies when "it is not possible to overturn or *completely* abrogate a pro-abortion law" – in which case one can "attempt to *limit* its evil aspects" (by implication, limit *any* of its evil aspects, and most obviously its permission of abortions).

[20] Thus Harte says ("Challenging a Consensus" p. 329, emphases adjusted): "One could try to prohibit some categories of abortion, not by introducing an Amendment Bill but by introducing separate legislation to prohibit some categories of abortion (i.e. the primary legislation). Such legislation might lower the time limit during which abortions could take place or prohibit 'social' abortions, but in so doing *it would tolerate if not specifically permit* earlier or 'hard case' abortions. Because such legislation would make an illicit distinction of persons – granting protection to some but not to others in a context which requires that the right to life of all the unborn should be safeguarded – it can be judged to be intrinsically unjust." By "can be judged intrinsically unjust" he means (as he confirms to me) "*is* intrinsically unjust."

leaves some abortions permitted,[21] the amending bill or law, according to Harte in 2001/2, is intrinsically unjust and can never rightly be voted for, however extensive the just and beneficial changes it makes to abortion's permissibility; what *EV* 73.3 so prominently makes (conditionally) decisive – namely, the fact that the amending law is *more* restrictive – is irrelevant. One is unlikely to come across a reading of *EV* 73 more misguided than Harte's.

Drawing a distinction which he admitted was unheard of "in any of the literature on the subject of abortion law reform", between *primary* and *secondary* abortion legislation, and a further, entirely unexplained distinction between "codified" and "UK-type non-codified" systems of law, Harte's 2001/2 paper "Challenging a Consensus..." claimed that in a UK-type system of law only one of the "four general ways in which one might attempt to limit abortion" is morally permissible: namely, "by enacting separate *secondary legislation* (i.e. legislation which is not an Abortion [Act] Amendment Bill)."[22] Harte's first of two examples of permissible secondary legislation was "Doctors have a right not to be involved in abortion procedures" – but it would never (he said) be permissible to vote for "Doctors have a right to decide whether or not to be involved in abortion procedures". For even "even though [this second measure] would have the same practical effect" as the first – indeed, it would have an identical impact on the juridical *content* and *effect* of the state's laws – it is, said Harte, a measure "predicated on the licitness of abortion, and can be judged to be [Harte meant: is] intrinsically unjust." His other example concerned funding: a measure stating that "Public money may not be used to fund abortions" is acceptable, but

---

[21] Thus Harte says (*ibid.*, emphases adjusted): "The key consideration is that the justness of any Amendment Act [for amending an Act like the Abortion Act in a UK-type non-codified system] is determined by judging the justness of the original act to which it refers, *as amended* by the Amendment Act. *If some abortions will still be permitted* or tolerated under the terms of a previous Abortion Act *after the enactment of an Amendment Bill*, the Amendment Bill can be judged to be intrinsically unjust..."

[22] Harte further specifies his notion of acceptable "secondary" legislation: not only is it not "predicated on the legality of abortion" (e.g. by being included in the statute permitting abortion) but it is itself "predicated on other rights and duties" (e.g. of doctors not to have to violate their own integrity). This too ignores *EV* 73.3's clear indication that the kinds of reforming legislation which it is legitimate to support are "not rare" and involve an attempt to limit not simply "the harm done by" the "pro-abortion law", and its "negative consequences at the level of public opinion and public morality", but also that law's own "evil aspects".

"Abortions can take place provided they are not funded by public money"[23] is intrinsically unjust.

The criteria and concepts used in Harte's paper to distinguish between what is and is not intrinsically unjust are foreign to *EV 73*; they cannot be found in, or legitimately imposed upon, the encyclical. *EV*'s criteria and concepts, being dynamic and comparative, concern (a) the bill's or new law's own aim (not simply the aims of any who promote or vote for it), and (b) the juridical circumstances or context (the permissiveness of the existing or otherwise imminent law, and the impossibility of overturning or completely abrogating it). The encyclical's judgment on this whole issue, like the course of episcopal statements it implicitly confirms, makes no use of non-dynamic, non-comparative concepts like "predicated on the licitness of abortion".[24] It is not interested in verbal distinctions of the kind that interest Harte,[25] distinctions that make no difference whatever to the propositional content of the state's law. It plainly rejects Harte's claim that a measure (bill/statute) is intrinsically unjust and cannot be voted for if, though itself "aimed at limiting the number of authorised abortions" and making the law "more restrictive" so as "to limit its [*that pro-abortion law's*] evil *aspects*", it would leave some abortions unprohibited.[26] Rejecting that kind of claim is indeed the obvious overriding purpose, intent and gist of *EV 73.3*.

---

[23] Remember, this is supposed to be "secondary legislation", in the context of "primary" legislation permitting abortion. So the phrase "Abortions can take place" would have no impact whatever on the juridical content of the state's laws, and the juridical as well as practical meaning and effect of Harte's two provisions about funding would be identical. In the realistic perspective adopted by *EV 73*, it is absurd to say that one is intrinsically immoral but the other not. (Neither of them is.)

[24] The 1974 Declaration's ambiguous phrase (sec. 22), "a law which would admit in principle the liceity of abortion" may have a comparative sense ("admit", meaning introduce), but in any event finds no counterpart in *EV 73.2/3*, a judgment made with the benefit of 20 more years of discussion.

[25] Harte, sec. 1, claims that it matters that my 24 to 16 week hypothetical might have been in the form "In Act X ... replace '24' with '16'" *or* in the form "Act X is repealed. Abortion is permissible up to 16 weeks and prohibited after 16 weeks." But of course it turns out that even on his own view these formalistic distinctions make no difference whatever to the (im)moral character of this sort of bill/statute. The first formula approximates to his Proposal G, the second to his Proposal C, both of which he claims are "obviously" intrinsically unjust.

[26] Harte (fn. 6) says that the opinion of William May (who was party to discussions with the CDF in relation to the drafting of *EV 73.3*) that the Pope clearly has taught [in *EV 73.3*] that legislators may vote for restrictive abortion legislation is "merely an 'interpretation'." Harte then says that "one cannot reasonably say that *EV 73* supports something 'clearly' when it is open to contradictory interpretations," and that May's interpretation of *EV 73* is open to contradictory interpretations because he, Harte, has challenged it. But *contradictory interpretations B, C... only cast a shadow on the clarity and correctness of interpretation A if they are reasonable.* Harte's interpretation of *EV 73* is not.

4. Codification, verbal separation, and use of the word "permitted" make no difference to intrinsic (in)justice

In his new paper Harte offers some examples of restrictive abortion legislation that would not, he says, be intrinsically unjust. They are all examples from a code in an imaginary country Littalia whose "laws are codified" and whose code, improbably enough, itemises each and every element of its extensive permission of abortion in separate numbered articles. Each article can be repealed by itself, without mentioning or tinkering with the others, and such a repeal, says Harte, is not intrinsically unjust even though it leaves undisturbed the other articles. (His examples of this are called Proposals D, E, and F.) But, he insists, any amendment to an *article* which leaves that article incompletely prohibitive, albeit more prohibitive, is intrinsically unjust because, even if the amending bill/statute does not mention permission, it "must be understood as ratifying and continuing some (though not all) of the permission that was previously included in the article."[27] Thus he sets himself against the approval given by the Italian bishops, and implicitly by the Holy See, to the 1981 pro-life referendum proposal to *amend* art. 6 of Italy's abortion law by repealing some but not all of that article's permissive phrases.[28]

Here we get close to the core of Harte's confusions about the nature of a law. A law is a "proposition of practical reason",[29] that is, a

---

[27] See sec. 3.1 in relation to "Proposal G".

[28] The pro-life referendum would have repealed art. 4 which extensively permits abortion during the first 90 days, and then would have repealed in art. 6 the phrases here italicised: "6. L'interruzione volontaria della gravidanza, *dopo i primi novanta giorni*, può essere praticata: (a) quando la gravidanza o il parto comportino un grave pericolo per la vita della donna; (b) quando siano accertati processi patologici, *tra cui quelli relativi e rilevanti anomalie o malformazioni del nascituro*, che determinano un grave pericolo per la salute fisica *o psichica* della donna." Those "remaining elements" of Italy's abortion law which are said by the Italian Bishops' Conference to be *not* morally licit can only be found *in art. 6 itself*, as amended.

[29] Aquinas, on the first page of his classic discussion of *lex* (law), states that laws are essentially "*propositiones* universales rationis practicae ordinatae ad actiones", universal propositions of practical reason directed to actions: *Summa Theologiae* I-II q. 90 a. 1 ad 2. "Universal" here is used in the logician's sense, to signify the picking out of a *kind* of action, however specific that kind (short of the pure particularity of e.g. a command directed to a single person, to do or abstain from a particular act on a particular occasion). As Aquinas goes on to say, a law "is simply a prescription of practical reason *in the ruler* governing a complete community" [and not, essentially, in statute-books or other documents, even though promulgation is essential to its validity]: I-II q. 91 a. 1c; also q. 92 a. 1c; both passages looking back to q. 90 a. 1 ad 2.

proposition[30] that by being (legally) true/valid is ready to direct and change the course of a subject's practical reasoning and deliberation towards choice and action. The state's law is the whole set of such propositions. No enactment or other pronouncement has juridical relevance unless it *introduces* into that set some proposition(s) not formerly part of the set, or *prevents* the elimination of some proposition which would otherwise have ceased to be part of the set, or *eliminates* from the set some proposition(s) formerly part of it. The concept of "ratification" has no juridical relevance except in special contexts where the very existence of a rule of law is in doubt (e.g. because of uncertainty about whether proper procedures were followed in enacting it). Except in such special contexts, a statute "ratifying" another statute *does nothing* juridically. That is, it leaves the state's law exactly as it was; the set of propositions of law (legally) applicable in that community remains unaffected. Ratification's only meaning and significance (the special contexts aside) are social – e.g. pedagogical and other effects on public opinion, party morale, and so forth. These effects are important, and alleviating them is one concern of restrictive reforms of the kind of approved by *EV* 73.3. But they are not the concern of the principle in *EV* 73.2.

The same must be said of Harte's notion that an amending statute which says "In article 91 replace '16 [weeks]' by '8 [weeks]'" *continues* (while restricting) the article's unjust permission. The truth is that the amending statute, in such a case, *does nothing* except prohibit abortion from the 8th week onwards. The amending statute introduces into the state's law the new proposition that abortion is prohibited between 8 and 16 weeks, to supplement the already (legally) true proposition that abortion is prohibited from 16 weeks to the end of pregnancy. The already existing proposition that abortion is permitted up to 8 weeks remains (legally) true. It continues to be

---

[30] As I use the terms "proposition" and "statement", one and the same proposition can be expressed in many different statements (e.g. in different languages), and one and the same statement can (where the statement is ambiguous) convey/express/mean and, if it is assertorically uttered, assert two or more propositions. This distinction is of vital importance to sound theology and sound legal thinking, but of course it too can be expressed in different language. When Aquinas says that law is *in* the practical reason and is a proposition of practical reason, he is certainly using the term *propositio* in the same way, to signify something that obtains at the level of understood meaning rather than at the level of text, word, expression, and so forth. And he clearly has in mind a position such as I am deploying in this paper: a *proposition of law* may be true even though there is no statement in the lawbooks which expresses or states it; the daily task of the law-student, legal practitioner, and judge is to reach a sound judgment about what proposition of law is (legally) true, in relation to a given problem, in the light of *all the sources of law*, including all relevant statements in applicable codes or statutes, understood in the light of other statutes, authoritative court decisions, professional and other customs and conventions, etc.

(legally) true, but not because of the amending statute. Juridically, the amending statute does *not* continue the existing permission. "Continue" has a juridical meaning and relevance if, and only if, some proposition of law *would cease* to be true *but for* the effect of the statute that continues it. And that is not the case in Harte's imaginary Proposal G.

Harte's confusion is this. He treats words and statements (e.g. in an amending statute) as identical with or equivalent to propositions. So he might object to what I say in the previous paragraph along the following lines. Before the amending statute there was, he might object, no proposition of law, *no law*, that abortion is permitted up to 8 weeks; the only relevant proposition was in article 91, namely that abortion is permitted up to 16 weeks. To which I would reply that the statements in article 91 and the other articles of the code are one thing and the relevant propositions of law are another. What every law student learns, and is second nature to every judge and lawyer, is that the law on a subject-matter is not what is stated in some relevant statute or code but rather, what is stated in the relevant code or statute *interpreted* or understood in the light of all relevant legal principles, written and unwritten, and all other relevant provisions of codes and statutes and the opinions of judges and other learned authorities. And every law student also comes to understand that there are as many true propositions of law as there are legally answerable questions that might be raised about the subject-matter. The following are at all relevant times (legally) true propositions of law in Harte's imaginary state Littalia: "Abortion is lawful at ten days", "Abortion is lawful at seven weeks", and so on, indefinitely (within the bounds established by the prohibition at 16 weeks).

Every competent lawyer, whether in a "codified" system or a "UK-type" (partially) uncodified system, understands the state's law as a vast sea of (legally) true propositions: "Abortion is permitted at 10 days", "Abortion is permitted at 12 days", "Abortion is permitted at seven weeks", "Abortion is permitted at eight weeks", "Abortion is permitted at 15 weeks", "Abortion is permitted at 16 weeks", "Abortion is prohibited at 17 weeks", and so forth.[31] Every competent lawyer understands that it is, legally/juridically, entirely irrelevant whether you amend this set (i) by assigning arbitrary numbers to the propositions making abortion non-prohibited (or affirming

---

[31] Despite their relative specificity, these are all "universal propositions" within the meaning of Aquinas's essential characterisation of a law as a universal proposition of practical reason. So they are all rules. This is not to say that there is much of importance in the distinction between, on the one hand, relatively specific universals (= rules) and, on the other hand, propositions about particulars (= applications of rules in particular propositions such as that Jane's abortion of her baby this week is/was/would be lawful/unlawful).

its permissibility) between 8 and 16 weeks and then declaring that all the propositions so numbered are hereby repealed, or (ii) by enacting that abortion is prohibited from 8 weeks on, or (iii) by enacting that in the code or statute permitting abortions "16" shall be replaced by "8"... And so forth – there are many other ways of making one and the same change in the law, and for each way many different form(ulation)s. Harte claims that amendments in forms (ii) and (iii) are intrinsically unjust, but form (i) corresponds essentially to his imaginary list of Littalia code articles 90–98 and his technique of repealing articles 92–96 and so, on his view, will not be intrinsically unjust.

If the Catholic Church and other reasonable people who support the right to life were to propose or defend such a distinction, they would be the object of ridicule, and the ridicule would be entirely justified. The whole matter is too serious to turn on distinctions which are, like Harte's, purely verbal or formalistic, in the worst sense – unhinged from reality and the relevant truths about a state's law.[32] Harte's focus is upon what bills and statutes *say*, rather than on whether those bills and statutes *make* (legally) true any (and if so which) proposition(s) of law not already true independently of them.[33] This focus results in a series of distinctions unknown to *EV* 73 and devoid of moral significance: for example, between codified and uncodified systems, between repealing a statute (but substituting an only partially changed alternative) and amending it (= partially repealing it), and between

---

[32] Harte's confusion – between (i) words and statements and (ii) the propositions that are conveyed by those words and statements when properly understood in the light of all other relevant words, statements and propositions – is closely analogous to the confusion involved in fundamentalist, e.g. early Protestant, biblical interpretation. Catholic faith and theology hold that every statement in the text of the Bible must be understood in the light not only of the language and idiom and thought-forms of the sacred writer (which both determine the range of propositions that might be expressed by that statement and indicate whether it is possible that one of these propositions is being not merely entertained but actually asserted by the writer), but also of all the other statements of that writer and of the other writers in all the books of the canon. Any theologian who fails to distinguish clearly between words/statements/expressions and the proposition(s) conveyed and perhaps asserted by them is doomed to misunderstand not only the Bible but also the magisterial teachings of the Church, in which, as both Vatican I (implicitly) and Vatican II (explicitly) explain, the "mode" in which truths of doctrine are "enunciated" is one thing and the truths themselves, their meaning as propositions asserted by the Church, are another thing. See e.g. Vatican II, *Gaudium et Spes* 62; Finnis, *Moral Absolutes*. Washington DC: Catholic University of America Press 1991: 7 n. 16; Finnis, "Saint Thomas More and the Crisis in Faith and Morals". 7/1 (2003) *The Priest*: 10 at 14–15.

[33] Or, of course, on whether the statute will *prevent* the ceasing to be true of some proposition of law which would otherwise cease to be true.

226

statutes that (supposedly) do and statutes that don't constitute "the whole abortion law" of the state.

In insisting that many of his imaginary abortion statutes constitute "the whole law of the state," Harte reveals his general misunderstanding not only of what laws are, but also of what is meant by "a law permitting" as that phrase is used in *EV* 73.2. No statute, indeed no code, could constitute the whole of a state's law on abortion (or any other topic). The law on any topic or issue is the proposition about that topic that is made legally true by the interaction of relevant statutory provisions with constitutional and other statutory provisions, with judgements of high courts, and with the general principles of law presupposed by all juristic thought. Among these general principles are: What is not prohibited is permitted, and What is permitted is a legal right unless, though not criminally or civilly prohibited, it (as English lawyers would say) is "contrary to [a judicially cognisable] public policy."[34] *Permission is the default position.* This is not a matter of logic[35] but of one of the "general principles of law recognised by civilized nations."[36] Trying to create a legal permission is redundant and futile (juridically, but perhaps not politically) unless the matter in issue is already prohibited or contrary to a legally recognised "public policy". At least in the eyes of the law, prohibitions exist like artificial islands in a boundless ocean of permission. In any modern state the default to permission is greatly strengthened, in the case of abortion, by constitutional principles protecting and enforcing the right to bodily or personal security, the right to privacy, equal protection of women, and so forth. Harte's repeated assumption that a short code or statute could comprise "the whole of a country's abortion law" is naive.[37]

In Littalia's "code" an article is amended by replacing "16" with "8". In my 1994/6 hypothetical case a statutory provision "Abortion is permitted up to

---

[34] Harte is right to hold that in relation to a matter of fundamental rights like abortion, any distinction between legal permission and legal toleration is beside the point. The point is taken for granted in my discussion, and in *EV* 73, though it may have been obscured somewhat in the CDF's Declaration of 1974, with deleterious effects on the decisions of the (West) German Constitutional Court thereafter.

[35] Logic is open to Aristotle's position that the default position is prohibition.

[36] I use the phrase used in the Statute of the International Court of Justice, art. 38, to pick out one of the principal elements in law, alongside law established by those instruments that establish laws (in the international context conventions, in the sense of agreements or treaties; in the intra-state context statutes and other enactments) and law existing by virtue of custom. See more generally Finnis, *Natural Law and Natural Rights*. Oxford: Oxford University Press 1980: 286–9.

[37] And this assumption is an essential premise for his central assertion (sec. 3.3) that "It is not possible to claim, without abandoning reason, that a vote for any one of the Proposals A or B or C is not a vote for an intrinsically unjust law."

24 weeks [and prohibited thereafter]" is amended (or repealed and substituted for) so as to read "Abortion is permitted up to 16 weeks [and prohibited thereafter]". It makes no difference. The effect of the change (repeal, partial repeal, amendment – draft the change as you please and call it what you will) is the same. A set of propositions (indefinite in number but bounded in meaning and effect) affirming abortion's legal permissibility cease to be (legally) true, and a new set of propositions *become* (are *made to be*) legally true, prohibiting abortion. The words of the amending statute(s) speak of permitting abortions up to 8 or 16 weeks, but their legal effect on the permissibility of abortion up to that point in gestation is nil. So Harte's line of argument entails that, except in the exotic and unheard-of case of a statute (he mysteriously insists, a "code") which conveniently frames a set of complete one-by-one permissions repealable one-by-one, all abortion statutes which are not completely prohibitive are intrinsically unjust and no reforming abortion statute can ever under any circumstances be voted for in a decisive ballot. *All or nothing* is the essence of his position.

EV 73's position is radically and rightly different. Statutes creating prohibitions which otherwise would not exist are just (in the sense of: not intrinsically unjust) in all that they juridically do.[38] What they juridically do or effect is make true a set of propositions of law, indefinite in number but bounded in meaning and effect. *Every* proposition of law that these amending or partially repealing statutes bring into being or make true is *nothing but prohibitive*. The state's law remains unjust to the extent that its permission of certain abortions remains in place and legally true. But that is not the result of anything in the amending statute. Appearances are misleading.

Harte says it is "self-evident" that legislators cannot rightly vote for a reforming bill which replaces a law permitting abortion up to 24 weeks with a law permitting it up to 16 weeks (or six weeks, or two weeks, or two days). For, he says, all such proposals "specifically 'permit' abortion." He is right to put the word *permit* in quotation marks. He is quoting the very wording of (one version of) such bills/statutes. But, as the Roman law *Digest* observes at its outset (I, 3, 17), "Knowing the law is not a matter of clinging to the wording [*verba*] of laws but of understanding their force and impact [*vim et potestatem*]" – what I have been calling their legal or juridical meaning and effect (logically prior to and distinct from any empirical effect they may have on the human behaviour they address). *The*

---

[38] There is a special kind of case where this is not so; I consider it near the end of sec. 6 below.

fact that a statute says that abortion is permitted does not entail that that is the statute's juridical effect. And in fact – that is, in legal truth – the reforming statute's only effect is prohibitive. So far from it being self-evident that the statute *permits*, i.e. makes permitted, some abortions, it is juridically and strictly speaking not true that a reforming statute of the kind just described permits any abortion, even one. What Harte thought self-evidently true is in legal reality false.

It is such legal realities that are the concern of *EV* 73. And, as it happens, there is an important element in *EV* 73.3 which makes doubly clear the Pope's indifference to all appearances and appearance-based distinctions of the kind that Harte relies upon. This element concerns the baseline against which any bill or amending statute is to be compared when assessing whether the amendment (or partial repeal) is permissive (and thus intrinsically unjust), or prohibitive and thus capable of being voted for by a Catholic or other pro-life legislator. In my own writings prepared for presentation in the Vatican during the preparation of *EV* 73, I treated the baseline as the law in force at the time of the putting of the proposal (bill) to the decisive vote. But the Pope takes the robustly common-sense approach that for the essential and crucial comparison there can also be another baseline, namely, the law that *will* be in force, not in some speculative future, but imminently – paradigmatically, I suppose, "tomorrow" – if the pro-life restrictive bill is not enacted. For, according to *EV* 73.3, the baseline may be "a ... law already passed" *or* " [a ... law [technically a bill]] *ready to be voted on.*" If this baseline law (legal position), already in force *or* virtually certain to be in force unless defeated by a pro-life alternative, is more permissive than that pro-life alternative, then the latter should be regarded, not as introducing into the state's law permissions, but rather as making valid certain prohibitions which would otherwise have been absent from the law tomorrow. As prohibitive, it is essentially just. True, it is conspicuously permissive by comparison with the old law. But the old law is no longer a relevant baseline for comparison; in situations of the kind the Pope is here considering the old law is doomed and practically speaking defunct. If the pro-life bill under consideration is not enacted, the state's law will tomorrow be completely or highly permissive. So: enacting the pro-life bill/statute introduces into the law certain propositions which tomorrow would have been excluded from the law, propositions each of which prohibits what would otherwise, tomorrow, have ceased to be prohibited. Despite the incompleteness of its prohibitions, the pro-life bill/statute is thus not a "permissive law" within the true meaning of *EV* 73.2's principle that one must never vote for a permissive law.

In short, not every statute that declares some abortions permitted is a permissive law in the sense intended by *EV* 73.2. For some such statutes permit – *make permitted* – nothing, but simply and exclusively prohibit.[39] And this is apparent not only as a matter of legal technicality. It is the common-sense of the matter.

5. The answer to Harte's challenge, and some causes of his mistakes

Harte's new paper sketches a number of hypothetical pro-life proposals and issues a challenge: Tell us first, he urges, whether these proposals – and the statutes they would enact – are just or unjust. Meanwhile he presses upon us his own answer: the intrinsic injustice of [these proposals] is self-evident, and cannot be denied without "abandoning reason" and "making an obviously incorrect factual judgment." My answer by now is clear. For the reasons I have indicated, proposals such as extending the prohibition of abortion from the 24th to the 16th week are not intrinsically unjust, and the statute or law they enact is not intrinsically unjust.[40] Indeed, in many

---

[39] In Harte's notation: in these cases, X2 (the reforming bill) and Y2 (the reforming statute), which both *say* that abortion is permitted up to 16 weeks (or that it is prohibited only up to 16 weeks, or that "16" is substituted for "24" – the differences of formulation don't matter) are not the cause of Z2, the (legally) true proposition of law that abortion is permitted up to 16 weeks. Despite their wording, X2 and Y2 permit nothing, but prohibit abortions from 16 to 24 weeks. They withdraw no part of the state's legal protection of unborn babies, they simply extend it. For the special case where some part of such a reforming bill diminishes that protection, see sec. 6 below.

[40] Proposal A is in substance the Polish law of 1992, enacted against the baseline of virtually complete permission; some permissions continue (*not*: are *given* continuing effect! What is already possessed by X cannot be given to X.). Proposal B is just (more precisely: not intrinsically unjust) compared with the baseline of existing law permitting abortion in any situation prior to the 24th week. Proposal B prohibits *all* abortions, from conception onwards, subject to only one exception where abortion is to remain permitted up to the 24th week. Pro-lifers should of course denounce the exception – an anti-Semitic one – as grossly unjust and vile. A refusal to prohibit motivated by racist contempt for some unborn babies may well be morally worse than a refusal to prohibit based on some muddled "balancing of interests" or some notion that life with handicap is not worth living. But in neither case are the pro-life legislators refusing to prohibit. It is their racist and/or muddled colleagues who are insisting that the final condition of the country's laws retain this exception to the just prohibition of abortion. If, in the alternative, the existing law is doomed and for practical purposes irrelevant, then Proposal B must be measured against Proposal C, which permits abortion in all cases (including Jewish babies) up to 16 weeks. As Harte's figures emphasise, it is reasonable to regard B as more restrictive than C, and thus as a proposal which in the circumstances is not intrinsically unjust, even though the final state of the country's law will, of course, remain grossly unjust because of the deadly combination of (a) the axiom that what is not prohibited is permitted with (b) the wicked refusal of some legislators to cooperate with pro-life/anti-racist legislators in prohibiting all abortions. In both cases Harte's

circumstances a statute of this kind is entirely just. Even though it does not do all that justice requires – completely prohibit abortion – everything it does is just.[41]

How did Harte come to think "obviously" and even "self-evidently" true what is in fact false? What mistakes induced this illusion? Some of them have already emerged, particularly his confusion between *statements* and *propositions*, and so between the law as the set of statements in documents such as bills and statute-books, and the law as the set of propositions (legally) true at a certain moment given all the legally relevant materials (such as statutes, judgments, and accepted assumptions and principles of law). This cluster of mistakes generates others, such as the insistence that "the whole of a country's abortion law" can be found in a single statute. Another related mistake of Harte's is his failure to keep in mind that prohibition and permission are not symmetrical, for the law's default position is always permission, never prohibition. This mistake leads, for example, to the incoherence that

---

notion that the proposed bill and statute will "be the whole abortion law" is the mistaken product of his thoroughgoing confusion between "the law" as what can be read in a book and the real law, the whole set of (legally) true propositions relevant to a subject-matter. And, for essentially the same reason, Harte's insinuation that it makes a difference that the proposals begin by repealing the old law (Abortion Act R) is completely mistaken. Abortion Act R is in substance completely permissive. And, in itself, the repeal of Act R leaves the law completely permissive. So the baseline for comparison in assessing the justice of (say) B is essentially the same, whether B begins by repealing R or is drafted as an amendment to R. Finally there is proposal G, to substitute 8 for 16 in Harte's Littalian code article 91. This too is not intrinsically unjust. The refusal of other legislators to substitute "0" for "16" is intrinsically unjust. The final state of Littalia's law is unjust. But the permission of abortion up to 8 weeks is not the result of article 91, whose whole juridical meaning is to prohibit abortion. The permission of abortion up to 8 weeks is the result of the axiom that what is not prohibited is permitted, enhanced (if need be) by other articles of the code or written or unwritten constitution and law of Littalia guaranteeing rights of liberty, privacy, bodily security, and so forth. Harte's formulation of G's *juridical* meaning is false insofar as (by the words "so that . . .") it insinuates that the permission of abortion up to 8 weeks is truly the juridical *effect* of article 91. The fact that Harte's Littalia's article 90 prohibits abortion "except where it is specifically permitted" does not affect the fundamental juridical position. The juridical position would be exactly the same if (i) article 90 instead said "abortion is prohibited except where it is described in an article of this code as a 'specified case'", (ii) old article 91 said "abortion up to 16 weeks is a specified case", and (iii) Proposal B's article 91 says "replace '16' by '8'." The whole juridical meaning of Proposal B, and of the amended article 91, is that article 90's *prohibition* is extended to protect babies from 8 weeks on. The permission of abortions up to 8 weeks comes, essentially, not from Harte's article 90's words "is specifically permitted" in combination with article 91, but rather, as I have said, from other liberty-favouring provisions, written and unwritten, of Littalia's law.

[41] But see fn. 4 above.

becomes evident when he claims that "A proposal to repeal an intrinsically unjust law can never... be intrinsically unjust." This claim is false if Harte's general thesis is true, namely his thesis that a statute which states that some abortions are permitted is an intrinsically unjust law. For simple repeal of a statute prohibiting abortion only after 24 weeks will leave the state with *no prohibition of any abortion at all* – a law intrinsically even more unjust. Such a repeal will be an intrinsically unjust measure. A real-life instance of such unjust action is the Canadian Supreme Court's invalidation of the Canadian abortion statute which had a few years earlier been unjustly amended so as to permit a wide range of abortions. This invalidation – in substance though not in form a repeal – has left Canada with a law on abortion which is certainly intrinsically unjust but can be given alternative descriptions, each of them correct and, despite appearances, consistent with the other: "no law at all", or: "a completely permissive law".[42] Harte's claim about repeal could only be true if the position proposed in *EV* 73.3 and defended in this paper is true, the position that to identify intrinsic injustice in a bill or statute about abortion one must ask what (if anything) it prohibits[43] and compare the extent of that prohibition with the extent of the prohibition (if any) which is in force or otherwise will tomorrow be in force.

But two other important mistakes have yet to be mentioned. The first is the assumption that "intrinsically unjust" means unjust regardless of context and circumstances, and intentions of any acting person. This is one of the central mainstays of Harte's whole position,[44] and it is thoroughly mistaken. In the case of intrinsically wrongful kinds of action, "intrinsically" means independently of context, circumstances and intentions *other than those circumstances and intentions* which are part of the "object" or "matter" by

---

[42] The fact that each of these *verbally* contradictory descriptions is correct should have warned Harte that simple theorems such as "if a law is intrinsically unjust you can never vote for it" need very careful handling – as *EV* 73.3 warned readers of 73.2.

[43] More precisely: one must ask what prohibiting propositions of law it makes (legally) true.

[44] Thus Harte sec. 3.3: "Whether or not the proposal is just does not depend on the circumstances of whether it is increasing permission from, say, 6 weeks or reducing permission from, say, 16 weeks. The view that the justness of this sort of proposal depends on the context or circumstances fails, fundamentally, to take into account what is meant by the concept of an *intrinsically* unjust law." And again, in sec. 5.3, he says: "... Finnis distorts the teaching that legislation cannot be supported because it is, objectively, in and of itself, always unacceptable, i.e. intrinsically unjust. He presents his own version of 'the always illicit vote', a version which appears to argue that the licitness of voting for legislation depends upon the context and one's reasons for doing so." Here Harte spectacularly overlooks the fact that every sentence and phrase in *EV* 73.3 "argues that the licitness of voting for legislation depends upon the context [comparison with existing or imminent law] and one's reasons for doing so."

reference to which this kind of action is identifiable (defined) as always wrong. So: all Catholic theologians have taught (and *EV* 75 recalls) that theft is intrinsically unjust, but theft is highly contextual and intention-relative: it is only those takings of another's property which are carried out without urgent necessity, and without a claim to be entitled to this property, and without a belief that the owner would consent, and so forth. Similarly, rape is intercourse in circumstances where one person is not consenting and the acting person lacks a belief that the other is consenting. No definition of lying is sound unless it includes the speaker's intent to assert, not merely state, a proposition, and his belief that what he is asserting is false. *Humanae Vitae*'s definition of wrongful contraception is in terms of the acting person's intention.[45] And so forth. So, similarly, it is one of the evident purposes of *EV* 73.3 to make clear that a statute or other law-making statement does not fall within the class of "intrinsically unjust" laws mentioned in *EV* 73.2 unless the legal and legislative context or circumstances are such that it *renders* (makes) non-prohibited what was or would otherwise tomorrow have been prohibited. These are matters of context and circumstance and intention ("aim") that enter into the very meaning of "permissive" as that term is used in *EV* 73.2 to identify a class of intrinsically unjust laws.

The second important mistake not yet mentioned is Harte's assumption that it makes no difference whether the legislator whose action we are considering is a member of a group (a legislature, a court, a referendum electorate...) or is a *sole ruler* with authority to make whatever law(s) he or she chooses.[46] But the difference is important in understanding the very

---

[45] Encyclical *Humanae Vitae* (1968), sec. 14: "any action which before, at the moment of, or after marital intercourse, is specifically intended – whether as an end or as a means – to impede procreation" {quivis ... *actus, qui*, cum coniugale commercium vel praevi-detur vel efficitur vel ad suos naturales exitus ducit, *id tamquam finem obtinendum aut viam adhibendam intendat, ut procreatio impediatur*}.

[46] Thus Harte sec. 1: "we are looking at the vote by which the law-maker – whether it be an individual with sole law-making authority, or a legislator in a parliament, or a citizen entitled to vote in a legally binding popular referendum ... expresses his or her will that a specific proposal (the bill for a law) be enacted as law." And sec. 5.2: "Whether lawmaking power is invested solely in a single person (say, a King), or in several hundred members of a legislature, or in the entire citizenship voting in referenda, those with that lawmaking power are 'making law'. ... Each lawmaker's act of voting represents what is willed. ... The will of the legislature in enacting legislation is indistinguishable from the will of the legislator voting for the enactment. What the legislature 'does' (in willing that certain permissions, tolerations, prohibitions, etc be enacted as law) is indistinguishable from what an individual legislator 'does' (in willing that the proposal with those very permissions, tolerations, prohibitions, etc. be enacted)."

meaning of a proposal to restrict abortion. In the case of a sole ruler who has the opportunity to choose what propositions of law shall be (legally) true in relation to abortion, the ruler's proposal to restrict abortions but not completely prohibit them is a choice that here prohibition shall end and permission shall begin. It cannot fail to be the expression of the unjust judgment that unborn children of a certain immaturity, or race, or condition of handicap are not entitled to the protection of the law. But in the case of statutes enacted by a group legislature, the very same bill and statute can be proposed and supported without making any such judgment.

This can be understood by reference to an analogy. Suppose a group of 20 stalwarts travelling in a desert region come upon a fortified camp. Observing it from outside its fence they discover that inside are hundreds of children being tortured to death, one by one, by the camp's evil guards. The group outside have no competing responsibilities capable of affecting their obvious responsibility to rescue the children if they can. And (they judge) they can, provided that *all 20* cooperate in a coordinated assault on the camp while the guards are mostly asleep. All but five of the group are determined to rescue every child. But those five insist that they are not willing to participate in the rescue, and indeed will positively block the rescue of any children at all, unless children of a race that (they say) persecuted the five's forebears are left behind; there are three such children, and they are the occupants of hut P. The fifteen protest at this unjust limitation on the rescue, but to no avail. The recalcitrant five veto all plans that include hut P. Reluctantly, but with all necessary vigour, the fifteen then carry out a rescue, acting together with the discriminatory five whose assistance proves to be as vital as was anticipated. Hundreds of children are rescued, but the five discriminatory rescuers block every attempt to go beyond the plan and liberate hut P.

The willingness of the fifteen non-discriminatory rescuers to carry out the rescue in no way expresses a judgment that the three children in hut P were not as fully entitled as the others to be rescued. That unjust judgment is made by the small minority of rescuers, whose judgments and willingness overlap and converge with but partially differ radically from the just judgments and will of the majority. The resultant "consensus" plan and rescue itself can be described as a group act, and that group act can be described as unjust – indeed, intrinsically unjust – insofar as from the outset it excluded three rescuable children. But more accurately the event can be described as two converging and overlapping but partially diverging group acts. One is the plan and act of the fifteen just rescuers. The other is the plan and act of the five unjust rescuers (whose act includes manifesting readiness to block any attempt by the fifteen to rescue the last three children). The accurate description of the fifteen's group plan and act is: "an attempt to rescue *every child* that it is within our power to rescue". That is a completely just kind of choice and act. The accurate description of the group act of the five is: "an attempt to rescue all the children within our power except three whom we choose to leave to certain death and to prevent others from rescuing." That is an unjust plan and act. The appearance of consensus and of a single group act is quite deceptive.

Harte, here as elsewhere in the toils of a fragile linguistic and legal positivism, insists that when a restrictive abortion law is enacted there is just one group act, "the act of the legislature".[47] That is a common way of talking which, though widely sensed to be something of a fiction, is accurate enough for many practical purposes. But it ceases to be accurate, or even reasonable, in the kind of context, and in relation to the kind of question, that we are considering. There should be no need to labour through a statement of the detailed applicability of the desert rescue analogy to situations of the kind dealt with in *EV* 73.2/3 and the present debate. Suffice it to say that if the fifteen were capable of carrying out the rescue without the cooperation of the five, their position would be like that of a single law-maker with sovereign powers (unshackled by any court or constitution), or like that of a *fully united controlling majority* in a legislature with authority to make what law "it chooses" in relation to abortion. And that is simply not the kind of situation under discussion.

It is not irrelevant to bear in mind the effect of Harte's mistakes. With a few ungrounded exceptions (based on his unsound notion of codification), he rules out any and every attempt to rescue the unborn through law unless all are to be rescued,[48] even though the limitations on the rescue result entirely from the unjust will of a sub-group within the larger group willing and able to mount a rescue, a sub-group who block the efforts of the pro-life sub-group who are willing and ready and *otherwise* able to rescue all. Confronted by a law which excludes from the law's prohibition of murder all persons under three or over 70, Harte's position evidently is that it is intrinsically wrong to vote for a bill which in its final form would extend the prohibition to those over 70 (but which says nothing about those under three), even though the bill as drafted and moved by its sincere pro-life promoters would have prohibited *all* murders by cancelling *both* of the vicious existing exclusion clauses, and even though it is clear that there will be no future opportunity to extend to those over 70 (let alone those under three) the protection of the law to which they (like those under three) are urgently entitled. To hold these views, in the face of *EV* 73.3 and all the episcopal and pro-life pastoral and

---

[47] See Harte sec. 5.2, immediately after the passage quoted in fn. 46 above.
[48] By condemning his hypothetical Proposal B as intrinsically unjust, he accepts that the 197,000 whom it would rescue must be left to die with the 3,000 whom – through no fault or omission of pro-lifers – it would fail to rescue.

political practice tacitly confirmed in *EV* 73.3, one would need grounds vastly more secure than Harte's.[49]

6. Intention is important but is not the primary issue in this debate

In my previous treatments of this whole issue I too failed to analyse it with all the precision that it calls for. As a result, my earlier discussions gave too much prominence to the distinction between intention and side-effect, and too little attention to the ambiguities in the phrase "unjust law" and "permissive law", ambiguities which the foregoing sections of the present paper try to bring to light.

Since my principal earlier treatment, written for the CDF's conference preparatory to *EV* 73.3, has been imprecisely reported and discussed by Harte and others, I shall quote its main passage at some length:

> The question *what* one is choosing to support (or not support, or oppose) is also conditioned by context, namely by the existing legal situation. For example: a *law* of the form 'Abortion is lawful up to 16 weeks' is an unjust law. But a *bill* of the form 'Abortion is lawful up to 16 weeks' might either (i) be proposed precisely as introducing a permission of abortions hitherto prohibited, or (ii) be proposed precisely as prohibiting abortions hitherto permitted between 16 and 24 weeks. The choice to support the bill in situation (i) is a substantially different choice from the choice to support the bill in situation (ii). For what is being chosen – the object of the act of supporting the bill – is different in the two cases. In case (i) it is supporting the permission of abortion. In case (ii) it is supporting the prohibition of abortions, indeed of all the abortions (let us suppose) that legislator at that moment has the opportunity of effectively helping to prohibit.
>
> To say this is not to embrace 'situation ethics' or proportionalism or any other theory which denies that there are intrinsically evil acts incapable of being justified by circumstances and/or intentions or ends. On the contrary, I take for granted that *supporting the making of legal permission of abortion (at any stage of pregnancy) a part of the law* and *supporting the retaining of such permission as part of the law* are intrinsically evil acts incapable of being justified by circumstances and/or intentions or ends or 'proportionate reasons', even 'to reduce the total number of

---

[49] One moment at which Harte gets beyond formalism is when he acknowledges that an improperly motivated *abstention* can be in reality a way of *voting for* a bad proposal (or against a good proposal).

abortions'.[50] I have been addressing the prior questions: What is *support*? What is *making permission a part of the law (or retaining it as part of the law)*?[51]

My discussion in the present reply to Harte simply unpacks the answer to that last question, which even as it stood made clear that a primary issue – in the present debate, *the* primary issue – is: What is it for a law to be – "objectively", if you like – "permissive"? Is that issue settled, as Harte supposes, by looking to see what a document, the bill or statute, *says*, regardless of the legal context or circumstances which may and usually will profoundly affect what *law* is brought into being or maintained in being by this bill or statute? But the rest of my discussion in that 1994/1996 essay in fact focussed upon the intentions of the voting legislator, and I loosely spoke, a couple of paragraphs later, of the restrictive reforming bill "continu[ing]" the unjust existing law. That way of putting it failed to keep in view the distinction between what the statute says and what it juridically means and does, a distinction I have spelled out above. The same failure is to be found in a 1997/8 address of mine, from which Harte has now quoted and relied upon the relevant loose sentence where I speak of the restrictive reforming statute as "a law which does in fact permit abortion",[52] even though the case I was discussing was of a statute which in law would neither create any permission nor keep in being any permission that would otherwise have ceased to be part of the state's laws.

---

[50] In his present paper (5.1) Harte alleges that voting for restrictive reforming legislation of the kind under debate is an unethical moral compromise. He provides no argument for this assertion save his general fallacious argument that every restrictive statute permits (= makes permissible) what it does not prohibit. And his distinction between the political and the moral is an unacceptable way of speaking. But he is right that the matter in debate excludes compromise. As I wrote to the Secretary of the CDF on 15 January 1995, "Permissible *obiecta* [for choice] do *not* include 'compromising with evil' or participating in the promotion of unjust or wrongful legislation. The only relevant *obiectum* which is permissible is *eliminating, or preventing, a wrongful law as far as concretely possible.* ... Support [for a restrictive reforming bill of the kind in debate] is not, in truth, a compromise with those seeking to maintain or introduce wrongful elements [of law]. There is a *material coincidence* between the upright Catholic legislator's or citizen's project and the wrongful project of those seeking to maintain or introduce wrongful elements. But this material coincidence is not appropriately describable as compromise, even if it is accompanied by certain agreements which the Catholic legislator may enter into in order to facilitate his project (e.g. the agreement to hold the vote at a specific time, or to 'pair' supporters and opponents who wish to be absent from the vote on legitimate business elsewhere." (emphases original)

[51] 71 (1996) *Notre Dame Law Review* at 599–600; J. Joblin and R. Tremblay (eds), *I Cattolici e la Società Pluralista: Il Caso delle 'Leggi Imperfette'*. Bologna: Edizione Studio Domenicano 1996: 99–114 at 106–8.

[52] Finnis, "The Catholic Church and Public Policy Debates...": 269 (where I say the same thing more than once).

The ambiguity which I was failing to keep steadily in mind is in substance the ambiguity (or one key aspect of the ambiguity) which has caused an interpretative problem for readers of Aquinas. Here is how I sketched that problem in 1991:

> Aquinas sometimes says that God can dispense from the Decalogue and sometimes (in the same works [works from both his early and his late writings]) says that God cannot.

I interject: interpretative methods like Harte's approaches to *EV* 73 and to the juridical meaning of statutes would here yield the confident conclusion that, self-evidently, one or other of these sets of texts should be abandoned, and that Aquinas was a bungler. But in fact, as I went on, the contradiction is only apparent, for:

> Insofar as the Commandments consist of *formulations* which can be taken as dealing with behaviour which is *conventionally* defined as murder, adultery, and so on, or which is behaviourally (physically) the same as murder or adultery defined *ex objecto* (i.e. in terms of intentions and choices), they *can* be dispensed from by God, since his special mandate so changes the circumstances that the chooser's [proximate] intention, the *object* of the act, can be different from what it is in all other cases to which the behaviourally *or conventionally* specified norm applies: cf. *In Sent.* I d. 47 q. 1 a. 4; *In Sent.* 4 d. 33 q. 1 a. 2; *De Malo* q. 3 a. 1 ad 17. But when the Commandments are considered as they should be, as *propositions* bearing on human acts understood in terms of their precise [and proximate] intentionality (*ex objecto*), they are altogether exceptionless and cannot be dispensed from by God: *In Sent.* 3. d. 37 a. 4; *Summa Theol.* I-II q. 100 a. 8.[53]

Early sections of the present paper amply illustrate the way in which talk of a "permissive" (and therefore unjust) abortion "law" has a similar systematic ambiguity. This ambiguity must be identified and cleared up before the *true principle* that *one must never vote for a permissive abortion law* can be rightly understood and applied so as to do justice, rather than the dreadful injustices that Harte's misunderstanding of it (in all innocence) would often cause.

Even though the intention/side-effect distinction should not have had the prominence it did in my former discussions of this issue, it is relevant and necessary for a correct understanding of two points. One is an element in

---

[53] J. Finnis, *Moral Absolutes* 39, emphases adjusted. I added: "For this interpretation, see Patrick Lee, 'Permanence of the Ten Commandments: St Thomas and His Modern Commentators', *Theological Studies* 42 (1981) 422–43." See also *Moral Absolutes*, 91.

the enactment of all restrictive abortion laws. The other is a special issue that may arise from time to time.

The general point is this. A restrictive bill or statute does in a culturally and pedagogically significant sense publicly "ratify" and "continue" (to use Harte's words) some of the existing unjust permission of abortion. It *appears* to do what Harte mistakenly thinks it legally or juridically does, and this appearance conveys the false and corrupting message (including to interpreters of the law) that some babies are not morally entitled to the protection of law. And, more fundamentally, it does leave some babies without the protection of law to which they have an urgent and overriding entitlement. Neither of these two broad classes of "effects" makes the statute a permissive law in the sense of *EV* 73.2. But both are very bad aspects of the enactment of the restrictive statute. Still, neither aspect is intended by a pro-life legislator. As *EV* 73.3 says, these legislators have a strict responsibility to make their "absolute opposition"[54] to abortion "well-known". If they can prevent or avoid the formulation of the restrictive statute in terms such as "abortion is permitted up to...", they ought to.[55] But the bad effects of seeming to withdraw legal protection from some of the unborn are *praeter intentionem*, side-effects, in relation to the choices of pro-life legislators whose intention

---

[54] The encyclical uses the unfortunate phrase "absolute personal opposition", unconscious of the way this sounds in the ear of English speakers who have heard Catholic politicians profess their "personal opposition" to abortion while in word and deed articulating and acting upon the view that legal prohibition of abortion is more or less improper or at least not a moral responsibility.

[55] In my paper prepared for the CDF conference and republished as "Unjust Laws in a Democratic Society", I took as my stock example a bill of that form. I was dealing with the issue proposed to the symposium by its organisers – the very same "problem of conscience" as is articulated in *EV* 73 – and I was deliberately framing it in a form *unusually difficult* for the Catholic or other pro-life legislator. The same problem of conscience can arise in forms which have all the appearance of being easier, and I could have made my argument rhetorically easier by using one of these. For example: if the existing permissive legislation read "Clause 1: Abortion is freely permissible up to 24 weeks of pregnancy", the reforming bill might simply read: "In Section 1, replace the word 24 with the word 16." Such a bill would *say* nothing about permitting abortion. Or the reforming bill might read: "Notwithstanding section 1, abortion after the end of the 15th week is absolutely prohibited." Such a bill would *say* nothing about permission and would articulate only a prohibition entirely appropriate and just in what it prohibited. But it was clear to me that the relevant problem of conscience does not turn on drafting formalities and differences. So, avoiding rhetorical advantages, I envisaged and discussed a bill whose *form(ulation)* was deliberately of the most unpromising and repellent kind, the bill with which you are now familiar from Harte's paper: "Abortion is lawful up to 16 weeks". Even when those formalities and differences have a public impact which the draftsman ought to avoid if possible, failure to live up to this obligation is not an intrinsic wrong.

in voting for the bill/statute is simply to prohibit all the abortions they can. As for the "leaving unprotected", this is not really an effect at all, but rather the absence of a desirable effect. It is like a pair of firemen who can carry only two persons leaving behind a third in a burning building. It is true that the firemen have a strong obligation to rescue each and every person in the building. But they are not at fault, and are not "choosing the lesser evil" or "compromising", when they rescue everyone they can, leaving behind those they cannot. That leaving behind is an important part of the story. Like its sequel or outcome, it is deeply regrettable, albeit in no sense culpable. If it is an effect at all it is certainly a side-effect, notwithstanding the certainty with which it can be foreseen. Common-sense has little difficulty in reaching right judgments in such cases.

The special point is this. Sometimes it will happen that pro-lifers who have initiated or supported a restrictive reforming bill whose only juridical effect would be prohibitive are confronted with an amendment to it which will make it in (say) one respect permissive. Imagine a one-clause pro-life bill to extend the prohibition of abortion from 24 weeks to three weeks[56] – thus saving 99% of all who would otherwise be aborted – onto which is tacked at the last minute (over the total but unavailing opposition of the pro-life legislators) a new clause B cutting back somewhat the existing comprehensive legal prohibition of abortion on grounds of the baby's gender. The bill thus amended is put to a final vote, and if it is not carried there will be no reform of abortion law for many years if ever (so far as human foresight goes). The bill is now, in one part (clause B), permissive within the meaning of *EV* 73.2 and the true principle that paragraph of the encyclical articulates. When asked by the Speaker to vote Aye or Nay, can the pro-life legislators vote Aye?

Positivist to the end, Harte's paper confidently declares:

> Legislators voting for proposals . . . are willing and choosing to enact precisely what is contained within those proposals. What the legislature "does" (in willing that certain permissions, tolerations, prohibitions, etc. be enacted as law) is indistinguishable from what an individual legislator "does" (in willing that the proposal with those very permissions, tolerations, prohibitions, etc. be enacted). Voting for the whole of the proposal which is presented as the matter of the vote is *the act of the legislator* just as the enactment of the whole of the proposal is *the act of the legislature*. (sec. 5.2)

---

[56] The pro-life legislators have floated a bill to extend the prohibition to 0 weeks (= from conception), but find that this has no support from those compromising legislators whose support is indispensable if there is to be any reform at all.

This sounds plausible, if one is in the grip of one's society's conventions, but as an action-description fit for moral analysis it is simply false.

The pro-life legislators each say "Aye" or walk through the "Yes" lobby. An effect of that behaviour is that, if enough others do likewise, the *whole* bill, and each of its parts, will be enacted. But what these pro-life legislators intend – both the proximate intention that each of them have (the precise object of their voting acts) and any further intention(s) or motive they have – is settled not by what other people or social conventions make of their behaviour but by their own course of deliberation, their own authentic practical reasoning (not to be confused with some inauthentic inner or outer story they might tell themselves or others to rationalise real and questionable or wrongful purposes). And it is their object, "the proximate end of a deliberate decision which determines the act of willing on the part of the acting person",[57] that settles the question *what they are doing*, the act(ion) which, thus accurately described, can then be subjected to moral analysis.[58] Their object in voting Aye is the enactment of clause A.[59] By virtue of the conventions (rules) of the legislature and the morally bad will and actions of the pro-choice and centrist legislators who secured the addition of clause B, the effect of their *voting for cl. A* will be that the whole bill, including cl. B, will be enacted. This effect is certain and inevitable, but (like many other certain and inevitable effects of what we choose to do) it is not part of what they intend or choose or do, in the senses of those words which are necessary for a true moral analysis (and for a Catholic analysis). The enactment of clause B is for these legislators a side-effect. (For others, of course, it is an important part of what these others intend and do.)

As we saw in earlier sections, a law is essentially a proposition of law, and one bill/statute can thus, whatever its verbal structure, enact many distinct laws. It follows that, in a case like this, precisely understood, the legislator who votes for the law made (legally) true by cl. A does not *vote for* the unjust law made (legally) true by cl. B. In the true principle articulated in *EV* 73.2, not only the phrase "permissive law", but also the phrase "vote for" must be understood with precision. One does not, precisely speaking, vote for what one does not intend to vote for.

---

[57] Encyclical *Veritatis Splendor* (1993) 78.

[58] "The morality of the human act depends primarily and fundamentally on the 'object' rationally chosen by the deliberate will, as is borne out by the insightful analysis, still valid today, made by Saint Thomas [fn. Summa Theol. I-II q. 18 a. 6]": *Veritatis Splendor* 78. Harte has sometimes suggested that the citation of q. 18 a. 6 somehow qualifies the obvious sense of *VS* 78. It does not. See fn. 62 below, and Finnis, *Moral Absolutes*, 65–74.

[59] "Why are you going through that lobby now – what's your immediate purpose?" "To do my bit towards enacting cl. A."

But it also remains true that, in the broader sense that counts for parliamentary procedure and its outcomes, one votes for the whole bill and all its parts. The enactment of the whole bill including its unjust part(s), here cl. B, is a side-effect for which the pro-life legislators are morally responsible, as one is always responsible for side-effects that one can or should foresee and could avoid. But the norms that govern the moral assessment of their willingness to cause that side-effect are not the strict and exceptionless negative moral norms which apply to what one intends, chooses and in that strict sense does. They are norms of fairness, commitment, role-responsibility, which are situation-relative,[60] and which allow for the judgment that *for these legislators*, who do not intend the enactment of clause B, the willingness to do what foreseeably and certainly has the effect of enacting clause B (and is conventionally *counted as* "intentionally voting for" and enacting the whole bill including clause B) is not unjust to the babies who will unjustly perish because of clause B's enactment.

This is a special and perhaps rather unusual kind of case. The more usual case is the kind discussed above, in which the reforming bill is – in law if not in formulation – nothing but restrictive. But the truth that precisely what a voter is doing in voting is settled by his or her actual course of deliberation, not by what is deemed in law or convention to be the effect of so behaving, is a general truth. So too is the truth that, whatever its verbal structure or drafting formalities, a bill/statute has the logical structure of a list of distinct propositions of law, rather like Harte's imaginary code, each of whose articles could be eliminated without mentioning or affecting the other articles – with the consequence that the object and intent of legislators in going through the "Aye" lobby can rationally be to enact some of these propositions of law, accepting the enactment of the others as a side-effect for which they are morally responsible but not in the uniquely stringent way that one is morally responsible for what one intends and chooses as an end or as a means. Thus my emphasis on the distinction between intention and side-effect in earlier analyses of the *general* problem of voting for restrictive abortion legislation was not so much mistaken as unnecessary and therefore misleading.

7. Cooperation: a reality but not important for the issue in debate

Going beyond classical theological ways of using the term "cooperation", *EV* 73.3 says that under the conditions as to circumstances and intentions that it specifies, a pro-life legislator who supports and votes for a restrictive statute is making "a legitimate... attempt to limit its [the unjust law's] evil aspects", and is not engaging in "an illicit cooperation with an unjust law".

---

[60] See fn. 1 above.

In my own writings on the matter, I have spoken of the pro-life legislator's vote for just restrictive legislation as "material cooperation" in the continuing legislative failure to rescue those who should be rescued. Harte, keeping a discreet silence about *EV* 73's non-traditional language, objects that I am departing from the traditional model of material cooperation. But this, and the rest of his discussion of cooperation, is quite beside the point. Even if everything he says about cooperation were correct – very little of it is – it would go no way at all to showing that the reforming statute itself and/or the act of a pro-life legislator in voting for it are unjust. So there is strictly no need to attend to the question of cooperation in order to answer the question in debate. My references to cooperation were by way of a concession, made in order to show that *even if* there is cooperation of pro-life legislators with unjust legislators in enacting just restrictive legislation, this cooperation does not involve the pro-life legislator in the wrongdoing of the unjust legislator, or any other wrongdoing.

Harte says that "Finnis appears to believe that though they are voting for the same legislation, at the same time, and within the same context, for some legislators the action is evil, and for others the action is good." I do "appear to believe this" – because I in fact plainly assert it.[61] The real possibility of identical behaviour being different descriptive and moral species of human acts is an immediate implication of a sound act-analysis. One finds such an analysis, for example, in Aquinas – not least in, amongst many other passages, *Summa Theologiae* I-II q. 18 a. 6, recalled in *Veritatis Splendor* 78 and from time to time mentioned by Harte himself as significant. As that passage puts it,[62] one's actually (interiorly) willed end or end – purpose(s),

---

[61] "*Behaviourally*, the [pro-life legislator's] support for the bill (e.g. the vote for it) is indistinguishable from the support given by a legislator who thinks unborn children have no rights or that their destruction is the lesser evil or that sacrificing some to save others is justified. Many people who observe the upright legislator's vote may misunderstand what he is doing, and think that he is supporting the permission of abortion for one or more of those or other bad reasons" – reasons which in the following sentence I describe as "serious sins, at least of thought and quite likely [as in the case of the compromising centrist legislator] of deed": "Unjust Laws in a Democratic Society" at 601–2.

[62] *S.T.* I-II q. 18 a. 6c: "So, just as one's external act gets its species or character from the object which it concerns, so one's internal act of will gets its species from one's end(s), as if that were its own object. But [or: And thus] whatever pertains to one's will stands as shaping and characterising in relation to whatever pertains to one's external act. For one's will employs one's members as its instrument in one's acting, and one's external acts only have moral significance insofar as they are willed. And so the species or character of a human act is formally [essentially] analysed by reference to one's end(s), and is analysed in terms of its matter by reference to the object of one's external act. Thus as Aristotle says in *Nicomachean Ethics* V, if one steals in order to commit

non-proximate intention(s) – stand(s) to the object (the proximate end) of one's exterior act as decisively characterising, *formale*, that is, as form stands to matter, namely as *making the thing what it is*. So, in the context of action, it is the ends and intentions of the acting person that make *the act* – what is *done* – what it is.[63] And they thus can make immoral what would otherwise be morally right. Two soldiers on a mission to rescue Jews and gypsies from an extermination camp are lying alongside one another, returning the rifle fire of the camp guards. One soldier intends his potentially lethal return fire to disable the guards from blocking the rescue mission. The other soldier intends to satisfy his lust to see or hear and gloat over men of a hated race dying in agony. The first's acts are acts of just defence of self and others, the second's identical *behaviour* is "materially" the same but formally (i.e., more really) and primarily (according to the teaching of Aquinas, following Aristotle) an act or set of acts of immoral lust.[64] At any rate, they are substantially different kinds of *act*, as that term is used in moral reflection. The same can and often does hold true of two legislators going through the voting lobby together: their behaviour is identical, their acts different, and one is acting uprightly, the other immorally.

This, says Harte, raises "some difficult questions and serious moral problems for pro-life legislators" who press for the compromising centrists' support in carrying a restrictive reforming bill/statute against the opposition of the pro-choicers. How can a pro-lifer press for support which would

---

adultery, one is, strictly speaking, more an adulterer than a thief." {Sicut igitur actus exterior accepit speciem ab obiecto circa quod est, ita actus interior voluntatis accepit speciem a fine sicut a proprio obiecto. *Id* [or: *ita*] *autem quod est ex parte voluntatis se habet ut formale ad id quod est ex parte exterioris actus*, quia voluntas utitur membris ad agendum sicut instrumentis, *neque actus exteriores habent rationem moralitatis nisi inquantum sunt voluntarii*. Et ideo actus humani *species formaliter consideratur secundum finem*, materialiter autem secundum obiectum exterioris actus. Unde Philosophus dicit, in V Eth., ut ille qui furatur ut committit adulterium est, per se loquendo, magis adulter quam fur.} In Aquinas's philosophy, "form" and *formale* refer to what is most essential to something being what it is – almost the opposite meaning from the modern idiomatic English "(mere) formality" etc. On what Aquinas means by speaking of an act's "matter", see Finnis, *Aquinas: Moral, Political and Legal Theory*. Oxford: Oxford University Press 1998: 142 nn. 43–4 with the citations especially to *De Malo*: in short, in this context "matter" and "object" and "close-in intention" are interchangeable.

[63] Elsewhere, and pervasively, Aquinas will remind us that good and bad are not symmetrical: good (further) intentions cannot make good an act made bad by its matter = object = proximately intended behavioural characteristics, but bad intentions (and/or inappropriate circumstances) make bad an act despite its being in its matter/object a good or not-bad kind of behaviour such as almsgiving or walking. See *S.T.* I-II q. 18 a. 4 ad 3; Finnis, *Aquinas*, 148.

[64] *Ibid.*

involve that centrist in the evil of willing the permission and ratification of abortion up to 16 weeks? But this is quite unreasonable scrupulosity, of a kind that would make social cooperation in the real world almost impossible. The pro-lifers press for support in *prohibiting abortion as far as possible*. They may foresee that some of this support will be given with very bad motives. They intend none of those motives, and their appeal for support is at least implicitly and often explicitly an appeal for a change of heart by centrists and pro-choicers alike. Harte's doubt – which in earlier writings he put forward with more vigour, as an assertion – would entail that if a commander notices that some of the soldiers essential to the mission of rescuing Jews and gypsies from extermination are carrying out their roles in the operation with seriously immoral motives of lust and/or hatred, the commander should abandon the rescue mission ("deferred pending moral conversion"), preferring to leave the victims to their fate rather than cooperate with immorally motivated soldiers in an operation which itself involves and calls for no immoral act whatsoever.[65] Which is absurd.

---

[65] Of course, the commanders should firmly attempt to prohibit the immorally motivated soldiers from committing any of the war crimes which would be possible and predictable outcomes of their immoral attitudes.

13

The opening up of a discussion: a response to John Finnis

Colin Harte

I welcome John Finnis' robust critique of my paper. The question we are disputing is a matter of life and death, and it is right that Finnis should have presented such a vigorous reply to my paper, enabling readers to consider carefully whether my view might be flawed and lead, as he fears, to "dreadful injustices."[1] It is right too that readers consider carefully whether Finnis' own argument might be flawed and lead, as I fear, to different, though also dreadful, injustices.[2]

Finnis' paper contains two main theses. The first is that a range of proposals, which can be bracketed under the label "restrictive abortion legislation," may be rightly supported, if failure to support them would result in a more extensive abortion law. Finnis' second thesis is not only that the first thesis is consistent with John Paul II's teaching in *Evangelium Vitae*, n. 73 (*EV* 73), but that it is the only possible interpretation of *EV* 73; and, furthermore, that the *very reasons* Finnis gives as justifying votes for restrictive legislation are also to be found in the actual teaching of *EV* 73. There is no inconsistency between his two theses; the problem for Finnis lies, I suggest, in their *excessive*

---

[1] Finnis, p. 238.

[2] A notable account of some of the injustices of restrictive abortion legislation, insofar as it excludes the most vulnerable of the unborn, is given in a paper describing attempts to restrict abortion in the UK. The paper has been published, so far, only in Polish. See Alison Davis, "Ofiara, Na Którą Można Się Zgodzić?" ["An Acceptable Sacrifice?"]. 61–62 (2003) *Ethos*: 214–231. See also Colin Harte, *Changing Unjust Laws Justly*. Washington DC: Catholic University of America Press 2005, Chapter 1, "A Denial of Solidarity".

consistency, with the two theses being so intimately intertwined that the unraveling of one thesis inevitably undermines the other. In this response I shall try, so far as it is possible, to comment on the two theses separately.

Although the discussion may be broadly characterized in terms of voting for "restrictive abortion legislation," Finnis' writings on the question (i.e. his papers of 1994, 1997, and his present one of 2003[3]) have referred to four different cases of legislative proposals, and it is helpful to keep each of these in mind in the following discussion:

> *Case 1* is what Finnis refers to as the "usual case"[4] (or the "general problem"[5]) of restrictive legislation, such as a restriction of abortion from 24 weeks by a bill/law, "Abortion is permitted up to 16 weeks." (Proposals A, B, C and G, rejected as intrinsically unjust in my paper, can also be regarded as "usual case" proposals.) *Case 1* proposals restrict abortion without introducing a "permission" for abortion that did not previously exist.

> *Case 2* refers to a law which *introduces* permissions for abortion (against, say, the background of a law *prohibiting all abortions*). Finnis recognizes rightly that if *EV 73* is to be interpreted as teaching that legislators can vote for *Case 1* proposals, *this interpretation necessarily entails* that even if the current law prohibits *all* abortions, legislators could vote for "Abortion is permitted up to 16 weeks" in order to prevent the imminent vote for a "24 week" bill which, almost certainly, would be enacted.[6]

> *Case 3* is Finnis' "special and perhaps rather unusual kind of case."[7] With these proposals, some abortions that were previously permitted are prohibited, others remain permitted, but *a new*

---

[3] In addition to Finnis' latest paper, I will refer back to his earlier papers that both he and I have cited. The first paper is the one given at the CDF conference in 1994, subsequently published in 1996 as "Unjust Laws in a Democratic Society...." The second paper was given at the Linacre Centre conference in 1997 and published in 1999 as "The Catholic Church and Public Policy Debates..."

[4] Finnis, p. 242.

[5] *Ibid.*

[6] Finnis, p. 229. See also, Harte, "Challenging a Consensus..." 337–338, which has been cited in my paper as well as Finnis'. Many people would regard it unconscionable to vote for the sort of *Case 2* proposal that introduces permissions for abortion against a background of prohibition. The fact that votes for such proposals are necessarily approved if *EV 73* approves votes for *Case 1* proposals should be sufficient reason to consider carefully what *EV 73* does in fact teach about voting for *Case 1* proposals.

[7] Finnis, p. 242.

permission is introduced for some abortions that were previously prohibited.[8]

Case 4 refers to a proposal like "the omnibus budget bill" mentioned by Finnis in his 1994 paper, details of which are cited in my paper.[9] *Case 4* proposals cover a range of matters, most of which would be unconnected to anything intrinsically evil like abortion and which, considered separately, would be just (e.g. just proposals concerning matters dealing with education, transport, or health, etc.); they would also, however, include something that would be intrinsically unjust (like permission for or funding of abortion).

1. Some points of contention with Finnis' first thesis

1.1. *"Permitting" abortion and "just" restrictive laws*

My paper presented the thesis that it is unethical, irrespective of the circumstances or consequences, to vote for legislation that is intrinsically unjust; legislators can only vote for just legislation. (I had previously argued that the teaching of *EV* 73 is entirely consistent with this thesis.[10]) It had seemed to me that Finnis had overlooked the question of whether the restrictive legislation was just or unjust, and the drawing up of Proposals A–H in my paper seemed to me a necessary way of establishing the point that was crucial to discussing the disputed question. The proposals that I presented as being intrinsically unjust (A, B, C and G) were, like Finnis' proposal "Abortion is permitted up to 16 weeks" (thereby lowering the abortion time limit from 24 weeks), examples of *Case 1* proposals. If they permit (or tolerate[11]) abortion, then they are necessarily unjust – indeed, intrinsically unjust – and cannot be supported.

I had not predicted whether Finnis would say that Proposals A, B, C and G were "just" or "unjust but not intrinsically unjust" or "intrinsically unjust" or "partly just and partly unjust" or that the question of their justness or

---

[8] Finnis' illustration of a *Case 3* proposal is on p. 240. To express it more simply: if abortion were legally permitted for any reason up to 24 weeks and all abortions prohibited thereafter, a *Case 3* proposal would be one specifying: "Abortion is permitted up to and not beyond 16 weeks, unless foetal disability has been detected, in which case abortions are permitted up to 26 weeks."

[9] Harte, p. 198, fn. 36.

[10] See Harte, "Challenging a Consensus . . . ," *passim.*

[11] I welcome Finnis' acknowledgement that "in relation to a matter of fundamental rights like abortion, any distinction between legal permission and legal toleration is beside the point" (p. 227, fn. 34).

unjustness was irrelevant. In his papers of 1994 and 1997 Finnis had adopted an "intention and side-effect" argument – i.e. an action-theory analysis – and argued that pro-life legislators could licitly vote for the restrictive "16 week" law which, he said, "does in fact permit abortion up to 16 weeks," because they would not intend to support the law's permission of pre-16-week abortions (this was, he said, a side-effect of their vote); the "moderate" pro-abortion legislators who were prepared to reduce the abortion time-limit to 16 weeks would nevertheless be doing moral evil because they also intended to support the law's *continued permissions* for abortions before 16 weeks.

Finnis' main argument now focuses not on that action-theory, but on a legal analysis that was entirely absent from his 1994 and 1997 papers.[12] Having previously asserted that the "16 week" bill "does in fact permit abortion up to 16 weeks," Finnis' revised opinion is that the restrictive legislation *does not in fact* permit abortion up to 16 weeks. Irrespective of its wording, he now says, "the new statute's *juridical* meaning and effect is simply pro-hibitive. The statute *does* nothing but prohibit abortions."[13] In short, the

---

[12] After quoting a main passage from his 1994 paper (pp. 236–237), Finnis says: "My discussion in the present reply to Harte simply unpacks the answer to that last question ["What is making permission a part of the law (or retaining it as part of the law)?"], which even as it stood made clear that a primary issue – in the present debate, the primary issue – is: What is it for a law to be – "objectively", if you like – "permissive"?" (p. 237). Though these comments may seem to imply that Finnis' present argument is rooted in his 1994 paper, such a claim (should it be made) would be indefensible. The argument of Finnis' 1994 paper was based on his action theory, not a legal analysis. Finnis is right to say that *the primary issue* in the present debate is "What is it for a law to be... "permissive"?" (Similarly, for me, the primary issue is the *character of the (restrictive) law*, though my presentation focuses on whether it is "just" rather than whether it is "permissive.") But this new question of Finnis' is not what he asked in 1994. The question asked in 1994 came at the end of a passage about action theory and referred to what preceded it: "*I have been addressing* the prior questions: What is *support*? What is *making* permission a part of the law (or *retaining* it as part of the law)?" (p. 237; emphases altered). The question "What is making permission a part of the law?" must be understood in the context of what preceded it, which were remarks about action theory. Indeed, in his published text, the question ends with a footnote reference drawing attention to the teaching of *Veritatis Splendor* n. 78, a foot-note which demonstrates, should there be any doubt about his point, that the question Finnis was addressing, in line with all his preceding (and following) remarks, had everything to do with *action theory* and nothing to do with *legal analysis*. It is also not credible that Finnis could have intended to present, in his 1994 paper, a legal analysis that the restrictive law does not truly permit abortions up to 16 weeks, whilst conveying the idea in that same paper, and stating more explicitly in his later 1997 paper, that the restrictive law "does in fact permit abortion up to 16 weeks."

[13] Finnis, p. 218.

restrictive statute is just.[14] Thus, Proposals A, B, C and G are just[15]: even if all the abortions within a country are performed with respect to what is permitted or tolerated *in a single statute*, like Proposals A, B and C, that statute (which is, substantively, the country's abortion law) is just.[16] Finnis acknowledges that "Proposal A is in substance the Polish law of 1993"[17] and his judgment that Proposal A can be judged to be *just*,[18] means that the same judgment applies to the Polish 1993 Act which was enacted as constituting *Poland's abortion law.*

I anticipate that Finnis' judgment that Proposal A in Noland (or, equivalently, Poland's 1993 Act) is "just" will surprise many people, including those who agree with him that legislators can vote for such restrictive legislation. With the full repeal of all previous legislation permitting or tolerating abortion in Noland (or Poland), the only law tolerating some abortions is, precisely, Proposal A (or Poland's 1993 Act). The former – now repealed – laws will have no relevance for any future judicial judgments or legislative changes. The law's toleration of some abortions *is fully specified* in the proposals for which legislators will have voted. Finnis' view that these tolerations of abortion are not "legally true" seems indefensible. Certainly, some tolerations are "legally true," and if it is not those specified in Proposal A (or Poland's law), where are those tolerations specified? If, in Noland or Poland, the legitimacy of aborting a disabled child were subject to judicial proceedings, any judgment would cite Proposal A or the Polish 1993 Act as the relevant legislation; there would be no citation of repealed laws that

---

[14] The view Finnis expresses at fn. 17, p. 218 is also mine. In the abstract, one cannot say that a proposal is "just," merely that it is "not intrinsically unjust," i.e., the judgment that any proposal is, in fact, just, depends, in a concrete situation, on a consideration of the circumstances. (The same applies to all human actions; in the abstract they cannot be labelled "good," merely "not intrinsically bad/evil/unjust.")

[15] Finnis, p. 230, especially fn. 40.

[16] Finnis says: "Harte's repeated assumption that a short code or statute could comprise "the whole of a country's abortion law" is naïve" (p. 227). It is unclear whether Finnis is objecting (unreasonably) because the codes or statutes, presented as simplified illustrations of what can be and is actually the case in different countries, are too "short", or because I am suggesting that a *single* code or statute could comprise the whole of a country's abortion law. The latter was virtually the case with the UK Abortion Act. Had it not been for the 1938 judicial judgment, *Rex v. Bourne*, under which some abortions were allowed, the unborn would have been fully protected by the law, and the Abortion Act 1967 would, alone, have specified under which conditions abortions could be procured. Poland's 1993 Act, cited on p. 181, fn. 8, in itself specifies which abortions are tolerated, whilst prohibiting all the others.

[17] Finnis, fn. 40.

[18] See fn. 14, above.

no longer exist or of general principles of law presupposing all juristic thought, such as "What is not prohibited is permitted."[19]

In many respects, Finnis' new legal analysis adds considerable weight to my argument that the teaching of *EV* 73, and the ethics of voting for restrictive legislation, focuses on the question of voting for *just* legislation.[20] Finnis appears to be saying that I am right in principle, but wrong in my legal analysis. If Finnis is right in saying that the sort of restrictive legislation to which I object does not actually permit or tolerate abortions and is in fact just, then my fundamental objection to voting for restrictive legislation like Proposals A, B, C and G necessarily falls. But is he right?

I will limit my remarks here to noting the novelty of the legal analysis that Finnis is now presenting, observing, first, that voting for restrictive legislation has been subject to so much debate and controversy because the legislation is commonly seen not to be straightforwardly or obviously, if at all, just. The very framing of the question in terms of voting for "*imperfect*" legislation reflects a general concern, if not an acknowledgement, that the legislation itself does in fact permit or tolerate abortions and is, thus, unjust. The underlying assumption that restrictive laws do in fact *permit* abortion was evident from the letter, sent by Cardinal Ratzinger, inviting participants to the 1994 symposium to focus on "the delicate problem of the collaboration of Catholics with imperfect laws (for example, laws *which permit abortion* in certain cases, but are more restrictive compared with exisiting laws)."[21] Robert George, Professor of Jurisprudence at Princeton (Finnis' doctoral student and a leading adherent of his ethical and legal theory), describes the "imperfectly just" law that is being supported as "an objectively unjust law."[22] Indeed, the standard view (of those who

---

[19] See Finnis, p. 227.

[20] This applies, at least, with respect to Finnis' argument for supporting *Case 1* and *Case 2* proposals. A focus on "justness" does not appear to support his view that *Case 3* and *Case 4* proposals can be supported, though it must be noted that Finnis does not appeal to the teaching of *EV* 73 to justify votes for proposals in these latter two cases.

[21] Emphases altered. See Finnis' fn. 15, and the passage of his text to which it refers (p. 217).

[22] "The Pope does not provide an extensive argument in behalf of his teaching about the permissibility of sometimes supporting imperfectly just laws .... While it can never be fair to will that members of a disfavored class – whether the unborn, the disabled, or members of some racial or religious minority group – be excluded from legal protections one wills for oneself and those dear to one, a legislator or voter is personally responsible for no unfairness to the victims of *an objectively unjust law where he supports that law* precisely, and only, because the alternative is even less protective of its victims" (emphasis added). See Robert P. George, "The Gospel of Life: A Symposium." 56 (October 1995) *First Things*: 32–38, viewed at http://www.firstthings.com/ftissues/ft9510/articles/symposium.html.

share Finnis' general interpretation of *EV* 73.3) has been that the teaching of *EV* 73.3 is *by way of exception* to the prohibition of voting for intrinsically unjust laws taught in *EV* 73.2.[23][*] The restrictive law has been regarded by many as a "legal evil" (and, therefore, not just), but a "lesser evil" in comparison to a law allowing more abortions.[24] In his previous papers, Finnis' view had not been simply that the restrictive law *gives the appearance of permitting* abortion, but that it *does in fact permit* abortion. Even though he thought legislators could vote for it, he acknowledged that *the law itself that was being voted for* was problematical, saying: "It is one thing for a legislator to vote for the law, quite another thing for Catholic bishops to be heard as saying that such a law is acceptable."[25] If the law, in a concrete situation, is judged to be just and desirable, then why should Catholic bishops or anyone else not say that it is acceptable? Indeed, in order to dispel any confusion about its justness and acceptability, there would be *more* reason for them to say it is acceptable.[26] And, to say that Proposals A, B, C and G are "just" is

---

[23] For example: "As a rule, Catholics are never supposed to vote for 'intrinsically unjust' abortion laws. But the encyclical identifies one exception to this rule; the Pope states that in some circumstances Catholic politicians may vote for laws that permit some abortion." See Leslie Griffin, *"Evangelium Vitae*: Abortion," in Kevin Wm Wildes sj and Alan C Mitchell (eds) *Choosing Life: A Dialogue on 'Evangelium Vitae'*. Washington DC: Georgetown University Press 1997: 159–173, at 170.

[*] [I accept Finnis' objection in his response to this paper that this is not rightly described as a "standard view" (pp. 272–273). When writing the sentence I had in mind Leslie Griffin's published remarks and the unpublished opinion commonly expressed in informal discussions when the unjustness of restrictive laws has been acknowledged. I accept that the frequent expression of an opinion does not make it a standard view. Though they have described as unjust the restrictive abortion proposals they think can be rightly voted for (according to *EV* 73.3), I knew that reputable writers, such as Archbishop Tarcisio Bertone (the former secretary of the CDF), Robert George and "the theologian [Mons. Angel Rodríguez Luño] whose study of the relevant issues was recently published at length in *L'Osservatore Romano*" (p. 272), do not share Griffin's view that the teaching of *EV* 73.3 should be regarded as an exception to *EV* 73.2's prohibition on voting for intrinsically unjust legislation. I regret that my sentence about the "standard view" suggested otherwise.]

[24] For a detailed discussion of this point, see Colin Harte, "Inconsistent Papal Approaches towards Problems of Conscience?" 2.1 (2002) *National Catholic Bioethics Quarterly*: 99–122.

[25] Finnis, "The Catholic Church and Public Policy Debates ..." 271.

[26] It would not be the ordinary role of Catholic bishops to intervene and direct legislators to support (let alone promote) any of the four (not intrinsically unjust) proposals, D, E, F or H, that I presented. But asked if the proposals are "acceptable," they should have no hesitation in saying yes. I agree with Finnis that Catholic bishops should not say that Proposals A, B, C or G are acceptable, but this is because they are intrinsically unjust and, fundamentally, unacceptable.

not consistent even with Finnis'current remarks about restrictive legislation, in which "restrictive" stands as shorthand for "prohibitive but less prohibitive than reason (justice) requires."[27]

Finnis' legal analysis is a new argument which neither he nor, as far as I know, anyone else has hitherto suggested as the main justification for votes for restrictive abortion legislation. This, in itself, does not mean that his analysis is incorrect, but it means that it has not been subject to the sort of rigorous examination that one would normally expect before such a view (which poses a significant challenge to what is commonly perceived as being "just," and which is of such far-reaching consequences) could be accepted.[28]

---

[27] Finnis, fn. 3, p. 210. By contrast, I think it is inappropriate to label Proposals D, E, F and H as "restrictive abortion legislation." Proposals D, E and F are simply proposals to repeal unjust law; the focus of Proposal H is specific to the prescription or distribution to, or the ingestion by, a pregnant woman of an abortion-inducing drug like RU 486; it does not deal with the general principle of abortion. The four proposals, in themselves, are entirely just.

[28] No doubt, Finnis' new analysis will now be the subject of much serious discussion. An initial test of its plausibility lies in whether such an analysis has ever been applied to any other instance of lawmaking, and it seems to me that it has not been, and would not be. Consider, for instance, a different legislative situation involving the repeal of a hypothetical Road Traffic Act 1950 which had specified, amongst other things, a maximum speed limit of 30 miles per hour within towns and cities. A new Road Traffic Act 2000 sets a maximum speed of 25 mph within towns and cities. Before the Act was passed various lobbyists called for a variety of limits: road safety campaigners wanted a 20 mph limit; ordinary motorists wanted no change; some businesses, eager to move their goods as quickly as possible, wanted a 35 mph limit. A Member of Parliament, Mrs Green, votes for the enactment of the Road Traffic Act 2000, and a year later is berated by a constituent for not voting for a lower speed limit: his son was killed by a car travelling at 25 mph and the police report indicated that the fatality would almost certainly have been avoided had the car been travelling even 3–5 mph slower. The constituent blames Mrs Green for his son's death, because she voted for the Act that specified that cars should be allowed to travel at speeds of up to 25 mph.

Mrs Green could reproach herself for voting for the Road Traffic Act 2000, or defend herself in a number of different ways, but in such an instance it is inconceivable that she or any other legislator would say, privately or publicly, in their defence: "In truth, *I did not vote to permit cars to travel at speeds of up to 25 mph*; the *juridical effect* of the Road Traffic Act 2000 is to prohibit cars travelling between 25 and 30 mph; the effect of the Act (with respect to this proposition of law) is solely prohibitive; the legislators responsible *for permitting* cars to travel between 0 and 25 mph are those who voted for the Road Traffic Act 1950 (if not those who voted for an even earlier Act)." Such a defence would be rightly rejected. Yet it would seem that this is what Finnis is now proposing should be accepted as the argument to justify voting for Proposals A, B, C and G.

1.2. An established or a changing baseline?

For Finnis, the justification of votes for *Case 1* proposals, presented in the previous section, also depends on what one regards as "the baseline" for assessing the proposal.[29] The permissiveness (and, thus, the justness) of proposals like the "16 week" bill depends, in Finnis' view, on the current law allowing abortions up to 24 weeks; measured against the "baseline" of the existing law the restrictive law is judged to be just. As noted, *Case 2* proposals (see above, p. 247) involve *the introduction* of permissions, supported to prevent the imminent vote for a law which would permit even more abortions. Finnis did not consider such proposals in his 1994 paper; at that time, he regarded the "baseline" as the law currently in force.[30] There is no indication whether, in 1994, Finnis would have supported *Case 2* proposals, but his analysis of *EV* 73 as supporting votes for *Case 1* proposals necessarily requires that it also teaches that *Case 2* proposals can be supported;[31] it may be on account of his (mistaken, I maintain) interpretation of *EV* 73 that he now believes *Case 2* proposals can be supported. But how can a legislator vote for *Case 2* proposals if, measured against the "baseline" of the current law, such proposals are permissive and therefore unjust? Finnis resolves the problem by arguing that in this situation there is a *different baseline*; in this situation, the baseline is not the existing law (which may prohibit *all* abortions) but the even more permissive law that will be enacted if the less permissive law is not supported. If one accepts this different baseline the "less permissive" law can be regarded as not "permissive" but "prohibitive" and, as Finnis maintains, "as prohibitive, it is essentially just."[32]

The UK's Abortion Act 1967, under which there are in the region of 170,000 abortions each year, is rightly judged intrinsically unjust. Finnis' argument would mean that if pro-life legislators had voted for the Act in 1967, in order to prevent a vote for a law that would permit even more abortions, then the very same Act would be "prohibitive" and "essentially just." Neither Finnis nor (to my knowledge) anyone else has previously advanced the view that he is now asserting, not only as being "true" but as being taught in *EV* 73. Indeed, there is a general reluctance amongst Catholic and other pro-lifers who support *Case 1* proposals to also support *Case 2*

---

[29] For Finnis, the baseline is the standard "against which any bill or amending statute is to be compared when assessing whether the amendment (or partial repeal) is permissive (and thus intrinsically unjust), or prohibitive and thus capable of being voted for by a Catholic or other pro-life legislator" (p. 229).

[30] Finnis, p. 229.

[31] See p. 247, above, especially fn. 6.

[32] Finnis, p. 229.

proposals, and a similar reluctance to acknowledge that if *EV* 73 authorizes votes for *Case 1* proposals, then it necessarily authorizes votes for *Case 2* proposals. Finnis is to be commended for admitting the implications of his interpretation of *EV* 73, but his interpretation with respect to *Case 2* proposals (and his argument to support it) highlights, in my view, the implausibility of his whole interpretation of the section and its application to *Case 1* proposals.

In my view, Finnis' establishment of one "baseline" for assessing *Case 1* proposals, and then a different one for assessing *Case 2* proposals, would mean that there is, in fact, *no baseline*. The whole of Catholic tradition, repeated in *Evangelium Vitae* itself, is that on "moral" (*ius gentium*)[33] matters, the baseline is the natural moral law, not a line which, because it changes according to the situation, can hardly be called a baseline.[34] John Paul II makes his own the teaching of Aquinas at *EV* 72: if a law is contrary to reason, if it violates the natural law, then it is an unjust law, indeed it is a corruption of law.[35] Finnis' notion of situation-changing baselines, enabling one to judge that *Case 1* and *Case 2* proposals can be judged "just", is contradicted by the firm baseline of the natural law, to which traditional Catholic teaching including the whole of *Evangelium Vitae* testifies, and with respect to which justness must be established.[36]

---

[33] Finnis states, without explanation, that my "distinction between the political and the moral is an unacceptable way of speaking" (p. 237, fn. 50). The distinction is the traditional distinction between matters that are contingent/negotiable (described by Aquinas as *ius civile*) and those that are fundamental/non-negotiable (described by Aquinas as *ius gentium*). There is no suggestion in the distinction that lawmaking on "political" matters does not involve moral/ethical considerations of justice, fairness, etc. A clear grasp of the distinction helps one to understand better why one cannot legislate to restrict abortion in the same way that one would legislate to lower a speed limit (see fn. 28, above).

[34] Finnis denies that he is embracing "situation ethics" (see p. 236, quoting from his 1994 paper), but his acceptance of changing baselines gives weight to the charge that he is.

[35] *EV* 72 cites Aquinas: "Human law is law inasmuch as it is in conformity with right reason and thus derives from the eternal law. But when a law is contrary to reason, it is called an unjust law; but in this case it ceases to be a law and becomes instead an act of violence" *Summa Theologiae, I-II*, q. 93, a. 3, ad 2. "Every law made by man can be called a law insofar as it derives from the natural law. But if it is somehow opposed to the natural law, then it is not really a law but rather a corruption of the law" *ST, I-II*, q. 95, a. 2.

[36] In my view, Finnis' promotion of situation-relative baselines, as opposed to the firm baseline of the natural law, is indicative of the "precarious legal positivism" inherent in support for restrictive abortion legislation that I cautioned against in "Challenging a Consensus..." (p. 342). I reject Finnis' labeling of my own position as "positivism" (pp. 235 and 240).

1.3. Intention and side-effects

Section 6 of Finnis' paper begins with an admission of a serious flaw in his former argument: "In my previous treatments of this whole issue I too failed to analyse it with all the precision that it calls for. As a result, my earlier discussion gave too much prominence to the distinction between intention and side-effect and too little attention to the ambiguities in the phrase 'unjust law' and 'permissive law'...."[37] I think it would be fair to say that Finnis' earlier discussions, in fact, gave no indication of "ambiguities" in the terms "unjust law" and "permissive law," and that they were concerned only with Finnis' action theory with respect to "intention and side-effect" (and, as I shall discuss below, "cooperation").

Finnis' earlier discussions (of 1994 and 1997) focused on a *Case 1* proposal (his "16 week" bill), and it is not a minor concession for him to admit that his "intention and side-effect" focus, with respect to such *Case 1* ("usual case") proposals, was misplaced.[38] It would seem that Finnis does not concede, however, that his "intention and side-effect" focus was entirely misplaced, because he regards it as relevant for *Case 3* proposals, i.e. proposals that would prohibit some abortions, but which introduce a new permission for other abortions (see above, p. 247). One assumes it would also be relevant when considering the sort of *Case 4* proposal he spoke of in 1994 (see p. 248).

In his current argument supporting votes for *Case 3* proposals, Finnis: (i) seems to be unconcerned with whether these proposals are just or unjust (though there is an indication that he acknowledges them to be unjust[39]); (ii) relies on his "intention and side-effect" action-theory analysis (not on a legal analysis); (iii) promotes a view that does not have clear magisterial

---

[37] Finnis, p. 236.

[38] Finnis does say now that *an* intention/side-effect distinction is "relevant and necessary" with respect to *Case 1* proposals insofar as a restrictive law's stated permission of abortions "*appears* to" permit abortion and this "appearance" is a "side-effect" which is "culturally and pedagogically significant" (p. 239). This is, however, a *new* notion of side-effect and entirely different from his analysis of 1994 and 1997 which maintained that the unintended side-effect was the law's *actual* permission of abortion. Finnis now says: "Thus my emphasis on the distinction between intention and side-effect in earlier analyses of the *general* problem of voting for restrictive abortion legislation [i.e. of *Case 1* proposals] was not so much mistaken as unnecessary and therefore misleading" (p. 242). Finnis is able to say that his earlier analysis was not "mistaken" because he has identified a *different* "side-effect," one that was absent from his previous argument.

[39] See Finnis, fn. 38 and the text to which it refers on p. 228.

support.[40] His 1994 argument that *Case 1* and *Case 4* proposals could be supported also bore these three features (and adds weight to my contention that he overlooked the question of the justness or unjustness of restrictive legislation). For Finnis, the "intention and side-effect" argument no longer applies to *Case 1* proposals; it does apply to *Case 3* (and, one assumes, to *Case 4*) proposals; it does not apply now to *Case 2* proposals, though Finnis has not said whether he ever thought that it did (and it is hard to see how it could). Finnis' acknowledgement that his previous analysis was significantly flawed lends weight to my paper's contention that the "first flaw" in his support for restrictive legislation lay in his "intention and side-effect" analysis,[41] and I continue to maintain that this analysis is inappropriately applied to any of the four cases.[42]

It seems that Finnis has settled upon a conclusion that legislation in each of the four cases he has presented can be supported, though the argument leading to that conclusion is uncertain. He switches between a (new) "legal analysis" and a (changing) "intention and side-effect" action theory, depending on the particular case he is addressing. His lack of consistency and non-identification of a principle that is applicable to all cases suggests, to me, a fundamental flaw in his whole argument.[43]

---

[40] Many people believe *EV* 73 authorizes votes for *Case 1* proposals. Fewer are willing to accept the possibility that *EV* 73 authorizes votes for *Case 2* proposals. To my knowledge, however, nobody has claimed that *EV* 73 authorizes votes for *Case 3* (or *Case 4*) proposals. It is unclear whether Finnis believes *EV* 73 authorizes such votes.

[41] Harte, sec 5.1, pp. 196–199.

[42] In his 1994 paper, Finnis said that pro-life legislators voting for the "16 week" law should explain that they are not choosing to abandon the pre-16 week babies, "nor trading them off as the price of saving the post-16 week babies" (p. 602). One can reasonably ask whether such "trade offs" are implicit in such "16 week" *Case 1* proposals. At any rate, a *Case 3* proposal which includes not only prohibitions, but also some new (even if limited) permissions, seems a definite case of a "trade off." It would seem that either *Case 3* proposals involve "trade offs" (and, therefore, would be ruled out by Finnis' other remarks), or Finnis' concept of intention is so broad that "trade off"considerations need never apply (which makes his 1994 remarks irrelevant).

[43] Given that Finnis maintains the "intention and side-effect" argument still applies to *Case 3* (and, one assumes, to *Case 4*) proposals, it is surprising that he did not stay with this argument for *Case 1* proposals. If he had done this he could have avoided committing himself to what would appear to be an "impossible position" of maintaining that *Case 1* proposals are just. *Case 2* proposals, however, appear not to fit at all into an "intention and side-effect" analysis, and only fit Finnis' "legal analysis" if one accepts his notion of the changing "baseline."

1.4. *Cooperation, rescuing and lawmaking*

Associated with his "intention and side-effect" analysis, the principles of "cooperation" were central to Finnis' former argument, but now they are "not important."[44] It would seem to be disingenuous for Finnis to claim that his previous "references to cooperation were by way of concession, made in order to show that *even if* [sic.] there is cooperation...." Why should Finnis regard this as a concession, and to whom is it a concession? Finnis' cooperation analysis was *his own argument*, an argument promoted without such qualification in his earlier papers.

Finnis' "cooperation" argument, promoted in his 1994 paper, preceded the publication of *Evangelium Vitae* in 1995. One of the least satisfactory ways in which Finnis has subsequently promoted or defended the argument is by claiming that it corresponds with the teaching of John Paul II in *EV* 73.[45] In his latest text, Finnis says that "going beyond classical theological ways of using the term,"[46] *EV* 73 regards the question of voting for restrictive legislation as a "cooperation" matter, and he challenges my "discreet silence about *EV* 73's non-traditional language," i.e. with respect to "cooperation."[47] The English, like the Italian, text of *EV* 73 does, of course, mention "cooperation," but the normative and authoritative Latin text omits all mention of "cooperation," as Finnis is aware.[48] The "discreet silence" of the authoritative Latin text on the question of "cooperation" says more than my own, and would seem to indicate, as does Finnis' new argument, that cooperation "is not important for the issue in debate."[49]

Because he now focuses on his new legal analysis, Finnis says "there is strictly no need to attend to the question of cooperation."[50] Finnis does

---

[44] Finnis, p. 242.

[45] Finnis, p. 243. See also his 1997 paper, at p. 269.

[46] Finnis, p. 243.

[47] *Ibid.*

[48] For a fuller account of this point, see Harte, "Challenging a consensus..." (cited in both of our papers) at p. 334. Though he has been made aware of the discrepancy between the normative Latin text and the English version, Finnis continues not only to cite the faulty English text, but, misleadingly, to use it as part of his argument. The English text "This does not in fact represent an illicit cooperation with an unjust law," reads in the Latin: "Hac enim agendi ratione officium suum non praestat illicitae vel iniustae legi." There is no mention of "cooperation." In footnote 16 Finnis observes, correctly, that *Evangelium Vitae* was drafted in Italian. However, the Italian text does not have "an authority" not shared by texts such as the English. As it is the language of the original draft, it is of particular interest, but the authoritative text is the Latin.

[49] Finnis, p. 242.

[50] Finnis, p. 243.

not address the points I made against his "cooperation" argument, and does not even explain what he had meant by his "cooperation" argument. Rather, he devotes most of his section on cooperation to addressing my point that an *adverse implication* of his argument is that it would be illegitimate to ask, or to put pressure upon, those legislators who are not in fact pro-life to vote for (unjust[51]) restrictive legislation, because (according to his analysis) they would be *doing evil*. To answer my point, Finnis turns to analogy, comparing legislators with soldiers on a mission to rescue Jews and gypsies (pp. 244–245). Earlier in his paper he had presented other "rescue" analogies, speaking of firemen rescuing some but not all people in a burning building (p. 240), and a group of 20 stalwarts rescuing many, but not all, children from a desert torture camp (p. 234). Such "rescuing" analogies have frequently been cited by pro-life campaigners – though rarely in print and, as far as I am aware, never as part of a serious academic argument. Though they may seem appealing, such analogies should be resisted, especially as there is a danger (to which Finnis appears to have succumbed) of regarding "rescuing" not simply as analogous but as descriptive of the legislator's action.[52] Legislators are either fulfilling a responsibility of *enacting law* (a basic presupposition of which is that the right to life of all is fundamental and not subject to negotiation or compromise) or they are *rescuing* (an action, which like all such human actions, depends on the circumstances so that it cannot be said that there is "a strong obligation to rescue each and every person in the

---

[51] I acknowledge that Finnis believes the legislation is not unjust, and my disagreement with him on this point is a key difference in our views. By describing the restrictive legislation here as "unjust," my purpose is to distinguish it from other legislation which may restrict abortion (e.g. by prohibiting the production or distribution of abortion-inducing drugs like RU486) without being unjust.

[52] Finnis speaks of "rescuing" not solely by way of analogy, but as if pro-life legislators themselves are "rescuers": "the correct answer to the problem is that voting Yes, to rescue those babies who can be rescued, is..." (p. 213, fn. 7); "With a few ungrounded exceptions... [Harte] rules out any and every attempt to rescue the unborn through law unless all are to be rescued, even though the limitations on the rescue result entirely from the unjust will of a sub-group within the larger group willing and able to mount a rescue..." (p. 235); "I have spoken of the pro-life legislator's vote for just restrictive legislation as 'material cooperation' in the continuing legislative failure to rescue those who should be rescued" (p. 243). "By condemning his hypothetical Proposal B as intrinsically unjust, [Harte] accepts that the 197,000 whom it would rescue must be left to die with the 3,000 whom – through no fault or omission of pro-lifers – it would fail to rescue" (p. 235, fn. 48). This last point seems particularly noteworthy. Proposal B either is or is not intrinsically unjust, and whether it is does not depend upon whether I or anyone else has "condemned" it to be. It almost seems as though Finnis has decided to label Proposal B "just" in order to "rescue" those babies who would be protected by it.

building" – as Finnis says of the firemen[53] – but rather, there must be "an attempt to rescue every child *that it is within our power to rescue*" – as Finnis says of the child rescuers[54]). The problem of "rescuing" analogies, and of regarding votes for restrictive legislation under the paradigm of "rescuing," requires a fuller treatment than it is possible to give in this short response, but the failure to understand the difference between lawmaking and rescuing is, in my view, largely responsible for the whole problem of voting for restrictive legislation.[55]

2. Some points of contention with Finnis' second thesis

2.1. Over-stating the teaching of EV 73

Finnis argues not only that *EV* 73 authorizes votes for *Case 1* and *Case 2* proposals, but, implausibly, that its few lines articulate "manifestly" and "plainly" and "clear[ly]" virtually all, if not all, of the different strands of his argument.[56] Particularly startling is the claim that his legal analysis, judging restrictive legislation like Proposals A, B and C to be "just," is clearly endorsed by the teaching of *EV* 73, and, what is more, that the teaching of *EV* 73.2 (that it is never licit to obey or vote for an intrinsically unjust law) is the foundation of his argument.[57]

---

[53] Finnis, p. 240.

[54] Finnis, p. 234.

[55] On other disputed questions, such as whether abandoned IVF embryos can be gestated (or "adopted") by a woman who is not the biological mother, there are also wider considerations than those of "rescuing." Whether it is ethical to "adopt" such embryos is not decided by judging the action to be a "rescue," and a judgment that it is ethical to "adopt" does not mean it should be regarded as a "rescue." For some brief remarks on the latter position see John Berkman, "Gestating the Embryos of Others. Surrogacy? Adoption? Rescue?" 3.2 (2003) *National Catholic Bioethics Quarterly*: 309–329, at 323–326.

[56] Finnis says, for example: "*Evangelium Vitae* 73.3 is manifestly intended to ratify what I have called the *dynamic and comparative* analysis of an amending bill or law. Phrase after phrase keep that analysis in the foreground" (p. 219); "In such cases, therefore, so 73.3 plainly teaches, voting for such a bill or new law need not be regarded – and indeed ... *should* not be regarded – as an instance of the kind of act declared by 73.2 to be always impermissible" (*ibid.*); "there is an important element in *EV* 73.3 .... This concerns the baseline against which any bill is to be compared .... For according to *EV* 73.3, the baseline may be ..." (p. 229); "it is one of the evident purposes of *EV* 73.3 to make clear that a statute or other law-making statement does not fall within the class of 'intrinsically unjust' laws mentioned in *EV* 73.2 ..." (p. 233).

[57] Finnis, pp. 209–211.

Two things, says Finnis, should be noticed about *EV* 73.2.[58] The first is that abortion laws typically permit some abortions, whilst prohibiting others, and *EV* 73.2's remarks about "obeying" (or rather, accommodating oneself to[59]) such "intrinsically unjust" laws can, in his view, refer only to the part that "permits" abortions and not to the part that prohibits others; otherwise, he says, police officers or judges could not prevent or punish the abortions the law prohibits. This leads to his conclusion that an abortion law can be unjust *insofar* as it is permissive, but just *insofar* as it is prohibitive.[60] Finnis' remarks do not necessarily reflect what would be the legal situation,[61] but even if they did, it would not follow, I contend, that police officers or judges *appearing to* accommodate themselves to "prohibitive" parts of a law (which, because it also permits abortions, is an intrinsically unjust law), would be acting wrongly; more importantly, it would also not follow that legislators would be entitled to vote to enact such a law to restrict abortion.[62]

---

[58] *EV* 73.2 is the one-sentence paragraph: "In the case of an intrinsically unjust law, such as a law permitting abortion or euthanasia, it is therefore never licit to obey it, or to 'take part in a propaganda campaign in favour of such a law, or vote for it.'"

[59] Finnis has previously noted that, though the English text speaks of "obeying," the Latin text speaks of "accommodating oneself to" an intrinsically unjust law ("eidem se accommodare"). See John Finnis, "Natural Law – Positive Law," in *'Evangelium Vitae' and Law* [Acta Symposii Internationalis in Civitate Vaticana Celebrati, 23–24 Maii 1996]. Vatican City: Libreria Editrice Vaticana 1997, 199–209, at 206.

[60] Finnis, p. 211.

[61] For example, after the enactment of the UK's Abortion Act 1967, police officers or judges attempting to prevent or punish abortions not tolerated by that Act could refer to pre-existing just legislation, and would not be obeying (or accommodating themselves to) the unjust Act itself. The inability of conscientious judges or police officers to prevent or punish abortions tolerated by the 1967 Act would not constitute "obedience" (or accommodation) to it. They should, however, refrain from judgments or activities that would seem to regard the Act's tolerations of abortion to be valid.

[62] The law gets into a terrible mess as soon it fails to protect some lives, especially when this leads to subsequent changes involving different permissions, tolerations or prohibitions. The messy situation now in Poland is that the 1993 Act (like Proposal A) specifies which abortions are prohibited or tolerated. That 1993 law is intrinsically unjust, and no conscientious police officer or judge should uphold as legally valid any abortions tolerated by it. Insofar as the Polish state regards the 1993 Act as a true law and citizens would expect violations of it to be prevented or punished, it seems reasonable and right for conscientious police officers or judges to do *what they are morally able to* in order to prevent or punish abortions. Their actions, understood from their perspectives as acting persons (even if misunderstood by some observers), could be regarded as upholding the moral law *insofar as they are able to*, rather than as obeying or accommodating themselves to the intrinsically unjust positive law. At any rate, the problem for judges or police officers is entirely different from that of legislators faced with a vote of *enacting a law* that permits or tolerates some abortions and is, thus, intrinsically unjust.

Of course, if there are many clauses or articles (i.e. laws) within a single statute (law), it is possible that some will be just and others will be unjust. But this does not mean that the law (i.e. statute) is just *insofar* as *x* and unjust *insofar* as *y*; as an entity it will be *either* just *or* (intrinsically) unjust. And it is precisely this judgment about the entire law which *EV* 73.2 is referring to, and which must be made, before any decision to vote for it.

The second point to be noted, says Finnis, is the quotation within the sentence of *EV* 73.2, taken from the Congregation for the Doctrine of the Faith's 1974 *Declaration on Procured Abortion*. Finnis says: "By making a key part of *EV* 73.2 a quotation, the Pope is indicating that in 73.3 he intends to pass judgment on a matter that for two decades had been causing disputes among Catholics... [and] had been left unsettled by the 1974 declaration...." In *Evangelium Vitae* there are 142 footnote references, and the quotation inserted in *EV* 73.2 is plainly typical of those found in the encyclical and other papal documents in indicating, not what Finnis suggests, but that the present teaching is built upon, and confirms, the authoritative teaching(s) that preceded it. It is worth recalling, not simply the few words from the 1974 *Declaration* quoted in *EV* 73.2, but those words in their fuller context:

> It must in any case be clearly understood that a Christian [*hominem*] can never conform to a law which is in itself immoral, and such is the case of a law which would admit in principle the liceity of abortion [*et hoc accidit, si lex feratur quae principium liceitatis abortus recipiat*]. Nor can a Christian [i.e., *homo*] take part in a propaganda campaign in favour of such a law, or vote for it (n. 22).

Finnis later acknowledges that the 1974 teaching about not conforming to a law "which would admit in principle the liceity of abortion" poses a problem for those contemplating support for restrictive legislation that does "admit in principle the liceity of abortion."[63] Finnis overcomes the difficulty for his view by dismissing the 1974 teaching as "ambiguous" and saying it "finds no counterpart in *EV* 73.2/3."[64] But the partial citation, in *EV* 73.2, of that very passage (i.e., n. 22 from the 1974 *Declaration*) is a strong indication of *the whole passage's* current validity and importance. Finnis seems to pick and choose as he wills: he rejects one clearly stated passage as "ambiguous," overlooks the plain sense of another, and attributes

---

[63] Finnis, p. 219.
[64] Finnis, p. 222, fn. 24.

"meanings" to sections of *EV* 73 that are known to nobody apart from himself.[65] It is simply not credible that *EV* 73, published in 1995, was intended to have the precise meaning that Finnis is now suggesting, when his legal analysis and some of the other arguments that he claims are "manifestly" present in the teaching have emerged, for the first time, eight years later in 2003.[66]

2.2. The CDF and EV 73

To support his argument, Finnis presents a series of statements and judgments made in the years prior to the publication of *Evangelium Vitae*. Some of these are a matter of indisputable historic fact; others fail to support the case he is trying to present.[67] Of more significance, however, are two recent documents, not mentioned by Finnis, from the Congregation for the Doctrine of the Faith (CDF), which bear directly on what is taught in *EV* 73. The first, the CDF's *Doctrinal Note on some Questions regarding the*

---

[65] A notably cryptic remark is to be found on p. 232, at fn. 42, where Finnis suggests that *EV* 73.3 warns readers of *EV* 73.2 of something.

[66] As has been noted, Finnis' 1994 paper was given at the CDF symposium addressing the question of "imperfect legislation." According to the volume of the symposium proceedings, nobody (including Finnis: see fn. 12, above) gave any indication of the sort of argument he is now presenting as justifying votes for restrictive abortion legislation. See Joseph Joblin and Réal Tremblay (eds), *I Cattolici e la Società Pluralista: Il Caso delle 'Leggi Imperfette'*. Bologna: Edizione Studio Domenicano 1996. Finnis' elaborate account of the detailed argument that he says is contained within *EV* 73 should be compared with Robert George's more realistic acknowledgement that "the Pope does not provide an extensive argument in behalf of his teaching" (see above, fn. 22). In my view, it is entirely implausible that, when approving *EV* 73 in 1995, the Pope had in mind the detailed analysis that Finnis is now presenting as the key to understanding *EV* 73, when there is no evidence that anyone (including the Pope) had that analysis in mind before its appearance in Finnis' paper of 2003. And it seems highly unlikely that the Pope would have taught something, in an authoritative encyclical letter, on such a disputed and momentous subject, if neither he nor anyone else had previously known the argument underlying what was being taught.

[67] For example, he refers at pp. 213–214 to a letter written by Cardinal Ratzinger in May 1982, part of which was cited in a 1989 article. Finnis says the letter was "implicitly accepting the moral permissibility" of voting for a particular amendment, but an unbiased reading of what is cited shows that Ratzinger was merely stating the relevant principles, leaving it (as would be quite proper) for the US bishops to apply the principles to their particular problem and to make *their* judgment. Clearly, Ratzinger does not impose a judgment on them. There is nothing in Ratzinger's statement of the principles with which I disagree.

Participation of Catholics in Political Life, dated 24 November 2002, says:

> As John Paul II has taught in his Encyclical Letter *Evangelium vitae* regarding the situation in which it is not possible to overturn or completely repeal a law allowing abortion which is already in force or coming up for a vote, "an elected official, whose absolute personal opposition to procured abortion was well known, could licitly support proposals aimed at lessening its negative consequences at the level of general opinion and public morality." [*EV* 73.3]
>
> In this context it must be noted also that a well-formed Christian conscience does not permit one to vote for a political program or an individual law which contradicts the fundamental contents of faith and morals ... (n. 4).

"In this context" refers precisely to what preceded it, i.e. the very situation considered in *EV* 73.3. In *this* context one is not permitted to vote for "a political program or an individual law which contradicts the fundamental contents of faith and morals." Does my Proposal A or the 1993 Polish abortion law constitute a law that contradicts the fundamental content of faith and morals? I say yes. Does the sort of "political program" mentioned in the text refer to the sort of *Case 4* proposal (the omnibus budget bill) presented by Finnis? I say yes. If Finnis' understanding of what is allowed by *EV* 73.3 were correct, the CDF's remarks would be entirely unnecessary and irrelevant, because, according to Finnis' analysis, legislators could vote for anything that was "restrictive," or generally regarded as "desirable", without being charged with supporting a law that was unjust (or, equally, a political program or an individual law which contradicts the fundamental contents of faith and morals). Finnis' analysis negates any purpose to the CDF's remarks, yet the CDF presents them as something that "must be noted."

The second document from the CDF, *Considerations Regarding Proposals to Give Legal Recognition to Unions between Homosexual Persons*, dated 3 June 2003, says:

> When legislation in favour of the recognition of homosexual unions is already in force, the Catholic politician must oppose it in the ways that are possible for him and make his opposition known; it is his duty to witness to the truth. If it is not possible to repeal such a law completely, the Catholic politician, recalling the indications contained in the Encyclical Letter *Evangelium vitae*, "could licitly support proposals aimed at limiting the harm done by such a law and at lessening its negative consequences at the

level of general opinion and public morality", on condition that his "absolute personal opposition" to such laws was clear and well known and that the danger of scandal was avoided [*EV* 73.3]. This does not mean that a more restrictive law in this area could be considered just or even acceptable; rather, it is a question of the legitimate and dutiful attempt to obtain at least the partial repeal of an unjust law when its total abrogation is not possible at the moment (n. 10).

After citing the teaching of *EV* 73.3 (that legislators can support proposals aimed at limiting the harm, etc.) the CDF comment is: "This does not mean that a restrictive law in this area could be considered just or even acceptable." Is this saying that legislators are allowed to vote for a restrictive law even though it *cannot be regarded as just* or acceptable? If it is, then the CDF would essentially be saying that it agrees with Finnis' conclusion that restrictive legislation (like Proposals A, B, C and G) can be supported, whilst rejecting as false his legal analysis that such legislation is just and, consequently, rejecting most of his analysis of *EV* 73.

I think it would be wrong, however, to believe that that is what the document is saying. The only sorts of proposals mentioned in the CDF's remarks, after the teaching of *EV* 73 is cited, are those referring to "the partial *repeal* of an unjust law." My paper judged votes for Proposals D, E, and F – proposals to repeal unjust law[68] – to be legitimate. The CDF document only mentions proposals that *repeal* an unjust law (with the question of repeal being precisely understood, and not called – or treated equivalently to – amendment, or anything else) and it is legitimate to support such proposals even though, after the partial repeal of an unjust law, there is in place a more restrictive law which can be considered neither just nor acceptable, and (crucially) which *has not been voted for* in the specifically focused proposal of repeal. Any document must be internally consistent, and just as any interpretation of *EV* 73 must be rejected that contradicts any other part of the encyclical, so too must interpretations of difficult passages be understood with respect to clearly articulated principles, like the one expressed in the 2003 *Considerations*: "Every humanly-created law is legitimate insofar as it is consistent with the natural moral law, recognized by right reason, and insofar as it respects the inalienable rights of every person" (n. 6).

---

[68] Each of Proposals D, E, and F can be labelled, without any contradiction, either a "proposal repealing unjust law" or a "proposal partially repealing unjust law." Insofar as what is repealed is "unjust law," there is a (full) repeal of unjust law; insofar as there is unjust law that is not repealed by the proposal, the repeal can be regarded as partial.

One notes too that on the two occasions it cites *EV* 73, the CDF cites only the part that I, too, have presented as the "teaching" and not the part describing the "problem of conscience" which John Finnis maintains is so crucial for understanding its (or, rather, his own) "dynamic and comparative analysis."[69]

2.3. Poland and EV 73

Concluding Section 2 on "the meaning and logic of *EV* 73.3," Finnis refers to events in the Pope's "much loved homeland" (i.e. the passing of Poland's 1993 law) as indicative of the correctness of his interpretation.[70] The facts, however, do not support his contention, not least because even those leading politicians who sided with Finnis in thinking that the 1993 law could be supported (and many others, it must be noted, did not) have given reasons for their support which Finnis would find wholly objectionable.[71]

Finnis is right, however, to look towards Poland as a source for understanding the meaning of *EV* 73, and the obvious place to look is the Catholic University of Lublin (KUL), where Karol Wojtyła held the position of Chair of Ethics for 22 years before his election in 1978 as Pope. No university compares with KUL in the contribution that has been made to understanding and promoting the thought of Wojtyła/John Paul II. And it may

---

[69] Finnis' remarks about the "dynamic and comparative analysis" are linked to his claim that I have ignored "entirely the Holy See's long tradition of teaching by answering questions whose terms are carefully devised or refined by the answer so as to define the answer's meaning and purport" (p. 220). This is yet another disputable assertion. For example, in *Humanae Vitae* Paul VI describes the problem of conscience as it was then being presented (*HV* 2) and asks whether it might be resolved by an application of the 'principle of totality' (*HV* 3). Perhaps this might induce the reader to think that the analysis was "dynamic and comparative" and clearly indicated that contraception was about to be approved. But the teaching of *HV*, like that of *EV* 73, is not the part expressed as the problem of conscience, but *the response* that is given – which did not approve the action that was the subject of the question.

[70] Finnis, p. 220.

[71] To my knowledge, no Polish politician or academic has presented the sort of analysis Finnis has given as justifying votes for the 1993 law. Finnis would entirely disagree with the views expressed in my paper by leading Polish politicians that the 1993 law tolerated or legalized abortions, or that the law could be supported as a "compromise." See Harte, p. 191, fn. 21. (Finnis denies that pro-life legislators are compromising (p. 237, fn. 50). However, he suggests, puzzlingly, that the "moderate" abortion-favouring legislators, *who are voting for what they believe in*, are compromising in their support for the restrictive legislation (see p. 240, fn. 56 and p. 244).) The Pope has never expressed any public support for the 1993 law, and, to my knowledge, he gave no informal advice that it was licit to vote for the bill that was finally enacted.

reasonably be assumed that amongst those who best understand the Pope's thinking are Professor Fr Tadeusz Styczeń SDS (who succeeded Wojtyła as Chair of Ethics in 1978) and Professor Fr Andrzej Szostek MIC (currently Rector at KUL), who have been singled out by the Pope as his "closest collaborators and disciples."[72]

In summer 2003, KUL made a notable contribution to the understanding of *EV* 73 by publishing (in Polish) an issue of its journal, *Ethos*, addressing the question of the meaning of *EV* 73. Whilst it includes papers representing both "sides" of the argument (including Finnis' 1994 paper, and my "Challenging a Consensus..." paper), the majority of papers, including all those written by Lublin philosophers – Styczeń and Szostek among them – broadly favour my view.[73] The issue of *Ethos* is entitled: "Imperfect Laws or Unjust Laws?"[74] There is no suggestion in the title or in any of the papers (from those of either side) that the restrictive laws are, as Finnis now claims, *just* laws.[75] The issue of *Ethos* rightly regards Finnis' paper, and the opinion of others who share his view, as worthy of serious consideration; however, it greatly undermines Finnis' claim that *EV* 73 teaches precisely what he says it teaches. If the teaching of *EV* 73 is as "clear" and "manifest" as Finnis has argued, it is inconceivable that the Pope's closest collaborators and disciples should either (a) ignorantly misunderstand it and promote a different view, or (b) deliberately and openly dissent from what has been authoritatively taught.

3. The opening up of a discussion

As I have noted, Finnis' paper has acknowledged flaws in his previous argument and introduced some notable arguments that have never before arisen

---

[72] John Paul II, *Crossing the Threshold of Hope*. London: Jonathan Cape 1994, 209.

[73] Supporting Finnis' "side" of the argument are papers by Archbishop Tarcisio Bertone SDB and Fr Angel Rodriguez Luño. Supporting my "side" of the argument are papers by Arthur F Utz OP, Claudio Vitelli, Damian Fedoryka, Alison Davis, and Lublin philosophers: Janusz Nagórny, Jarosław Merecki SDS, Barbara Chyrowicz SSpS, Andrzej Szostek MIC, and Tadeusz Styczeń SDS. Though I speak broadly of two "sides" of the argument, there are some differences of opinion between writers on each of the two sides.

[74] "Prawo Niedoskonałe Czy Niesprawiedliwe?" 61–62 (2003) *Ethos*.

[75] I assume that Finnis gave permission for his paper to be translated into Polish and published (as I did for mine). It is remarkable that he should have given permission, fairly recently, for the re-publication of a paper which promotes an argument that he now acknowledges to be deficient, without, at least, indicating, in the re-published text, its deficiencies. It suggests that Finnis' new legal analysis has been devised since Finnis gave permission for the re-publication of his 1994 paper.

in discussions on the *EV* 73 question. Whilst expressing my disagreement with much of Finnis' argument, my response has not attempted to answer fully each of his points but has tried, rather, to indicate some questions that require particular consideration, such as: Is restrictive legislation, like Proposals A, B, C and G, or Poland's 1993 law, just or unjust? What is the "baseline" from which one judges whether *Case 1* and *Case 2* proposals are just? Is it ever licit to vote for intrinsically unjust proposals? Are *Case 3* and *Case 4* proposals just, and, if not, can they be licitly supported? Is an "intention and side-effect" analysis – by means of which legislators might be said to vote not for "the whole" of a bill but only the parts they "intend" to support – legitimate or fundamentally flawed? Are traditional principles of "cooperation" relevant to the question, and if so, how are they properly applied? Are legislators voting for restrictive legislation "lawmaking" or "rescuing"? There are further matters, raised by Finnis' paper, which limitation of space has prevented me commenting upon in this response, and which lead to further questions, such as: Can a law be judged "intrinsically unjust" if enacted by a sole ruler, but "just" if enacted by a group of lawmakers (such as members of a legislative assembly or the populace in a referendum)? Do votes for restrictive legislation involve "compromise" and, if so, who is compromising and is it legitimate? These are just some of the questions that have been raised by our discussion.

On the one hand, Finnis' paper suggests that nothing is open to discussion and that all relevant considerations are addressed in the teaching of *EV* 73. On the other, his paper has introduced some new arguments which, by virtue of their very novelty, require further consideration and discussion. The opinion of the Lublin philosophers seems to concur with mine that there is in fact much more that needs to be discussed, not only about the precise meaning of *EV* 73 but also about the ethics of voting for restrictive abortion legislation. Notwithstanding the fact that Finnis and I maintain that our conflicting interpretations "fit" what is taught and are appropriate and correct, the precise meaning of *EV* 73, being subject to such dispute, cannot be regarded as clear. Far from being the last word on the question, *EV* 73's value may well be that it has helped to open up such an important and necessary discussion.

14

"A vote decisive for... a *more* restrictive law"

John Finnis

1. Introduction

Colin Harte's response remains inattentive both to the nub of the discussion between us, and to the clear intent and meaning of *Evangelium Vitae* 73.

My first paper in this volume, "Restricting legalised abortion..." ("the 2003 paper"), showed how *EV* 73.3 ratifies nearly two decades of episcopal teachings embracing what I call a "comparative" analysis of the circumstances and potential object of a legislator's vote. Where the vote, as *EV* 73.3 puts it, "would be decisive for the passage of *a more restrictive* law... *in place of* a more permissive law already passed or ready to be voted on" – one that "it is not possible to overturn or completely abrogate" – then the vote can be "legitimate and proper [*doveroso* – a matter of duty]".[1] To spell out what is involved in this sort of comparison, I spoke of "baselines". Take a bill stating that abortion is permitted up to 5 weeks and prohibited after 5 weeks. The baseline for this change might be existing law prohibiting all abortion. In that case, the bill is simply one for "a law permitting abortion", and can never be supported (*EV* 73.2). But a bill with identical wording might be introduced from the different baseline of a law permitting abortion up to (say) 24 weeks. In that case, the bill when enacted *does nothing except prohibit* abortion between 5 and 24 weeks. It neither introduces any permission nor continues in force any permission which would otherwise have expired. In what it does, it (a) is untainted by any inherent injustice, (b) is not "a law permitting abortion" in the sense of *EV* 73.2's use of that phrase, and (c) can in many circumstances be supported, even though the law of the land will still, after the reform effected

---

[1] All emphases in quotations are by me, unless otherwise indicated.

by the bill's enactment, remain seriously unjust in permitting abortion up to 5 weeks.

My use of the metaphor "baselines" is, I think, sufficiently clear. It is nothing more than a shorthand for the fact that comparisons can have different comparators. One and the same bill may have to be compared with a more permissive law (baseline A), or, in a different time and place, with a less permissive law (baseline B). Depending on the baseline, the necessary comparative analysis differs in result. Against baseline A, the bill can be judged supportable. Against baseline B it will necessarily be unjust and insupportable.[2]

It goes without saying that the *standard* of or *measure* for the comparison is not the baseline but the *moral norm* constantly upheld by the Church and reaffirmed in *Evangelium Vitae*, which demands that the protection of the law of the state against homicide include the unborn with the born. That moral norm entails that a bill whose effect is to permit abortion is unjust and cannot be supported. Whether a bill has that effect, however, can only be determined by comparing it with the baseline, the existing law.[3]

Colin Harte has misunderstood all this. Proclaiming that the "the baseline is the natural moral law", he asserts that my talk of different baselines "gives weight to the charge that" I embrace situation ethics. That is a false ethics, condemned by the Church, and contested in my writings for decades, as false to the natural moral law.[4] Sensible discussion is impossible when participant B makes participant A's words mean what B wants them to mean, not what A plainly meant by them. Harte is free to say that the baseline

---

[2] There are other, more complex baselines, *e.g.* where the existing law is a dead letter, and is about to be replaced by one or other of two specific proposals, "ready to be voted on". In such a situation, as *EV* 73.3 plainly implies, it is possible that the real baseline is the more permissive of the two proposals.

[3] More precisely, it can only be determined by comparing the set of prohibitory or permissive propositions legally true before the enactment with the set of prohibitory or permissive propositions legally true after that enactment.

[4] See particularly John Finnis, *Moral Absolutes* (Washington, DC: Catholic University of America Press 1991). The claim stated in Harte's talk (fn. 36) of "Finnis' promotion of situation-relative baselines, *as opposed to* the firm baseline of the natural law" is mere calumny. Moreover, as Harte is well aware, the notion of situation-relative baselines is at the heart of *EV* 73.3's teaching about "cases where a legislative vote would be decisive for the passage of a more restrictive law ... in place of a more permissive law *already passed or ready to be voted on* ...." The polemic in his papers against Finnis, promoter of a long-condemned ethics, only thinly veils Harte's interest in what seems his real target, the magisterium whose carefully meditated (and since reiterated) resolution of a long-disputed question in *EV* 73 he declares is "far from being the last word on the question", and has for him precisely this "value": "that it has helped to open up such an important and necessary discussion" (the one in which Colin Harte is prime discussant). That is his final sentence, and perhaps the most revealing statement in all his papers.

for judging laws and bills is the natural moral law, and in the sense in which he is using the term "baseline" that is a correct proposition. He is not free to assert or presume that that was how I (in line with a common scholarly jargon) was using the term "baseline(s)".[5]

Nor is he free to use the Church's documents in a manner which conceals the fact that they use (in my jargon) a "comparative" and "baselines" analysis. But that is what he does in his response. Confronted by the CDF's June 2003 document about homosexual unions, deploying just such an analysis, Harte quotes no less than thirteen lines of that analysis but entirely omits the sentences, in the very same passage, with which the CDF makes it clear that the moral judgment can and should differ *according as the baselines differ.* Here is the relevant passage from section 10 of the CDF's 2003 document, with my explicatory jargon inserted in brackets:

> When legislation in favour of the recognition of homosexual unions is proposed for the first time in a legislative assembly [= *baseline 1*], the Catholic law-maker has a moral duty to express his opposition clearly and publicly and to vote against it. To vote in favour of a law so harmful to the common good is gravely immoral.
>
> When legislation in favour of the recognition of homosexual unions is already in force [= *baseline 2*], the Catholic politician must oppose it in the ways that are possible for him.... If it is not possible to repeal such a law completely, the Catholic politician, recalling the indications contained in... *Evangelium Vitae,* "could licitly support proposals aimed at limiting the harm done by such a law and at lessening its negative consequences at the level of general opinion and public morality", on condition that "his absolute personal opposition" to such laws was clear and well known and that the danger of scandal was avoided.[6]

---

[5] He constructs (fn. 29) a paraphrase-with-selective-quotation to make me seem to speak like him: "For Finnis, the baseline is the standard 'against which any bill or amending statute is to be compared... [*etc., etc.*]'". But the phrase "is the standard" has been inserted by him, and has no counterpart in the sentence he purports to be quoting and paraphrasing. Such mishandling of texts is frequent in Harte's writings on these matters.

[6] The passage continues: "This does not mean that a more restrictive law in this area could be considered just or even acceptable; rather it is a question of the legitimate and dutiful attempt to obtain at least the partial repeal of an unjust law when its total abrogation is not possible at the moment." The first nineteen words correspond to my statement, above, that "the law of the land will, after the reform effected by the bill's enactment, still remain seriously unjust in permitting abortion up to 5 weeks." See further sec. 9 below.

Harte has suppressed the first two sentences. This omission is part and parcel of his failure, in each of his two papers in this volume, either to take seriously *EV* 73.3 *as a whole* (and as following immediately on *EV* 73.2), or to face up to the sequence of episcopal teachings which *EV* 73.3 tacitly ratifies. The failure is a failure to advert to the comparative or baselines analysis characteristic of all those teachings.

Astoundingly, Harte claims that "the standard view (of those who share Finnis' general interpretation of *EV* 73.3) has been that the teaching of *EV* 73.3 is *by way of exception* to the prohibition of voting for intrinsically unjust laws taught in *EV* 73.2." (Those who share my general interpretation include, as he concedes, not only the archbishop who was at the relevant times Secretary of the CDF, but also the theologian whose study of the relevant issues was recently published at length in *L'Osservatore Romano*.) Harte identifies only one person as holding or even mentioning this alleged "standard view", Leslie C. Griffin – who notoriously dissents from the Church's position on a number of related moral matters[7] – writing a foolish critique of *EV* 73 in a book of essays of proportionalist cast.[8] Proportionalists (situation ethicists) commonly imagine that the Church's specific moral teachings are wholly or largely a matter of ecclesiastical legislation ("rules", "prohibitions", "bans", which we are "supposed to" follow) to which Church "rulings" can make exceptions. But that is opposed to the moral doctrine reiterated by John Paul II, and to everything I have written on ethics over the past forty years. The idea that *EV* 73.2, teaching that one may *never* support or vote for intrinsically unjust laws (including laws

---

[7] See Leslie C. Griffin, "Good Catholics Should be Rawlsian Liberals". 5 (1997) *Southern California Interdisciplinary Law Journal*: 297; "The Problem of Dirty Hands". 17 (1980) *Journal of Religious Ethics*: 31–61; "American Catholic Sexual Ethics 1789–1989", in Charles Curran and Richard McCormick (eds), *Dialogue about Catholic Sexual Teaching: Readings in Moral Theology No. 8*. New York: Paulist Press 1993: 453–484; Charles Curran and Leslie Griffin (eds), *The Catholic Church, Morality and Politics: Readings in Moral Theology No. 12*. New York: Paulist Press 2001.

[8] Kevin Wm. Wildes SJ and Alan C. Mitchell, *Choosing Life: A Dialogue on* Evangelium Vitae. Washington DC: Georgetown Univeristy Press 1997: 159–173 at 170. The quality of Griffin's discussion can be seen from the following excerpts from her conclusions about *EV* 73 (*ibid.*, 171). Her exposition of the encyclical's teaching: "*Evangelium Vitae* forsakes the natural law and asks Catholic politicians to enact a theological teaching into law... [and] impose the Church's teaching on non-Catholics. For pragmatic reasons, Catholics may vote for less restrictive abortion laws when their absolute ban on abortion cannot be passed. Catholics may vote only to restrict abortion rights or to ban abortion altogether.... Moral error has no rights." Her own position: "*Evangelium Vitae* imposes a theological doctrine upon the Church's faithful, but theological doctrine should not be imposed on non-Catholics by the state and politicians, not even by Catholic politicians." And so forth.

permitting abortion), might be immediately followed in 73.3 by an *exception* (= not never) is outlandish. Harte's claim that this idea is a standard view shows how far he is from understanding the encyclical, or the most authoritative and "standard" commentaries on it, or those who like Robert George and me and other more authoritative writers defend its moral teachings.[9]

Harte thinks (fn. 43) it is "impossible" for *Case 1* proposals, like those adopted in Poland in 1993, to be anything other than unjust. The supposed impossibility is an illusion. The law of Poland about abortion, as it exists since reformed in 1993, is *gravely unjust* insofar as it permits abortion, and at the same time is *just* insofar as it prohibits many kinds of abortion that before 1993 were legally permitted and – by virtue of general principles of Polish law presupposed by, but not articulated in, the 1993 statute – would remain permitted to this day but for the enactment of the 1993 proposals. Those proposals introduced into Polish law (i.e. the whole set of propositions of law applicable in Poland) nothing but new prohibitions, all of them just. That is why the proposals embodying those new prohibitions were not contrary to the truth subsequently articulated in *EV* 73.2, and could rightly be voted for even though they failed to introduce as many pro-

---

[9] [In the light of this paragraph, Harte has added a footnote withdrawing the claim that the standard view treats *EV* 73.3 as articulating an exception to *EV* 73.2. (See p. 252 above.) That is welcome, but the footnote muddies the waters yet again by raising another issue, namely, whether it is the "standard view" that the proposals which *EV* 73.3 says can rightly be voted for are to be "described as unjust". He concedes that the "reputable writers" I mentioned in the above paragraph do so describe such proposals, and that that description is also "commonly expressed in informal discussions". But he then remarks that, nevertheless, "I [Harte] accept that the frequent expression of an opinion does not make it a standard view" – as if I was objecting to calling *standard* the view of these reputable writers (that such proposals are unjust). But the fact is that these writers, *like me* and (I imagine) most if not all who speak to Harte in informal discussions, describe such proposals *both as unjust, and as just.* And they can do so without contradiction for the reasons set out in both my present papers (see for example the next paragraph in this one). Proposals of this kind are unjust in what they *say* is permissible, and against a different baseline of law they would be unjust in what they legally do. Considered as statements of policy, independent of the context created by existing law, they articulate a very unjust policy. No-one who had the power to introduce into law a wider prohibition could justly be content with proposing only the limited prohibition spoken of in these proposals. But in relation to the kind of context (baseline) identified in *EV* 73.3, they do not in fact or in law *introduce any permission or maintain any permission that would otherwise have expired*, but instead *introduce new and just prohibitions of abortion.* So they are just in all they do, and therefore, despite appearances, in all that they propose to do in the adverse circumstances which prevent their just proposers from doing all that justice requires.]

hibitions as justice requires, and even though at the level of words they articulated various (unjust) permissions and/or tolerations (marking the boundaries, so to speak, of the prohibitions). Some of those who voted for the 1993 proposals were acting morally uprightly, having made it plain that only the recalcitrance of their fellow legislators (if not also of constitutional judges) prevented them from enacting the wider prohibitions which justice requires. Others of those who promoted and voted for the 1993 proposals were acting morally wrongly insofar as their stance included their persistence in blocking the adoption of those wider prohibitions. That is the obvious way to read and apply *EV* 73.3, giving full weight to *EV* 73.2's condemnation of voting for unjust laws (including laws that permit abortion), and bearing in mind that the encyclical was published in the aftermath of the 1993 reforms in Poland. It is utterly improbable that a Polish pope who thought (like Harte) that the 1993 proposals *could not* be rightly voted for would have published *EV* 73.3, in which not even one phrase hints at that thought.

At the root of Harte's mistaken arguments is his failure to grasp that the phrase "a law permitting abortion" in *EV* 73.2 is not self-explanatory, and that the most authoritative resource for understanding and interpreting it correctly is *EV* 73.3, each of these two paragraphs being taken in the light of the other.

2. The Principle and the Primary and the Secondary Arguments

What I have said in section 1 is really all that need be said in response to Harte's reply. The issue is what the Church teaches and reason confirms and explains, not what I have said or not said in the past. Still, since Harte distorts, misstates, and misunderstands my writings as much as he distorts and misunderstands the teachings of the magisterium, I shall attempt some further clarifications.

Implying that my position is different from his (and the Church's) on the point of fundamental principle, Harte says (sec. 3) that one of the points under discussion between us is *"Is it ever licit to vote for intrinsically unjust proposals?"* But that is a question which my 2003 paper unambiguously answered six times. The summary at the head of the paper affirms "the true principle that permissive abortion laws are intrinsically unjust and may never be voted for". (I shall call this the Principle.) The headline of the paper's first paragraph is "Permissive abortion laws are unjust and never to be voted for." The first sentence itself quotes *EV* 73.2, and says it will be the foundation of my reflections: "In the case of an intrinsically unjust law, such as a law permitting abortion..., it is... never... licit to... vote for it." The last sentence of section 2 refers to "the seriously immoral act of voting for a bill or law unjust by its very nature."[10] In section 4, I recall "*EV* 73.2's principle that one must never vote for a permissive [abortion] law",[11] and in section 6 it is referred to, with emphasis, as "the *true principle* that *one must never vote for a permissive abortion law*".[12]

My 1994/6 paper already stated the same position and affirmed the Principle. Having defined "support" as including casting a final vote *for*, I said (with emphases): "I take for granted that *supporting the making of legal permission of abortion (at any stage of pregnancy) a part of the law* and *supporting the retaining of such permission as part of the law*[13] are intrinsically evil acts incapable of being justified by circumstances and/or intentions or ends or 'proportionate reasons', even 'to reduce the total number of abortions'."[14]

What, then, determines whether a vote is being cast in violation of the Principle? My first paper in this volume argues that there are two main considerations.

The primary question is whether the proposal (proposed bill) itself *permits* – makes permissible – any kind of abortion.[15] "Restricting legalised abortion" is devoted mainly to showing how this question can and must be answered by comparing the proposal with the existing law so as to establish whether or not the proposal introduces any new permission, or continues in being any existing permission which otherwise would have ceased to be in force. The argument shows that many proposals which refer to permission, and appear to institute a permission or to continue and modify one, are

---

[10] "by its very nature" (*sua natura*) is the Latin used in *EV* 73.2 to signify "intrinsically", the word used in all the modern language versions (Italian, French, English, Spanish, Portuguese, *etc.*).

[11] In my papers, a law permits abortion not only if it removes any prohibition of it but also if it "tolerates" it in the sense of Harte's use of that word, *viz*, exempts it from punishment. So the Polish and "Nolandish" laws treating some categories of abortion as not punishable articulate an unjust position and would be unjust laws if they had the *effect* of doing what they say. But against the baseline of the law they replaced, that was not their effect; they did not *introduce* or *cause* any permission, and in that precise sense (needed to reconcile *EV* 73.2 with *EV* 73.3) were and are not permissive.

[12] As I mention in my earlier paper, *EV* 73 uses "law" very broadly (loosely) to refer also to bills and proposals not yet enacted.

[13] Readers will notice that already in 1994 my discussion took for granted that short phrases like "a law permitting abortion" are ambiguous and need to be understood with the kind of precision which the italicised sentence here was attempting to provide, and which my present two papers articulate more fully as the Primary Argument.

[14] Quoted in "Restricting legalised abortion . . ." text at fn. 51.

[15] Here one must recall that not every operation which has the effect of terminating a pregnancy is an abortion in the sense relevant to the judgment of Catholic faith and doctrine. See "Restricting legalised abortion" fn. 4.

actually not doing anything but prohibit. That argument, deployed but too tersely in my 1994/6 and 1997 papers, is the 2003 paper's Primary Argument.

But the 2003 paper also deploys an argument distinguishing what is intended from what is accepted as a side-effect, in casting a vote in relation to a proposal. That Secondary Argument was deployed more fully in my 1994/6 and 1997 papers, and is expressly reaffirmed in "Restricting legalised abortion". Harte's repeated statements that this is an argument which I now acknowledge to be "serious[ly] flaw[ed]", "significantly flawed", etc., are all wrong. The Secondary Argument is not, I believe, flawed. What was flawed was my exposition of the questions at issue, and the flaw was not in using a bad argument, but in failing to articulate sufficiently clearly, and give primacy to, another good argument, what I now call the Primary Argument. What I say in my 2003 paper, and say again, is that in most cases where the Principle is at stake, it is *unnecessary* to deploy the argument from intention *to show that the reform statute in question, considered precisely as changing the law, is not intrinsically unjust.*[16] But the argument distinguishing intention from side-effect, the Secondary Argument, remains correct (and relevant) even where it is not needed for the purpose of testing whether the Principle is being violated. And the Secondary Argument is relevant and needed, as I showed, in two other ways. (i) In all cases of voting for restrictive abortion laws the Secondary Argument is relevant in showing that it is not necessarily unreasonable to cause the bad effects of *seeming* to approve of permitting abortion[17] – the reason being that these bad effects are side-effects and are therefore subject to different moral requirements, strong and demanding but not absolute. (ii) In a few cases (of the kind now labelled by Harte *Case 3* and *Case 4*) the Secondary Argument is relevant also to determining whether a particular act of voting violates the Principle, given that one or more of the provisions of the reform bill or statute is permissive in the *EV* 73.2 sense of "permissive", by repealing or partially

---

[16] Here as always one must bear in mind that the law of the land after the reforming statutes under consideration have taken effect remains gravely unjust to the extent that it continues to contain permissions of abortion.

[17] Harte asks (text at n. 33): "If the law, in a concrete situation, is judged to be just and acceptable, then why should Catholic bishops or anyone else not say that it is acceptable?" The answer is obvious. The justice and acceptability of the proposals in question is entirely relative to the baseline which they replace. That justice and acceptability can and should be affirmed by Catholic bishops. But the *text* of the proposals articulates an unjust position, and so Catholic bishops must take very great care that they not be misunderstood as meaning that what the bill or statute *says* (articulates) *about permissibility or tolerability* is true (or just). (Harte, for one, will go on insisting that that is what they must be meaning – until he sees the point of the Primary Argument – and so will regard them as false teachers. Others of those who similarly misunderstand will regard them as true teachers and so be led into evil.)

repealing an existing prohibition or by continuing in force an existing permission which would otherwise have ceased to be in force.[18]

3. A secondary issue: Why *Case 3* and *Case 4* proposals can sometimes be voted for

"*Case 3*" proposals are proposals with more than one part or provision. One part introduces by clause A a new prohibition of a class (perhaps a vast number) of abortions currently permitted, but another part, clause B, introduces a new permission by repealing the current prohibition of a class (perhaps a tiny number) of abortions. As I stated unambiguously, clause B is unjust. Clause A, however, is just. In this special and rather unusual kind of case, the Secondary Argument becomes of primary importance in showing that legislators can vote for clause A even though their votes will also be counted as a vote for clause B: their intention can be simply to enact clause A, accepting the bad side-effect that their votes will help enact clause B. They are responsible, as we always are, for the bad side-effects, but their responsibility is to be assessed by moral norms more circumstance-relative than the exceptionless negative norms which govern what one *intends*. Nor is it reasonable, or compatible with *EV* 73.2, to argue that *Case 3* must be either just as a whole or unjust as a whole. For if that were so, it would have to be counted as unjust as a whole, and therefore its welcome and beneficial prohibition would have to be counted morally invalid and *never to be obeyed* and no police officer or judge could rightly enforce it.[19] Which would be absurd. The general analysis of propositions of law, in the Primary Argument, shows why it is right, and commonsense, to give the question this answer: a *Case 3* proposal or bill is just in one of its parts and unjust in another.

---

[18] There is also a relevant argument about cooperation in wrongdoing. For if voting for a restrictive abortion law were formal cooperation in the evil acts of those legislators who intend that abortions be permitted and done, it could never be justified. So in earlier papers I included arguments about the nature of the cooperation involved in casting votes for, or counted as for, restrictive proposals. *But Harte agrees that there is no formal cooperation*, and claims that in all the cases we are considering there is not even any material cooperation by pro-life legislators with the acts of the unjust legislators! So arguments about cooperation are simply not relevant *in a debate with him*, and it is odd that he gives them the prominence he does. In setting them aside, I have not abandoned any of my arguments about cooperation, and my concession, in earlier articles, that there is indeed cooperation with the unjust legislators was and remains relevant in debate with those who argue that it is precisely such cooperation that renders the relevant legislative activities of pro-life legislators wrongful.

[19] See the text of "Restricting legalized abortion" in the paragraph which includes fn. 5.

Harte's position is (fn. 42) that in every instance a vote for a *Case 3* proposal involves "trading off" the lives of the babies who will be killed under the new permission in order to save the lives of the babies who will be protected by the new prohibitions. In the *Case 3* scenario that I described,[20] there is no such trading off; the pro-life legislators do no deal in order to secure the votes of other legislators for this or any other measure, or for any other benefit. They simply vote for their own prohibitory proposals, knowing that, as a result of other people's actions, those votes will now have the bad side-effect of counting as support for the obnoxious new permissive proposal tacked onto it against their will by other legislators. They may in some circumstances judge that it would be unfair to incur that bad side-effect. But in other circumstances they may rightly judge that it is not unfair or in any other way wrong to cast the vote that has that bad side-effect. The moral norms applicable to the incurring of side-effects are never exceptionless.[21]

The same goes for *Case 4* proposals.[22] In the real world, such proposals are unlikely to involve provisions changing the criminal law and thus increasing the permissibility of abortions, but rather matters such as the funding of abortions. Still, it is always wrong to support or vote for the funding of abortion, for one who funds wills that the funds be used for successful abortions.[23] The question, then, is whether it is permissible to vote for, say, a budget bill which, besides its funding support for the state's many worthy and necessary activities for the relief of poverty and sickness, includes certain provisions for funding the state's immoral counter-population nuclear deterrent policy and the carrying out of abortions in state facilities. The question is not whether it would be better, all things considered, for pro-life legislators to abstain or vote against the budget: it may often be right and morally necessary for them to do so, in witness to the moral truth which the bad clauses of the budget ignore or defy. The question is whether it is *ever* permissible to vote for the good clauses in the budget, accepting as a bad side-effect that these votes will – as these legislators in voting foresee but do not intend – be counted as also supporting the budget's bad clauses. For the reasons stated above, and in "Restricting legalised abortion", in relation to *Case 3*, it can be.

---

[20] In describing this *Case*, which he ascribes to me, Harte omits features that were important in my account of it, notably that the new permissive provision is not introduced or proposed by the pro-life legislator.

[21] See *Veritatis Splendor* 78–9, 82; Finnis, *Moral Absolutes*, 67–77.

[22] See "Unjust Laws in a Democratic Society". 71 (1996) *Notre Dame Law Review*: 595 at 603 (the main discussion of abortion law is on pp. 599–601).

[23] In discussions with the CDF in 1993/4, I urged the condemnation of all support for the funding of abortions, and that remains my position.

4. Voting for prohibitions on abortion is one way of rescuing unborn babies[24]

Those who are doing what *EV* 73.3 approves, on the conditions that *EV* 73.3 specifies, are doing all they can do, as legislators, to rescue the unborn babies whose abortions they prohibit (by an act of prohibition which would in almost every case[25] be condemned by Colin Harte). Their rescue effort is by means of law-making. Once it is realised that their means of rescue is precisely the making of a prohibitive law more prohibitive than the current law, the commonsense Primary Argument shows – quite independently of the Secondary Argument – that the only proposition of law they *make* is an entirely prohibitive one.[26] So their rescue-effort, so far as it goes, is an entirely just one. Only the bad will of their pro-choice or compromising[27] opponents prevents them carrying out the complete rescue – enacting the completely prohibitory law – which justice demands. Some babies remain unrescued – their abortion remains permitted – but these legislators cannot be morally required to do what is impossible, and so their rescue-effort, despite the limits unjustly imposed upon it by others, remains just.

Harte backs himself into the false dichotomy, legislating or rescuing, because he wants to assert – or at least, to suggest – that "enacting law" is a kind of action which somehow transcends circumstances, whereas "rescuing" is "an action, which like all *such* human actions, depends on the circumstances". The responsibility of rescuers, he rightly says, is only to do what is within their power in the circumstances. But because the right to life is "not subject to negotiation or compromise", the responsibility of legislators, he implies, is not subject to circumstances. But this whole

---

[24] *Cf.* Harte, *Response* 1.4: *"Legislators are either fulfilling a responsibility of enacting law ... or they are rescuing ...* the failure to understand the difference is ... to a large extent responsible for the whole problem of voting for restrictive legislation." Harte gives no hint of a reason for thinking that this blank assertion is not a false alternative, somewhat like "either despatching a helicopter or rescuing".

[25] Harte's approved Proposals D, E, F and H, involving complete repeal of one or more entirely separate provisions of a code, correspond to nothing that I know of or expect to come across in the real world.

[26] This statement applies without qualification in the usual cases, which Harte calls *Cases 1* and *3*. The Secondary Argument shows that in *Case 2* or *4* situations, the only law they need *intend* to make is an entirely prohibitive law, and they can reasonably regard the fact that their vote will be counted as also supporting a new permission as no more (and no less) than a bad side-effect.

[27] Harte (fn. 71) thinks it "puzzling" that I call some or all of these legislators compromising. But there is no puzzle here. Whether or not their vote is in line with their moral opinion, their moral opinion is typically an unstable compromise ("happy mean") between respect for human life in each human person and some kind of "pro-choice" ideology.

position of Harte's is absurd. The moral character, not simply of "all *such* human actions", but rather of every kind of positive human act, every kind of fulfilment of a positive responsibility *to do something*, is subject to the circumstances. To say this is not to deny that the negative responsibility of legislators, *not* to enact unjust laws (including laws permitting abortion), is absolute, exceptionless, not subject to circumstances. In this, it is just like the responsibility of more ordinary rescuers *not* to choose to kill hostages as a means of rescuing others, however many more numerous these may be than the hostages.

5. Is the Primary Argument a new one?

The gist of the Primary Argument is that, as acts or items of law-making, bills and statutes restricting abortion can be entirely just because they do nothing to the law except introduce new prohibitions in place of permissions. Even a bill as repellent in its formulation as my old hypothetical, "Abortion is permitted up to 16 weeks", is not intrinsically unjust if it simply amends (= partially repeals)[28] an existing law which permits abortion up to 24 weeks.

The emphasis that I put on the Primary Argument in the conference paper and in "Restricting legalised abortion" was new. Reflecting on Harte's condemnation of the actions of most pro-life legislators in, for example, his draft conference paper,[29] I had come to think that the Primary Argument deserves to be primary because it captures a part of *what commonsense pro-life legislators*, with some understanding of what law is, *have always taken for granted*. In all usual kinds of case, the restrictive proposals they support do not introduce any permission into the law. Pro-life legislators have always been aware that, given their context and (sometimes) despite their wording, these proposals are in law and in reality *not permissive*. Such a proposal, if enacted, is not "a law permitting abortion" within the meaning of

---

[28] See sec. 8 below.

[29] On the last page of his conference paper itself he said: "my critique of Professor Finnis' argument suggests that the view I am opposing leads to an *abandonment of principle* ... for restrictive abortion legislation typically entails that the *right to life of the most vulnerable* of the unborn – those who are younger, disabled, or conceived after rape or incest – *will be overlooked* in the interest of protecting others. This was the case in Poland in 1993 .... All *votes to enact* the legislation, and not only the legislation itself, *can be judged to be intrinsically unjust* .... The continuation of abortions that could be prevented by unjust restrictive legislation like the Polish law indicates that a high price may be the result of sticking to principle. The abandonment of principle, however, is the abandonment of ethics, which in itself is *an abandonment of humanity*." (emphases added except for "votes to enact"). See sec. 10 below.

EV 73.2. For that reason alone, even apart from distinctions between intention and side-effects, such proposals (bills and statutes) cannot be called intrinsically unjust as that term is used in *EV* 73.2.

But those who take this commonsense approach may find their position hard to articulate when confronted with objections such as Harte's, which take the legal formulae out of their context of amending (by partially repealing) permissive law, and recite the formulae to show that they say something unjust: "abortion is permitted up to 16 weeks"! So it is worthwhile spelling out in full detail, as I did in my 2003 paper "Restricting legalised abortion", just why such objections can and must be rejected as confusions between laws as sets of words and sentences, and laws as propositions made (legally) true by all the sources of law taken together. I do not claim that the spelled-out argument was present to the mind of anyone involved in drafting *EV* 73 or the subsequent CDF documents reiterating the Church's teaching. But the common-sense position which the spelled-out argument does no more than unpack and explicate certainly was.

To see how the spelled-out Primary Argument unpacks thoughts contained both in my 1994 paper and in *EV* 73 itself, not to mention most if not all of the episcopal statements between 1974 and 1995, consider first the central statement in my 1994 paper, already quoted in "Restricting legalised abortion":

> The question *what* one is choosing to support (or not support, or oppose) is also conditioned by context, namely *by the existing legal situation*. For example: a *law* of the form "Abortion is lawful up to 16 weeks" is an unjust law. But a *bill* of the form "Abortion is lawful up to 16 weeks" might either (i) be proposed precisely as introducing a permission of abortions hitherto prohibited, or (ii) be proposed precisely as prohibiting abortions hitherto permitted between 16 and 24 weeks. The choice to support the bill in situation (i) is a substantially different choice from the choice to support the bill in situation (ii). For what is being chosen – the object of the act of supporting the bill – is different in the two cases. In case (i) it is supporting the permission of abortion. In case (ii) it is supporting the prohibition of abortions, indeed of all the abortions (let us suppose) that legislator at that moment has the opportunity of effectively helping to prohibit.

Though calling for some refinement, that statement articulates the substance of the Primary Argument. Its distinction between "a law" and "a bill" needs to be clarified. A more refined and adequate way of expressing it would be: (i) the proposition of law "Abortion is lawful up to 16 weeks" is an unjust (proposition of) law; but (ii) a bill *or statute* which uses the statement

"Abortion is lawful up to 16 weeks" may, depending on the legal context, be either (a) unjustly introducing a new proposition with that content, replacing a current prohibition, or (b) justly prohibiting all abortions currently permitted between 16 and (say) 24 weeks. But this more adequate way of stating the matter does not change the substance of what was being said in the old, less adequate formulation, and introduces nothing novel.[30]

EV 73.3, too, makes best sense (and harmonises most smoothly with 73.2) on the basis that the Primary Argument, though not articulated, is being presupposed. The alternative[31] is to say that *EV* 73.3 relies on the Secondary Argument, which distinguishes between the voting pro-life legislators' intentions and the side-effects of their acts. It might be thought that there is some trace of the Secondary Argument in 73.3's references to "aim", but these are to the aim of the reforming bill/statute rather than of the voting legislator. At most one can say that 73.3 leaves the field open for the Secondary Argument.

So 73.3 must presuppose some reason for judging that its teaching – that it is sometimes acceptable to vote for a bill which reforms permissive abortion law by prohibiting some abortions while more or less expressly leaving others permitted – is consistent with 73.2's teaching that it is never acceptable to vote for a law permitting some abortions. A reading of 73.2/3 as a whole, against the background of the dynamic and comparative or baseline analysis deployed in the episcopal statements from 1974 to 1992, leaves no doubt that its primary presupposition is that the "more restrictive" reform bills which it regards as supportable do not *permit* abortion in the sense of "permit"

---

[30] The common-sense distinction between (a) bills/statutes/laws which are permissive in the sense that their enactment leaves some abortions unprohibited (and/or that they refer to some abortions as permitted) and (b) bills/statutes/laws which are permissive in the sense intended by *EV* 73.2, in that they introduce some legal permission or maintain a legal permission that would otherwise have expired, is also made in my 1997 paper: see fn. 43 below.

[31] To say that this is "the alternative" assumes, of course, that Harte's unhistorical interpretation, presuming contradiction where there is only distinction, is set aside. It is to be observed that he does not repeat (though he does not visibly abandon) his previous Linacre Conference claims about what kind of permissible reforming legislation *EV* 73.3 had in mind, and has made no effort to respond to the arguments proposed in "Restricting legalised abortion" for an interpretation which harmonises all the elements of 73.3 not only with 73.2, but also with the literary methods of the Holy See, with the history of ecclesiastical teaching and pro-life practice from 1974 to 1994, with the CDF's preparatory conference, and with the entire body of interpretation put out with the Holy See's approval since *EV*. To say that "the alternative" to the Primary is the Secondary Argument also assumes, of course, the falsity of Harte's bizarre thought that "standard" interpretations of *EV* 73.3 regard it as stating an *exception* to *EV* 73.2: see sec. 1 above.

intended by 73.2. The fact that the reforming bill/statute expressly or impliedly treats some abortions as still permitted (or even, in the extreme case, states that some abortions are permitted or non-punishable) does not show that the bill/statute *does* anything to the law of the land other than introduce one or more new prohibitions. So 73.3 can be understood correctly as an application of 73.2 (not an exception to it), once 73.2's use of the term "permitting" is understood in the way proposed in the Primary Argument, that is, as referring to acts of cancelling prohibitions by bringing new prohibition-cancelling propositions of law to bear upon on the wider subsisting set of propositions that make up the law of the land.

6. Harte has no tenable argument against the Primary Argument

Only in a footnote (fn. 28) does Harte attempt to meet the Primary Argument deployed in "Restricting legalised abortion." He does so by proposing an alleged analogy.

Recall, yet again, what the Primary Argument says and presupposes. A law, properly understood, is a proposition of law which is valid because, and for as long as, it has the validating kinds of relationship to sources of law such as enactments, customs, judicial application and interpretation, and so forth. The law of the land is the whole set of such propositions of law. Change in the law of the land is made by legislative approval of the introduction of some new proposition or propositions into the set. A legislature's utterances amount to law-making only when and insofar as they change the law in some way. In particular, *legislating to permit* means *changing the law by cancelling some prohibition which exists or will be in force by virtue of some existing law.* What a reforming bill/statute *says* does not settle what it *does*. And a bill's or statute's *statement that* some abortions are permitted does not entail that that bill or statute introduces any permission into the law or preserves any permission which would otherwise have ceased to be in force.

Instead of pointing to some error in the premises or reasoning of the Primary Argument, Harte counters with an analogy: a legislator has voted – with what motives and in what legislative circumstances, he does not say – for a 2000 Act replacing a 1950 speed limit of 30 mph with a new one of 25 mph, and is now accused of helping cause a death by preferring 25 to 20 mph. She would never conceivably, he says, offer the defence that she did not vote to permit driving at speeds up to 25 mph, that the effect of the 2000 Act was solely prohibitive, and that the permission to drive up to 25 mph was created in 1950 or before. "Such a defence would rightly be rejected. Yet it would seem that this is what Finnis is now proposing should be accepted as the argument to justify voting for Proposals A, B, C and G."

For such a legislator to offer such a defence would indeed be absurd, because Harte has made her situation profoundly unlike the situation of the legislators envisaged in *EV* 73.3 or in Proposals A, B, C, and G as I understand them.

The situation of pro-life legislators envisaged in *EV* 73.3[32] is in important respects similar to the situation which Harte's road traffic legislators would confront if everything were as he describes it except in one respect: there was also a 1935 constitutional provision, not amendable without a nine-tenths legislative majority, laying it down that the speed limit might be fixed by the legislature at any level *from 25 mph upwards*. In circumstances such as *these*, the legislator accused of voting for an excessive speed could, and probably would, defend herself by pointing out that, despite appearances,[33] her vote did not help to permit cars to travel up to 25 mph, that the sole juridical effect of her vote and of the 2000 Act was to prohibit driving between 25 and 30 mph, that the lethal permission to drive up to 25 mph was created in (at latest) 1935, and that those morally responsible for the continuance of that permission were the tiny minority (12%) of the legislators who refused to amend the Constitution so as to allow the majority to choose the speed limit they judged appropriate. This modified version of Harte's analogy is decisively closer to the situation of pro-life legislators envisaged in *EV* 73.3 because it shares with their situation the key feature that it is *simply outside their voting power* to extend the law's prohibition to the degree that it should be extended.

That is why my 2003 paper "Restricting legalised abortion" stressed that Harte is mistaken to treat the situation discussed in *EV* 73 as equivalent to the situation of a monarch with supreme and untrammelled legislative power, or to the position of a *united majority* in a constitutionally untrammelled legislature like the United Kingdom's. It would indeed be absurd for an all-powerful monarch or united majority to defend themselves by saying that their statute permitting abortion up to 16 weeks (in place of 24) is purely prohibitive. For the existing permission would itself exist and persist *by the sheer permission* of the monarch or united majority!

The situation in *EV* 73.3 is also similar to that of a legislator in the unmodified Harte scenario who believes and moves in Parliament that the

---

[32] Or in Proposals A, B, C and G as I understand them.

[33] The 2000 Act could read, for example, "The maximum speed at which cars are permitted to drive is 25 mph." Or it might read "In the 1950 Act '30' is replaced by '25.'" Or "Driving above 25 mph is prohibited." "Or the 1950 Act is repealed. The maximum speed limit is henceforth 25 mph." Or "The 1950 Act is amended by repealing section 4 and substituting '4. The speed limit is 25 mph.'" And so on and on. Such drafting differences are of no interest whatever for purposes of legal or moral analysis.

relevant speed limit should be reduced to 10 mph. Her motion is rejected and despite all efforts by the pro-safety lobby, only two proposals remain live: 25 or 35 mph (the old 30 mph limit has no prospect of surviving the night's voting). She accordingly votes for 25 mph and that prevails over the 30 and 35 mph alternatives. She could and probably would defend herself against reproaches by pointing out that the juridical effect of the new law is purely prohibitory (of driving at 25–30 mph), that the permission of driving up to 25 mph was introduced in 1950 and (despite her best efforts) *continues*, and that for her to vote No or abstain in the vote on 25 mph (on the ground that a 25 mph limit is 15 mph higher than it should be) would have been procedurally and morally tantamount to voting for 35 mph.[34]

7. Harte's present position yields absurdity

Harte does not respond at all to the arguments by which "Restricting legalised abortion" demonstrates that it is coherent to hold both (i) that a restrictive[35] abortion law is unjust and (ii) that a bill or statute which uses the same words to prohibit abortions currently permitted is not unjust. He says nothing about the key distinction between statements and propositions, nothing about the "contradictory" texts of Aquinas on dispensation from divine laws, nothing about the distinction between the words of a statute and their legal effect *if any*. My position is that "permitting" means permitting, but that *saying* "is permitted" does not always have the *effect* of permitting, even when the statement is in a statute.

The kernel of Harte's counter-position is that a law which permits abortion is unjust and *therefore* a statute which prohibits some currently permitted abortions while in some way *stating or indicating or revealing by its own formulation* that others *remain* permitted is unjust. I agree with the premise but deny the conclusion. *EV* 73.2 articulates the premise, but *EV* 73.3 teaches that bills/statutes making a current (or imminent) permissive law more restrictive are not intrinsically unjust, and gives no hint that it matters whether or not one can tell from the wording of the bill/statute that some permission remains. Harte has entirely failed to prove that

---

[34] It should go without saying that in pointing out the weakness of Harte's arguments from analogy, I am not saying that one can legislate to restrict abortion in the same way that one would legislate to lower a speed limit. In legislating about abortion one must always be supporting complete prohibition, and voting for incomplete prohibition only when complete prohibition is impossible.

[35] Here as always in these discussions, "restrictive" means restricting but not prohibiting to the extent required by true justice.

EV 73.2's phrase "a law permitting abortion" means something other than: a law which introduces a permission or continues in force a permission which would otherwise have ceased to be in force. Indeed, his reply to my "Restricting legalised abortion" makes no effort to show that that common-sense interpretation of *EV* 73.2 is mistaken. His whole position continues to *assume* precisely what I deny: that a statute which uses the words "is permitted", or in some other way mentions or signals the existence of an ongoing permission, *must* be introducing a permission or continuing in force a permission which would otherwise have ceased to be in force. As has been amply shown, there is no such necessity.

So there is no contradiction in holding both parts of the position I defend as in line with *EV* 73.2/3:

(1): A proposition of law accurately expressible in the formula "*Abortion is permissible up to 5 weeks*" is an unjust (proposition of) law.

(2): A bill or statute which partially repeals the existing legal permission of abortion up to 24 weeks, by prohibiting abortions after 5 weeks, is not an intrinsically unjust statute, whether it uses the formula
> F1: "Abortion is prohibited after week 5",
or the formula
> F2: "In Criminal Code art. 165, replace '24' with '5'",
or the formula
> F3: "*Abortion is permissible up to 5 weeks*".

Each of these statutes is enacted for its legal effect, its legal effect is exclusively prohibitory, and so the statute is not intrinsically unjust. In *each* case, including Act F3, the statute, and the enactment of its formula, is *not the reason why*[36] the unjust proposition of law "Abortion is permissible up to 5 weeks" remains legally true as part of the law of the land in force after as before the statute's enactment.

It is easy to see why Harte has confusedly assimilated or equated the reforming statute, visible and persisting in the statute book, with the ongoing unjust proposition of law which is expressible in the same words as may (as in F3, but not F1 or F2) be used in the statute. But they are two different things, and the statute, even Act F3, is not even the cause of the unjust proposition's (legal) truth. In any of its forms, this reform Act F1, or F2, or F3 is the cause only of the legal truth or validity of the (countless) new propositions of law that now prohibit all abortions at 7 weeks, 10 weeks, 16 weeks, 17.5 weeks and so on.

---

[36] That is, the unjust proposition would remain legally true even if the reforming statute were not enacted.

Remember: Harte regards *each* of these reforming statutes as intrinsically unjust, apparently because in each case[37] you can tell from its wording that abortion is going to remain to some extent (5 weeks) permitted. However, according to him the very same reform as is made by Acts F1, F2, and/or F3 would not be unjust if the previous generation of abortion lawmakers were kind and foolish enough to word their law in discrete statements (articles), one or more of which is now being repealed, separately, *without verbally signalling* the fact – obvious, however, to everyone – that the remaining permissive articles are being left to remain fully in force. So: suppose that the Criminal Code had the form:

273. abortion from 1 to 5 weeks is permitted if 2 doctors agree.
274. abortion from 5 to 24 weeks is permitted if one doctor agrees.
275. abortion for handicap is always permitted.
276. abortion of a fetus of Jewish parentage is always permitted.
277. subject to arts. 275 and 276, abortion after 24 weeks is prohibited.

Then, according to Harte, a reform bill/statute of the form

F4: "article 274 is repealed"

would not be unjust: for from that enactment, read by itself, you cannot tell whether any abortions remain permitted. On Harte's view, Act F4, despite leaving articles 273 and 275 untouched, not only does not permit but *does not even tolerate abortion!*[38] Moreover, the legislature itself that approves F4 *and leaves articles 273 and 275 untouched* does not, on Harte's view,[39] choose to tolerate abortion!

Test this a little further. Suppose that a (different) Criminal Code has the form:

354. abortion is permitted
   (a) from 1 to 5 weeks if 2 doctors agree;
   (b) from 5 to 24 weeks if one doctor agrees;
   and otherwise is prohibited.

---

[37] So he condemns as intrinsically unjust his Proposal G: "In art. 91 replace '16' by '8'".
[38] See "Problems of principle" sec. 6: ". . . Proposals like D or E or F or H [see *ibid.* sec. 2.3] . . . neither tolerate nor permit abortion and are not intrinsically unjust."
[39] For Harte says (*ibid.*) that "those voting for Proposal D (in Littalia) [see *ibid.*, sec. 2.3] cannot be charged with voting *to permit* (or, more precisely, *to tolerate*) abortion if the unborn child has been conceived after rape, and is disabled, *etc.*" and (*ibid.*, sec. 5.2) that "The will of the legislature in enacting legislation is indistinguishable from the will of the legislator voting for the enactment."

It is unclear what, on Harte's position, should be said about the justice or intrinsic injustice of:

F5a: "Art. 354 is amended by deleting (repealing) sub-clause (b)"

or

F5b: "In art. 354 sub-clause (b) is repealed."

Neither of these reforming statutes *mentions* that clause (a) remains in force.[40] But nor does Act F2 *mention* that abortion is permitted – it mentions nothing but two numerals – and Harte is certainly not satisfied to leave it at that. He says that proposals like Act F2 have a "juridical meaning" which refers to abortion being permitted up to 5 weeks, not 24.[41] So by parity of analysis, the "juridical meaning" of Reform Acts F5a or 5b presumably refers to abortion being permitted up to 5 weeks. So F5a and 5b, like F2, F1, and F3, but not F4, are (on Harte's account) intrinsically unjust. Harte's method of analysis thus leads to absurd results. There is no difference, either in legal analysis or commonsense, between Act F4 and Acts F5a or 5b. Indeed Act F4 could be analysed into its "juridical meaning", too: "The Code provisions on abortion[42] are amended by repealing the article permitting abortion from 7 to 24 weeks, leaving abortion permitted up to 5 weeks under art. 273, and in all cases of handicap or Jewish parentage under arts. 275 and 276."

The truth is that there is no legally significant distinction between Reform Acts F1, F2, F3, F4, and F5a or F5b. There are differences between them that might have some relevance to their cultural side-effects among a population in the grip of words. But a moral analysis that judges some but not others of them *intrinsically* unjust is deeply mistaken, and finds no support in *EV* 73. All of them *leave* some abortions wrongfully permitted. All of them *in that sense* "permit" abortion. But when one looks to their legal effect, it is also true that none of them permit abortion in the sense of "permit" used in

---

[40] Would it make a difference to Harte if the statute repealing sub-clause (b) also stated that sub-clause (a) is no longer numbered "(a)"?

[41] See "Problems of principle" sec. 2.3 on Proposal G. Harte's preferred version of Act F2's "juridical meaning" would be "Amend art. 165 so that abortion is permitted up to 5 weeks, not 24 weeks". The "so that" assumes what I deny, namely that the reforming statute has the *purpose* and/or *effect* of permitting.

[42] In order to bring his analysis into line with the CDF's 2003 *Considerations*, Harte now says (*Response*, fn. 68) that each of his Proposals D, E and F can be called proposals "partially repealing [an] unjust law" (he reveals his unease by unwarrantably omitting, twice, the CDF's word "an"). He thus effectively concedes that his imaginary Code provisions on abortion can be regarded not only as a whole law, but also as one which can be amended by having part(s) subtracted from it by repeal.

EV 73.2, for none of them make legally permissible what would otherwise have become or remained forbidden by the state's law.[43]

8. Partial repeal is a form of amendment, and amendments of the relevant kind are partial repeals

Not all amendments repeal. Some amendments add new provisions or new words which supplement the meaning without subtracting any existing meaning. So "amendment" and "repeal" are not synonymous. But in all the kinds of cases I have discussed in this debate, the amendments under consideration have been by way of partial repeal.[44] Sometimes the repeal is

---

[43] As Harte tirelessly observes, I said in my 1997 paper ("The Catholic Church and Public Policy Debates . . .", in *Issues for a Catholic Bioethic* (London: Linacre Centre 1999), p. 269), that a law (bill/statute) saying abortion is lawful up to 16 weeks, in the context of an existing or imminent law saying it is lawful up to 24 weeks, "does in fact permit abortion up to 16 weeks". As the last three sentences in the text to which the present footnote is appended make clear, that statement of mine remains true, and contradicts nothing in my subsequent papers showing that it is also true that such a bill/statute/law does *not* permit. Indeed, I implicitly indicated the ambiguity of the word "permit" – which makes the pair of apparently contradictory statements non-contradictory – before the end of the very paragraph from which Harte quotes, when I said that Catholic legislators must "never vote to permit it [abortion], *i.e.* to make it more permissible" (that is, more permissible that it has hitherto been or would, but for the bill/statute, become). Though the rapid treatment of *EV* 73 in the relevant one and a half pages of the 1997 paper leaves unsaid much that could usefully be said – it was discussing *EV* 73 solely in order to illustrate the difference between formal and material cooperation – I think it is correct so far as it goes, with one qualification: I would not now concede or say unqualifiedly that voting for a bill/statute restricting the permission of abortion from 24 weeks to 16 weeks has the "side-effect of permission". The vote, like the bill/statute itself, leaves abortion up to 16 weeks permitted, but since there is here no *making permitted* of what was (or would otherwise have become) prohibited, there is strictly speaking no *effect*. Or if there is an effect (as we might say that the continuance of the suffering of the man who fell among thieves was an effect of the passing by of the priest and the Levite on the other side, or that the withering of the unwatered plants was an effect of the gardener's neglect of duty), it is the effect of those whose wrongful unwillingness to vote for a law restricting all abortion prevents such a restriction, and not an effect of the 16-week bill/statute, still less of those who vote for it only because it introduces new prohibitions and eliminates the permissions it eliminates.

[44] In the kind of case I consider in sec. 10 below, where there is substantially no law prohibiting abortion, and it is regarded as a matter of legal right (privacy, bodily security, or whatever), the introduction of a constitutionally valid law restricting abortion (say, by prohibiting it during all but the first five weeks) would not be described by most lawyers as a *partial repeal* of the existing law, nor as an *amendment*. But this would be because these terms are habitually used in relation to statutes and other enactments. In substance, what would be happening would indeed be the amendment of the

express, in others it is what lawyers call implied repeal.[45] In all cases where a later statute overrides part of the meaning of an earlier statute, the later statute is said to impliedly repeal that part (provision, or part-provision) of the earlier – unless it has expressly done so. All such cases can also be called amendment.[46] Even where a whole statute is repealed, lawyers will say that the law on the matter in question has been amended. It is usually no more than arcane conveniences of parliamentary procedure, or draftsman's whim, that determine whether or not the earlier statute will be expressly repealed as a whole or in part, in the way that Harte postulates in setting up his Cases *A, B, C, D, E,* and *F.* Such differences correspond to nothing that could affect the moral issues at stake in *EV 73.*

9. The CDF's statements in 2002 and 2003 reject positions held by Harte

The 2002 *Doctrinal Note* leaves matters where *EV* 73.3 left them, in relation to situations where "it is not possible to overturn *or completely repeal* a law allowing abortion which is already in force *or coming up for a vote.*" It thus reminds us that incomplete (= partial) repeal is permissible, and that the baseline for assessing whether a reform *reduces* the cases of unjustly permitted abortion can be either the law already in force or a "law" coming up for a vote. (This is the "shifting baseline" which excites Harte's

---

existing law of the land on the matter by partially repealing (overriding, eliminating from the *corpus juris*) those of its provisions (say, common law rights of privacy, or constitutionally protected rights of bodily security) that made abortion's legal permissibility legally true. "To repeal an Act is to cause it to cease to be a part of the *corpus juris* or body of law." "Statutes", *Halsbury's Laws of England* (Fourth ed. revised), vol. 44(1), para. 1296 ("Meaning of 'repeal'").

[45] "The rule is, therefore, that one provision repeals another by implication if, but only if, it is so inconsistent with or repugnant to that other that the two are incapable of standing together." "Statutes", *Halsbury's Laws*, vol. 44(1), para. 1299 ("Implied repeal"; in general), text at n. 4.

[46] "*Meaning of 'amendment'.* To amend an Act or enactment is to alter its legal meaning, whether expressly or by implication .... Amendment may take the form of, or include, repeal [3] [fn. 3] A substitution is a repeal in so far as it removes words .... If a provision of an Act is deleted, it can be said that the provision is 'repealed' but that the Act is 'amended'. In so far as an amendment also constitutes a repeal, the rules relating to repeals will apply." "Statutes", *Halsbury's Laws of England* (4th ed.), vol. 44(1), para. 1289; see also para. 1290: "*Implied amendment.* Where a later enactment does not expressly amend (whether textually or indirectly) an earlier enactment, but the provisions of the later enactment are inconsistent with those of the earlier, the later by implication amends the earlier so far as is necessary to remove the inconsistency between them. [1] [fn. 1] .... Similarly, a part of the earlier Act may be regarded as impliedly repealed where it cannot stand with the later."

uncomprehending protests about *Case 2*, his suggestion that I am a closet subscriber to "situation ethics", and so forth.)

The 2002 *Doctrinal Note* adds that one must never vote for "an individual law which contradicts the fundamental contents of faith and morals". Harte hastens to assume that the laws to which the CDF refers are laws of the kind which, *in situations where they introduce new prohibitions*, I have defended. He assumes (2.2) that otherwise the CDF's statement would be "entirely unnecessary and irrelevant": its purpose would be negated because there is nothing for it to refer to except statutes of the kind I have defended![47] He forgets the large category of statutes which cannot be defended, above all those statutes whose point and substance and effect is to cancel existing prohibitions which would otherwise have remained in force, or to sustain permissions which would otherwise have ceased to be in force. That is precisely the category which a key sentence in the CDF's 2003 *Considerations* should have recalled to Harte's attention.

But, as I showed in section 1 above, Harte has decided to omit that key opening sentence from his otherwise ample quotation from section 10 of the 2003 *Considerations*. As I have recalled above, this sentence, taken with the rest of the passage, lays out the entire structure of analysis which the Church now regularly uses, and which I have labelled dynamic and comparative or baseline analysis.

The final sentence of the passage, which I shall quote again, implicitly makes the distinction to which the Primary Argument draws attention, and which I have amplified a little in section 7 above. It is the distinction between the propositions of law which will be in force after the reforming, "more restrictive" statute, and the formulations whose enactment in the reforming statute will have the legal effect of eliminating *some* unjust propositions of law:

---

[47] Harte grossly misstates the class of reform statutes I defend: "according to Finnis' understanding of what is allowed by *EV* 73.3, legislators could vote for anything that was 'restrictive', or generally regarded as 'desirable'...". This has no basis in my text or my argument, which, like *EV* 73.3's, holds that one of the necessary conditions for a bill or statute to be supportable is that it be *more* restrictive than the baseline law. He forgets that, because we are talking about intentional killing of defenceless innocents, the requirements of justice and fairness, even in respect of side-effects, are strong: see, *e.g.* my "Unjust Laws in a Democratic Society". 71 (1996) *Notre Dame L. Rev.* at 601–2, 604. He also forgets the stringent requirement, articulated in all my papers, that the legislator exclude all motivations of the "generally... desirable" kind – *e.g.* "I need to vote this way to get re-elected and go on benefiting people generally", "Poor people deserve the same availability of abortion as the rich", "It's best overall not to impose one's personal opinions on people who disagree", *etc.*, *etc.*

This does not mean that a more restrictive law in this area could be considered just or even acceptable; rather it is a question of the legitimate and dutiful[48] attempt to obtain at least the partial repeal[49] of an unjust law when its total abrogation is not possible at the moment.

There is no hint here or anywhere else that the words of the supportable[50] reforming statute must exclude anything acknowledging that some homosexual unions will remain legally valid and available [or that some abortions remain legally permitted]. The CDF's attention is exclusively on the question identified by the Primary Argument as the decisive question: What is being *done to* the law itself (the set of propositions of law in force before, and the set of propositions of law in force after the reforming statute takes effect)? More specifically: If the law (the set of propositions of law in force before the reforming statute) is not completely repealed or totally abrogated, are at least *some* of its unjust propositions abrogated? If so, the attempt to abrogate those unjust elements may be not only legitimate (not intrinsically unjust) but actually a matter of duty.

In short: the sentence I have just quoted from the CDF's 2003 *Considerations* is a clear rejection of Harte's whole strategy. For he insists that if a bill or statute, considered in abstraction from any baseline, articulates an unjust law, then *EV* 73 forbids any support or vote for it, whatever the baseline,

---

[48] Notice that the CDF uses the Italian *doveroso* (and its English equivalent) – the word used to make the same point in *EV* 73.3 – in preference to the Latin *opportunus* [= appropriate] used in the Latin version of *EV* 73.3. Contrast fn. 48 in Harte's *Response,* claiming that the English (and thus the Italian, French, German, Spanish, *etc.*) is "faulty" because *only* the Latin is authoritative. The CDF thinks otherwise. (And in any case, the discrepancy Harte alleges is non-existent: "cooperate" and "*officium praestare*" are acceptable translations of each other.)

[49] This causes an acute difficulty for Harte, who had maintained that his Proposals D, E and F repealed [whole] laws: see sec. 3.3 of his "Problems of Principle", where he describes the articles about abortion in his imaginary Littalia code as "a series of *laws.*" See also his fn. 68 in "Opening up a Discussion", where he attempts to cover over his difficulty by omitting the CDF's word "an" when seeming to quote its phrase "partial repeal of an unjust law". Note also his (accurate) observation in that footnote (and earlier in sec. 3.3 of "Problems of Principle") that there is no contradiction in saying that a proposition is both a [whole] law and part of a law. If he were to apply the same standards of flexibility and justifiable complexity to my own analysis, he would find how unwarranted are all his claims and suggestions that my position (that laws permissive in formulation need not be permissive in legal effect) contains "contradictions".

[50] This is just shorthand for a proposal that right-minded legislators can vote for if no more prohibitory alternative is available, provided that their opposition to its remaining permissions or authorisations is public and authentic.

and permits no repeal of any of its unjust permissions or authorisations unless all are repealed (except in the fantasy case of complete, free-standing permissions within a set of artificially separate unjust permissions). The CDF's sentence tells us *not* to ask whether the law of the land in place after the proposed reform is just or acceptable, but whether the *change* effected by the reform is an at least *partial* repeal of the baseline law's unjust elements.

10. Final reflections on Harte's position

The arguments that I brought against Harte's position, in my "Restricting legalised abortion", have been met with nothing more than unargued denial or, in one case, a lame analogy. Most of those arguments have been redeployed or recalled, above. So they need not be repeated in this final section, but they all remain important and intact. I add two final reflections.

Pro-life legislators and authenticity: In his conference paper Harte spoke as if Polish pro-lifers (and I) were abandoning ethics and humanity, and he suggested that in Poland in 1992/3 the pro-lifers who had voted for the eventual statute had "overlooked" the right to life of the most vulnerable of the unborn in the interest of protecting others.[51] He made no acknowledgement of the fact that thoroughgoing pro-life legislators whose votes helped give the bill its majority, but who had overlooked nothing about the rights and fate of the victims of the unjust permissions or tolerations remaining in Poland's amended abortion law, were *prevented* from giving effect to their just purposes of saving all the vulnerable. They were prevented by the bad will or confused thinking of other legislators (if not also of the constitutional court). It is true that the Church's position in *EV* 73, like its position on all the other moral absolutes – exceptionless but defined by the object of the relevant act, and thus to some extent by the deliberations of the acting person – is open to misapplication, lip service, inauthenticity. *EV* 73.3's acknowledgement – bolder than my own pre-*EV* arguments – that an imminent permissive enactment can be properly regarded as a baseline is obviously open to abusively lax (mis)interpretation or (mis)application. But none of that is ground for impugning the truth of the position stated in *EV* 73.3, any more than the abuses sometimes or often associated with annulment of marriage are ground for impugning the teaching that – presupposing the absolute indissolubility of consummated sacramental marriage – some marriages contracted in the Church can be ecclesiastically recognised to have been morally invalid *ab initio*.

---

[51] See fn. 29 above.

Words, propositions, and sophisms. The routine statement that a certain long-standing marriage was void *ab initio* is equivalent to saying that what seemed to be (and in some respects was) a marriage was not really a marriage – not a marriage within the meaning of the true teaching that marriage is indissoluble. The routine manner of speaking involves a silent shift in the application of the word "marriage", and though *verbally* or *apparently* contradictory involves no contradiction at the level of propositions. This is all well known to commonsense, though commonsense can find itself flat-footed when challenged to explain itself – and sophists exploit this weakness. (Many sixteenth-century attacks on traditional teaching are riddled with such sophistry.) Something rather like this is true of the position set forth in *EV* 73, in the sense explained in the Primary Argument. The statement that certain bills/statutes/laws which are permissive (because incompletely prohibitive) are entirely restrictive (given the relevant baseline) is equivalent to saying that they are not really permissive – not permissive in the sense of the Principle and the teaching in *EV* 73.2. Harte's focus on words at the expense of a consideration of propositions is unsound and, in the last analysis, sophistical.

It meets a particular nemesis in situations, such as Canada or the United States, where the existing law on the permissibility of abortion is essentially, one may say, *no law.* For in such jurisdictions there are, for all practical purposes, no statutory words validly declaring abortion sometimes prohibited and sometimes not. Harte's candidate for acceptable restrictive abortion reform ("pure" repeal of neatly separate existing items of articulated permission) – a solution rarely if ever available in the real world – is out of the question in such a situation: the form of the universal permission in such countries being silence (total absence of any prohibition), there is no "law" capable of being partially repealed *in Harte's sense.* Yet Harte is content to think that the Catholic Church *obviously* teaches – just read the words of *EV* 73.2! – that in such countries nothing can be done, ever, under any circumstances, to introduce any legal prohibition, however extensive and beneficial, unless it is the complete prohibition demanded by the justice whose demands are truly identified in the Church's teaching on abortion – a justice whose demands are unlikely ever to be fully accepted in any political community foreseeable this side of Judgment Day.[52]

---

[52] Harte's position entails that in circumstances such as Canada's or the United States', the notion of incomplete "abrogation" used in *EV* 73.3 and of "partial repeal" and "(non)total abrogation" used in the CDF's 2003 *Considerations* simply has no application. There are no words there to be abrogated or repealed! But it is mere commonsense that even an entirely silent and universal permission can be wholly or partially abrogated, not by complete or partial repeal in Harte's formalistic sense (for that is unavailable here), but by complete or partial prohibition.

Confronted by serious argumentation to show that, in (amongst others) a country so situated, a more (albeit incompletely) restrictive law can indeed be introduced without in any way violating the Principle stated in *EV* 72.2, Harte's response is not to welcome the possibility that millions of abortions could thereby be prevented, and therefore to assess and weigh the merits of the argument with some care and interpretative understanding. Instead he intimates alarm at the possibility that Catholic pro-life legislators will feel free to embrace a "situation ethics" and do whatever they think "desirable" (what?); and reiterates, always question-beggingly, the assumption whose falsity is made clear by the arguments in "Restricting legalised abortion ..." – the formulaic assumption that if the words of a statute introducing prohibitions say or in any way acknowledge or imply that some kinds of abortions (however few) will *remain* permitted, the statute must be a law that violates the Principle against legally *permitting* abortion, so that any who vote for it will be doing something intrinsically evil.

To repeat: if Harte were right, pro-life legislative effort to restrict abortion in states with completely permissive abortion law would be pointless at best, and generally immoral. For in those states (i) there is no real-world possibility of complete prohibition, (ii) Hartean partial repeal is logically impossible because at the level of words there is no law about abortion available to be repealed, and (iii) every kind of partial amendment or incomplete abrogation of the universal permission (the permission at the level of propositions) is, Harte claims, forbidden. Of course, if that really were the upshot of a sound moral analysis, we should all accept it, whatever the consequences. The Church's teaching in *EV* 73 is very different, however, and directs us towards a different and entirely sound position.

Meanwhile, analyses such as Harte's, accusing most pro-life activists of doing or favouring intrinsic moral evil, and promoted with vehemence and over-confidence, have done not a little to block the pro-life efforts of legislators and voters (and Catholic bishops) in the United States and Canada and elsewhere. Hence the unwelcome length of this incomplete commentary on some of the logical, legal, and theological mistakes in those analyses.[53]

---

[53] [For a relatively short account of the whole matter, focusing on the key arguments without reference to the ins and outs of Harte's writings, see now my "Helping Enact Unjust Laws without Complicity in Injustice". 49 (2004) *American Journal of Jurisprudence*: 11–42.]

15

US law and conscientious objection in healthcare

Richard S. Myers

The problem of rights of conscience in health care is one of the most serious religious freedom issues that now exists in the United States. In many ways, there are profound ironies about this. The legal system in the United States has been characterized as "A Republic of Choice."[1] Appeals to choice (and personal autonomy) tend to dominate public policy debates. The rhetoric of choice is exceedingly powerful, and it is difficult to resist its appeal. I think this point is evidenced by the way "choice" is invoked by all sides of the political spectrum. It is no accident that those in favor of abortion rights and those in favor of school vouchers both refer to themselves as movements of "choice."[2]

Appeals to "choice" are very common in bioethics. Perhaps the most infamous judicial example occurred in the Supreme Court's decision in *Planned Parenthood v. Casey*.[3] There, the Court noted: "matters involving the most intimate and personal choices a person may make in a lifetime, choices central to personal dignity and autonomy, are central to the liberty protected by the Fourteenth Amendment. At the heart of liberty is the right to define one's own concept of existence, of meaning, of the universe, and of the mystery of human life. Beliefs about these matters could not define the attributes of personhood were they formed under compulsion of the

---

[1] Lawrence M. Friedman, The Republic of Choice (1990).

[2] For a discussion of choice in education, see Richard S. Myers, School Choice: The Constitutional Issues, 8 Cath. Soc. Sci. Rev. 167 (2203). It is noteworthy that in early 2003, one of the major abortion rights organizations, The National Abortion and Reproductive Rights Action League, changed its name to NARAL Pro-Choice America. See http://www.naral.org.

[3] 505 U. S. 833 (1992).

State."[4] This line of thinking has also played a role in the assisted suicide area. In the mid-1990s, one of the lower court opinions addressing the constitutionality of the State of Washington's ban on assisted suicide stated: "This Court finds the reasoning in *Casey* highly instructive and almost prescriptive on the... issue [of a terminally ill person's choice to commit suicide]. Like the abortion decision, the decision of a terminally ill person to end his or her life 'involv[es] the most intimate and personal choices a person may make in a lifetime' and constitutes a 'choice [...] central to personal dignity and autonomy.'"[5]

In its 1997 decisions on assisted suicide,[6] the Supreme Court did reject reliance on this broad language from *Casey* in concluding that there was no federal constitutional right to assisted suicide.[7] The Court's majority there seemed to confine the use of the language to the limited context of abortion.[8]

Somewhat surprisingly, however, the United States Supreme Court resurrected this language in its June 26, 2003 decision in *Lawrence v. Texas*.[9] In *Lawrence*, the Texas case involving homosexual sodomy, the Court relied on *Casey*'s more expansive approach without so much as mentioning the assisted suicide cases.[10] As Justice Scalia pointed out in his *Lawrence* dissent, this language (which he described as the Court's "famed sweet-mystery-of-life passage"[11]) threatens the constitutionality of nearly

---

[4] 505 U. S. at 851.

[5] Compassion in *Dying v. Washington*, 850 F. Supp. 1454, 1459–1460 (W. D. Wash. 1994) (quoting Casey, 505 U. S. at 851), rev'd, 49 F. 3d 586 (9th Cir. 1995), rev'd, 79 F. 3d 790 (9th Cir. 1996) (en banc), rev'd sub nom. *Washington v. Glucksberg*, 521 U. S. 702 (1997).

[6] See *Washington v. Glucksberg*, 521 U. S. 702 (1997); *Vacco v. Quill*, 521 U. S. 793 (1997).

[7] Glucksberg, 117 S. Ct. at 2270–2271.

[8] Id. The Glucksberg Court seemed to adopt a far more restrained approach to judicial review. See Richard S. Myers, Physician-assisted Suicide: A Current Legal Perspective, 1 Nat'l Cath. Bioethics Q. 345, 349 (2001); Michael W. McConnell, The Right to Die and the Jurisprudence of Tradition, 1997 Utah L. Rev. 665.

[9] 123 S. Ct. 2472, 2481 (2003).

[10] In Justice Kennedy's majority opinion, there is neither a citation to nor a discussion of the assisted suicide cases. In his dissenting opinion, Justice Scalia noted that "Roe and Casey have been equally 'eroded' by *Washington v. Glucksberg*... which held that *only* fundamental rights which are 'deeply rooted in this Nation's history and tradition' qualify for anything other than rational basis scrutiny under the doctrine of 'substantive due process.'" 123 S. Ct. at 2489 (Scalia, J., dissenting). For a detailed discussion of the ways in which Lawrence departs from Glucksberg, see Robert C. Post, Foreword: Fashioning the Legal Constitution: Culture, Courts, and Law, 117 Harv. L. Rev. 4, 91–107 (2003).

[11] 123 S. Ct. at 2489 (Scalia, J., dissenting).

all morals legislation.[12] We see, yet again, the almost overwhelmingly powerful appeal of the language of choice and of "an autonomy of self."

The idea here is, of course, that the state must remain neutral on these basic moral choices. In fact, some even celebrated the statement in *Casey* as support for the idea that moral relativism is a constitutional command.[13] Under this view, morality is purely private, purely subjective. The state must remain neutral about the content of the individual's choice. The state must remain indifferent toward whether the pregnant woman chooses life or death.[14] It is considered a sufficient answer to these questions to leave these matters entirely to the realm of subjective choice. You see this on bumper stickers: "Don't like abortion, don't have one" – as if that adequately resolved the underlying moral question.

Yet this is a false neutrality. On the issue of abortion, for example, the state must decide whether an unborn child is a person entitled to the full protection of the law. This is not a matter that can adequately be dealt with by falsely pretending not to decide whether an unborn child is a human being entitled to legal protection.[15] For as Pope John Paul II stated in *Evangelium Vitae*, "when freedom is detached from objective truth it becomes impossible to establish personal rights on a firm rational basis;

---

[12] Justice Scalia noted that the Court's approach "effectively decrees the end of all morals legislation." 123 S. Ct. at 2495 (Scalia, J., dissenting).

[13] See Stephen G. Gey, Is Moral Relativism a Constitutional Command?, 70 Ind. L. J. 331 (1995).

[14] See Myers, supra note 8, at 346.

[15] This error is common. In *Roe v. Wade*, 410 U. S. 113 (1973), Justice Blackmun noted: "We need not resolve the difficult question of when life begins. When those trained in the respective disciplines of medicine, philosophy, and theology are unable to arrive at a consensus, the judiciary, at this point in the development of man's knowledge, is not in a position to speculate as to the answer." 410 U. S. at 159. In a recent article, Professor Whitman makes the same error. She stated: "The constitutional question posed by abortion cannot be 'when does life begin.' Legal analysis cannot answer that question, so it cannot be the test or doctrinal structure on which the right to abortion hinges." Chris Whitman, Looking Back on Planned Parenthood v. Casey, 100 Mich. L. Rev. 1791, 1995 (2002). The problem with this false gesture of humility is that a decision is being made about the status of the unborn. The Roe Court later noted that "we do not agree that, by adopting one theory of life, Texas may override the rights of the pregnant woman that are at stake." 410 U. S. at 162. The Court reached this conclusion because it had its own theory of human life that it enshrined into the law. The Court in Roe was in fact concluding that the unborn child could not legally be regarded as a human person entitled to the full protection of the law. Whatever this is, it is assuredly not a failure to decide the question. For a critique of Professor Whitman's article, see Richard S. Myers, Reflections on "Looking Back on Planned Parenthood v. Casey," in Life and Learning XIII: The Proceedings of the Thirteenth University Faculty for Life Conference (J. Koterski ed. 2003) 3–19.

and the ground is laid for society to be at the mercy of the unrestrained will of individuals or the oppressive totalitarianism of public authority."[16] In 1991, then-Cardinal Ratzinger made this point with great force. He stated: "[A] state which arrogates to itself the prerogative of defining which human beings are or are not the subject of rights and which consequently grants to some the power to violate others' fundamental right to life, contradicts the democratic ideal to which it continues to appeal and undermines the very foundations on which it is built. By allowing the rights of the weakest to be violated, the State allows the law of force to prevail over the force of law. One sees, then, that the idea of an absolute tolerance of freedom of choice for some destroys the very foundation of a just life for men together. The separation of politics from any natural content of right, which is the inalienable patrimony of everyone's moral conscience, deprives social life of its ethical substance and leaves it defenseless before the will of the strongest."[17]

We see this playing out in the United States. What begins with an appeal to "choice" and to freedom quickly moves to the will of the strongest prevailing, in large part by certain powerful individuals turning to the "oppressive totalitarianism of public authority."

We've seen this in dramatic fashion with regard to abortion. Defended first as a private choice, we quickly saw moves to require that taxpayers (even those with a moral objection) pay for abortions.[18] Although the United States Supreme Court rejected the view that this was required by the Constitution,[19] it has been mandated by a number of states.[20] We've also

---

[16] Pope John Paul II, Evangelium Vitae 96 (1995), available at http://www.vatican.va/holy_father/john_paul_ii/encyclicals/documents/hf_jp_ii_enc_25031995_evangelium-vitae_en.html. [hereinafter *Evangelium Vitae*].

[17] Joseph Cardinal Ratzinger, Doctrinal Document on Threats to Life Proposed, 20 Origins 755, 757 (1991), available at http://www.priestsforlife.org/magisterium/threatstohumanlife.htm#ratzinger.

[18] John T. Noonan, Jr., A Private Choice: Abortion in America in the Seventies 191 (1979).

[19] *Harris v. McRae*, 448 U. S. 297 (1980); *Maher v. Roe*, 432 U. S. 464 (1977).

[20] In *Humphreys v. Clinic for Women, Inc.*, 796 N. E. 2d 241 (Ind. 2003), the Indiana Supreme Court concluded that the Indiana Constitution required the funding of abortions in certain limited cases. One Justice, who thought that the majority's opinion did not go far enough, noted that "[t]welve of the seventeen state courts that have considered the issue in published opinions have concluded that denial of benefits to indigent women for medically necessary abortions is a violation of their state constitutions. Under prevailing constitutional doctrine in this state, I would reach the same result." Id. at 264–265 (footnote omitted) (Boehm, J., concurring in part and dissenting in part). As Justice Boehm notes, this conclusion has been rejected by some states. See, e.g., *Bell v. Low Income Women of Texas*, 95 S. W. 3d 253 (Tex. 2002).

increasingly seen moves to make participation in or facilitation of abortion mandatory.[21] We now see "choice" becoming compulsory.[22] These efforts to violate conscience are becoming increasingly widespread.

I'll provide just a few recent examples. There are, of course, many examples that could be cited.[23] There is a concerted effort throughout the United States to mandate that employers provide coverage for contraceptives, even contraceptives that commonly act as abortifacients.[24] This mandate typically extends to religious employers. Catholic Charities of Sacramento challenged California's contraceptive mandate but its religious freedom objections were rejected by the California courts.[25] The United States Supreme Court refused to intervene.[26] New York's law was passed at the end of 2002 and religious groups have challenged the constitutionality of this law, which mandates that employers provide coverage for contraceptives even when these employers have a religious or moral objection to providing such coverage. On 25 November 2003, a trial court in New York upheld the constitutionality of the New York law.[27]

On 12 June 2003, newspapers in Massachusetts reported on a proposed law that would require all hospitals, including Catholic hospitals, to provide the so-called "morning-after" pill to rape victims.[28] A supporter of the proposed law was quoted as saying, "We've had problems with Catholic hospitals not offering [the morning-after pill]."[29] In 2005, Archbishop

---

[21] See, e.g., The Campaign to Force Hospitals to Provide Abortion (September 2003), Fact Sheet prepared by United States Conference of Catholic Bishops, Secretariat for Pro-Life Activities, available at http://www.usccb.org/prolife/issues/abortion/andaindex.htm.

[22] Lynn Vincent, Compulsory "choice," 18 World Magazine, January 18, 2003, available at http://www.worldmag.com/world/issue/01-18-03/cover_3.asp.

[23] For a more comprehensive listing, see Lynn D. Wardle, "For the Sake of Conscience": The Case for Legal Exemptions for Religious Objectors (August 19, 2003) (copy of paper on file with author) [hereinafter cited as Wardle Paper].

[24] See Peter J. Cataldo, Compliance with Contraceptive Insurance Mandates, 4 Nat'l Cath. Bioethics Q. 103 (2004); Susan J. Stabile, Religious Employers and Statutory Prescription Contraceptive Mandates, 43 Cath. Law. 169 (2004). See generally http://www.covermypills.org. This website, which is sponsored by Planned Parenthood, contains a detailed review of developments on this issue throughout the United States.

[25] *Catholic Charities of Sacramento, Inc. v. Superior Court*, 109 Cal. Rptr. 2d 176 (Cal. Ct. App. 2001), aff'd, 32 Cal. 4th 527 (Cal.), cert. denied, 125 S. Ct. 53 (2004).

[26] The United States Supreme Court denied a petition for writ of certiorari on October 4, 2004.

[27] *Catholic Charities of the Diocese of Albany v. Serio*, No. 8229–02 (N. Y. Sup. Ct. Nov. 25, 2003) [hereinafter Catholic Charities of the Diocese of Albany].

[28] Julie Mehegan, Bill would force hospitals to dispense "morning-after" pill to rape victims, Lowell Sun, June 12, 2003.

[29] Id.

Charles J. Chaput protested when a Colorado state legislator objected to the Catholic Church's resistance to a law that would require all hospitals in Colorado, including Catholic hospitals, to provide "emergency contraception" to rape victims. Archbishop Chaput argued "At a minimum, Catholic hospitals – which provide their services based on moral and religious convictions about the dignity of the human person – should not be obligated to perform or refer for procedures which violate Catholic teaching. This doesn't involve 'preaching' to anybody. It involves fidelity to principle and conscience – the same principles and conscience that animate Catholic service to the poor."[30]

There have been a variety of proposals over the last several years that would require hospitals to provide and doctors to be trained to perform abortions and other "reproductive services". In 1995, the Accreditation Council for Graduate Medical Education passed a requirement that would have mandated that every OB/GYN residency program in the country include induced abortion training.[31] This effort with regard to abortion was defeated,[32] although the programme requirements mandate clinical training in contraception and sterilization.[33] In 2000, the American Medical Association considered a resolution that would have committed the AMA to support legislation that would have required that all hospitals receiving federal funds provide a full range of reproductive services, including services such as contraceptives and sterilizations that violate the religious teachings of many of these hospitals.[34] The issue has been particularly contentious when Catholic hospitals have merged with or acquired hospitals that formerly provided these services.[35] Catholic leaders, including Cardinal Francis George, testified against the resolution, which they accurately characterized as an effort to abolish the Catholic health care system in the United States.[36] The AMA's House of Delegates defeated this resolution (by a 247–184 vote), although the Delegates approved a milder resolution that

[30] Archbishop Charles J. Chaput, Emergency contraception: What the words mean, Denver Catholic Register (March 2, 2005). See http://www.archden.org/dcr/news.php?e=119&s=2&a=2751.
[31] For detailed discussion of this controversy, see Michael J. Frank, Note, Safeguarding the Consciences of Hospitals and Health Care Personnel: How the Graduate Medical Education Guidelines Demonstrate a Continued Need for Protective Jurisprudence and Legislation, 41 St. Louis L. J. 311 (1996).
[32] Id. at 327–328.
[33] The programme requirements are available at the ACGME website. See http://www.acgme.org.
[34] Bruce Japsen, AMA Approves Compromise on Sterilization Proposal, Chicago Tribune, June 16, 2000.
[35] See generally Wardle Paper, supra note 23, at 28–32.
[36] See supra note 31.

supported access to a full range of reproductive services while stopping short of calling for legislation that would mandate that result.[37]

Nurses and pharmacists are increasingly being forced (at the threat of disciplinary measures or the loss of their jobs) to dispense contraceptives (with abortifacient effects) and the morning-after pill, even when they have conscientious objections to such conduct.[38] For example, in Wisconsin, a pharmacist was sanctioned by the state pharmacy board for refusing to dispense contraceptives. Among other sanctions, the pharmacist was required to pay $20,000 and was also required to take continuing education classes in pharmacy practice.[39]

These pressures arise in other areas of health care as well. On occasion, religious hospitals have been forced to withdraw life support or the provision of food and water, even when so doing violated the hospital's religious beliefs.[40] To the extent the Oregon situation – where assisted suicide is legal[41] – becomes more widespread, these pressures are likely to become worse. As perhaps a forerunner of things to come, there have been recent reports in the press that Belgium is thinking about requiring that all hospitals be ready to provide euthanasia. According to press reports, this proposal to force all hospitals to make euthanasia available is designed to counter opposition by some Catholic hospitals that have refused to permit assisted suicide on their premises.[42]

As one can see from this brief survey, the trends in this area are quite troublesome. While some of these initiatives have been defeated and while some of these measures contain exemptions for those with an objection to being forced to participate in the procedures in question, there is increasingly pressure to conform to the secular vision of heath care and morality. While there may be a value in seeking exemptions from these mandates in terms of providing a moral witness and while there may be certain benefits to professional or institutional martyrdom, the plight of those who adhere to a moral

---

[37] Id.

[38] See generally Wardle Paper, supra note 23, at 24–28; Bryan A. Dykes, Note, Proposed Rights of Conscience Legislation: Expanding to Include Pharmacists and Other Health Care Providers, 36 Ga. L. Rev. 565 (2002).

[39] See Steven Ertelt, Wisconsin Board Sanctions Pro-Life Pharmacist on Script Refusal. http://www.lifenews.com/state 990.html.

[40] For discussions of this issue, see J. David Bleich, The Physician as a Conscientious Objector, 30 Fordham Urb. L. J. 245 (2002); Katherine A. White, Note, Crisis of Conscience: Reconciling Religious Health Care Providers' Beliefs and Patients' Rights, 51 Stan. L. Rev. 1703, 1720–1724 (1999).

[41] See Myers, supra note 8, at 345 (noting the Oregon situation).

[42] See http://www.consciencelaws.org/Conscience-Archive/Conscience-Breaking-News-Archive/Conscience-Breaking-News-20033-02.html. See news item of June 23, 2003.

vision that was widely shared a hundred years ago is becoming more and more serious.

We are increasingly witnessing a comprehensive assault on religious freedom in health care. The protection for religious freedom under US law is, perhaps surprisingly, not comprehensive. The United States is associated with religious freedom. For example, Judge John Noonan goes so far as to describe the free exercise of religion (and here he has in mind the idea of inscribing in fundamental law an ideal of freedom of religion) "as an American invention."[43] Yet, in most of the situations described above, constitutional protections for religious freedom in the United States provide little protection in practice.

To demonstrate this point, I will provide a brief summary of the law in the United States on religious liberty, with a primary focus on the Constitution of the United States. In general, the free exercise clause of the First Amendment provides very little judicially enforceable protection against federal or state laws that mandate conduct that might be viewed as interfering with the religious liberty of an individual or an institution. If the federal or state requirement is a "neutral law of general applicability," then (under current law) there is no realistic argument that the Constitution provides any basis to resist the mandate.

The leading case here is *Employment Division v. Smith.*[44] *Smith* involved two individuals who were denied unemployment compensation because of work-related misconduct. The workers were fired from their jobs with a drug rehabilitation organization due to their use of peyote, an illegal drug, even though they used peyote for religious purposes. The United States Supreme Court, in an opinion by Justice Scalia, concluded that Oregon could "include religiously inspired peyote use within the reach of its general

---

[43] John T. Noonan, Jr., The Lustre of Our Country: The American Experience of Religious Freedom 2 (1998).

[44] 494 U. S. 872 (1990). The Smith decision was tremendously controversial. For support of the outcome in Smith, see Gerard V. Bradley, Beguiled: Free Exercise Exemptions and the Siren Song of Liberalism, 20 Hofstra L. Rev. 245 (1991); Lino A. Graglia, Church of the Lukumi Babalu Aye: Of Animal Sacrifice and Religious Persecution, 85 Geo. L. J. 1 (1996); Philip A. Hamburger, A Constitutional Right of Religious Exemption: An Historical Perspective, 60 Geo. Wash. L. Rev. 915 (1992); John Harrison, The Free Exercise Clause as a Rule about Rules, 15 Harv. J. L. & Pub. Pol'y 169 (1992); William P. Marshall, In Defense of Smith and Free Exercise Revisionism, 58 U. Chi. L. Rev. 308 (1991). For criticism, see, e.g., Douglas Laycock, The Remnants of Free Exercise, 1990 Sup. Ct. Rev. 1; Michael W. McConnell, Free Exercise Revisionism and the Smith Decision, 57 U. Chi. L. Rev. 1109 (1990); Michael W. McConnell, The Origins and Historical Understanding of Free Exercise of Religion, 103 Harv. L. Rev. 1409 (1990).

criminal prohibitions on use of that drug...."[45] To allow an exemption from laws prohibiting "socially harmful conduct"[46] would allow an individual with a religious objection to such laws '"to become a law unto himself."'[47]

Under this approach, so long as the federal or state mandate is a neutral law of general applicability, then there is no prospect of a court finding that someone with a religious objection to the mandate is exempted from the mandate. One seeking an exemption from such a mandate would be limited to seeking an exemption from the legislature. Justice Scalia noted that "leaving accommodation to the political process will place at a relative disadvantage those religious practices that are not widely engaged in; [he concluded, though]... that [that] unavoidable consequence of democratic government must be preferred to a system in which conscience is a law unto itself or in which judges weigh the social importance of all laws against the centrality of all religious beliefs."[48]

This analysis is easily applied to the contraceptive mandate issue. As noted above, some states have required that employers that provide their employees with health insurance or disability insurance coverage that includes prescription drug benefits must include prescription contraceptives in the coverage. These laws typically apply even to most employers with a religious objection to providing such coverage. As long as the contraceptive mandate is applied across the board, those employers with a religious objection to providing such coverage do not have much of a chance of resisting these mandates under the United States Constitution.

If the mandate is not viewed as a neutral law of general applicability, then the state must satisfy the "strict scrutiny" test, which means that the mandate must be narrowly tailored to meet a compelling government interest. How to decide whether a law fails this "neutral law of general applicability" requirement is an unsettled question under US law.[49] The one Supreme Court case on the issue – *Church of the Lukumi Babalu Aye, Inc. v. City of Hialeah*[50] – involved local laws that were directed at outlawing animal sacrifice as practiced by the Santeria religion. Under the local laws, one could kill an

---

[45] Id. at 874.

[46] Id. at 885.

[47] Id. (quoting *Reynolds v. United States*, 98 U. S. 145, 167 (1879)).

[48] 494 U. S. at 890.

[49] See generally Christopher C. Lund, A Matter of Constitutional Luck: The General Applicability Requirement in Free Exercise Jurisprudence, 26 Harv. J. L. & Pub. Pol'y 627 (2003). This article provides citations to the voluminous literature on this topic.

[50] 508 U. S. 520 (1993).

animal for almost any reason except for a religious one,[51] and the laws therefore, were treated and invalidated as a transparent effort to shut down a religion.[52]

Some have argued that these contraceptive mandates could similarly be regarded as transparent efforts to target particular religions (principally the Catholic Church), and that therefore employers with religious objections to these mandates ought to be entitled to an exemption.[53] There are two basic arguments here, and the arguments are so closely related that they are really just different versions of the same argument. One argument arises in situations where the contraceptive mandates contain legislative exemptions, and so arguably the laws fail the "neutral law of general applicability" requirement.[54] The other argument is a "legislative intent" argument; according to this view, these contraceptive mandates (with or without legislative exemptions) are in reality efforts to attack the Catholic Church and should be viewed as failing the "neutral law of general applicability" requirement.[55]

Both aspects of this argument were considered in the lawsuit involving California's contraceptive mandate.[56] The law requires that employers that provide their employees with health insurance that includes prescription drug benefits must include prescription contraceptives in the

---

[51] The Supreme Court stated: "[T]he ordinances are drafted with care to forbid few killings but those occasioned by religious sacrifice." 508 U. S. at 543.

[52] The Court stated: "We conclude, in sum, that each of Hialeah's ordinances pursues the city's governmental interests only against conduct motivated by religious belief. The ordinances 'have every appearance of a prohibition that society is prepared to impose upon [Santeria worshippers] but not upon itself.'" Id. at 545 (quoting *Florida Star v. B. J. F.*, 491 U. S. 525, 542 (1989) (Scalia, J., concurring in part and concurring in the judgment)). There is a great deal of debate in the literature about whether laws will fail the "general applicability" requirement only in cases that are as extreme as Lukumi. For example, Professor Gedicks interprets Smith and Lukumi narrowly. He has stated: "a religiously neutral law does not fail the test of general applicability merely by being modestly or even substantially underinclusive; rather, the law must be so dramatically underinclusive that religious conduct is virtually the only conduct to which the law applies. The Court will tolerate a tremendous amount of underinclusion before finding that a law is not generally applicable, so long as the underinclusion stops short of religious targeting." Frederick Mark Gedicks, The Normalized Free Exercise Clause: Three Abnormalities, 75 Ind. L. J. 77, 114 (2000) (footnote omitted). Others take a far broader view. See Richard F. Duncan, Free Exercise is Dead, Long Live Free Exercise: Smith, Lukumi and the General Applicability Requirement, 3 U. Pa. J. Const. L. 850 (2001).

[53] *Catholic Charities of Sacramento, Inc. v. Superior Court*, 32 Cal. 4th 527, 550–556 (Cal.)(describing and rejecting this argument), cert. denied, 125 S. Ct. 53 (2004).

[54] Catholic Charities of Sacramento, Inc., 32 Cal. 4th at 550–552.

[55] Id. at 552–556.

[56] Id. See also Catholic Charities of the Diocese of Albany, supra note 27.

coverage.[57] The law does contain an exemption for religious employers but the exemption is basically a smokescreen. In order to qualify for this exemption, an employer needs to satisfy each of the following requirements: (1) the inculcation of religious values is the purpose of the entity, (2) the entity primarily employs persons who share the religious tenets of the entity, (3) the entity serves primarily persons who share the religious tenets of the entity, and (4) the entity is a non-profit organization pursuant to the Internal Revenue Code.[58] It is quite clear that this exemption, which has been characterized as "narrow" by those supporting such mandates,[59] would cover very few – if any – Catholic organizations. It is doubtful, for example, whether many Catholic organizations that provide social services would be able to maintain that the purpose of their entity was to inculcate religious values. Many of these organizations do not employ or serve primarily persons who share the religious tenets of the entity. Think about a hospital or a parish elementary school in the inner city or a soup kitchen or a homeless shelter, none of which likely serves primarily persons who share the religious tenets of the entity. Moreover, the exemption would be very difficult to administer – is the Capuchin soup kitchen supposed to inquire whether the individuals it serves "share the religious tenets of the entity?"[60]

Catholic Charities of Sacramento filed a lawsuit challenging the constitutionality of the California law. As the suit explained, Catholic Charities is not covered by the law's religious exemption. The suit contended that the strict scrutiny test ought to apply because the law should not be treated as a "neutral law of general applicability" since the law, unlike Oregon's prohibition on peyote use involved in the *Smith* case, does contain an exemption and since the law allegedly [was] "gerrymandered" to reach only Catholic employers.[61] The California courts rejected these arguments,[62] and the United States Supreme Court refused to intervene.[63]

---

[57] Catholic Charities of Sacramento, 32 Cal. 4th at 537–538 (describing California's statute).

[58] Id.

[59] See Protecting the Rights of Conscience of Health Care Providers and a Parent's Right to Know: Hearing on H. R. 4691 Before the House Committee on Energy and Commerce, 107th Cong. (2002) (statement of Catherine Weiss, Director, ACLU Reproductive Freedom Project), available at http://energycommerce.house.gov/107/hearings/07112002Hearing632/Weiss1088print.htm.

[60] In the California litigation, the California Supreme Court explained that "Catholic Charities does not qualify as a 'religious employer' under the... [Act] because it does not meet any of the [statutory] definition's four criteria." 32 Cal. 4th at 539. Catholic Charities admitted that it didn't qualify for the exemption. Id.

[61] Id. at 550.

[62] Id.

[63] 125 S.Ct. 53 (2004).

The California court rulings are not in any way idiosyncratic. I think most courts in the United States would reach the same conclusion.[64] Most courts would agree that the contraceptive coverage mandate is a "neutral law of general applicability,"[65] and therefore would fall outside First Amendment protection altogether. Even if a court found that a mandate failed this test (because of the way it evaluated the relevance of any exemptions, for example), it might still conclude that a law passed the strict scrutiny test.[66] This is a test that sounds demanding but did not prove to be so in the religious freedom area prior to the *Smith* case in 1990. As one commentator described the situation, during this era this test was "strict in theory, but ever-so-gentle in fact . . . ."[67]

An important reason why the religious freedom claims are likely to fail is that courts in the United States tend to have a very restricted view of religious liberty, even in those situations when the Constitution provides any protection at all. Religion only receives much protection in areas such as religious belief and worship. But when religion is out in the world – running schools or hospitals or homeless shelters – the courts tend to say that it must be treated just like any other entity. Under this view, there is very little room for religious entities to be faithful to their religious identities when they venture out into the public realm; these entities must bow to the demands of the secular state.

The opinions of the California courts in the Catholic Charities case are good examples. For example, the California Supreme Court was untroubled by the statement of the law's sponsor who noted that the law's narrow exemption was intended to cover only the "religious" activities of employers. As the sponsor explained, "The more secular the activity gets, the less religiously based it is, and the more we believe that they should be required

---

[64] The recent New York case confirms this prediction. See Catholic Charities of the Diocese of New York, supra note 27. For discussion of the New York situation, see Edward T. Mechmann, Illusion of Protection?: Free Exercise Rights and Laws mandating Insurance Coverage of Contraception, 41 Cath. Law. 145 (2001).

[65] Catholic Charities of the Diocese of New York, supra note 27, slip op. at 11.

[66] Id. at 12. For additional discussion of this issue, see Inimai M. Chettiar, Comment, Contraceptive Coverage Laws: Eliminating Gender Discrimination or Infringing on Religious Liberties?, 69 U. Chi. L. Rev. 1867 (2002). See also Catholic Charities of Sacramento, 32 Cal. 4th at 564–566 (finding that the California statute survived strict scrutiny).

[67] Ira C. Lupu, The Trouble with Accommodation, 60 Geo. Wash. L. Rev. 743, 756 (1992). See Richard S. Myers, Curriculum in the Public Schools: The Need for an Emphasis on Parental Control, 24 Val. U. L. Rev. 431, 436 (1990); see also Frank, supra note 31, at 328–337 (discussing a case in which the court rejected the religious freedom arguments of a Catholic hospital that had its accreditation withdrawn because it refused to provide abortion or sterilization training for its ob/gyn residents).

to cover prescription drug benefits for contraception."[68] Although the courts typically will say that they will assume that religious individuals and institutions are sincere in claiming a religious basis for objection to a government mandate, the underlying tone of the opinion is that Catholic Charities is not really engaged in a religious practice at all. This is apparent from the testimony at a legislative hearing dealing with rights of conscience in health care. An ACLU official stated: "When, however, religiously affiliated organizations move into secular pursuits – such as providing medical care or social services to the public or running a business – they should no longer be insulated from secular laws that apply to these secular pursuits. In the public world, they should play by public rules."[69] The ACLU has issued an official report on this topic entitled "Religious Refusals and Reproductive Rights," and the choice to characterize claims of conscience with the far less appealing label of "religious refusals" was surely no accident.[70] This Report says that it supports "protecting the religious practices of insular, sectarian institutions while insisting on compliance with general rules in the public, secular world."[71] This is obviously far from any sort of broad acceptance for hospitals and individuals maintaining a strong sense of their religiously informed identities.

Although this separation between religious and secular sides of life is foreign to the self-understanding of many religious men and women, the courts commonly draw this distinction. We have seen this in areas outside the health care context. Thus, landlords have been forced to rent to unmarried couples, even when so doing violates the landlord's religious beliefs.[72] The courts that have ruled against these landlords reflect the view that this kind of "commercial" activity is not really religious, or is at any rate not entitled

---

[68] Catholic Charities of Sacramento, 32 Cal. 4th at 556. Justice Brown's dissenting opinion objected because she correctly concluded that "[t]he government is not accidentally or incidentally interfering with religious practice; it is doing so willfully by making a judgment about what is or is not religious." Id. at 578 (Brown, J., dissenting).

[69] Protecting the Rights of Conscience of Health Care Providers and a Parent's Right to Know: Hearing on H. R. 4691 Before the House Committee on Energy and Commerce, 107th Cong. (2002) (statement of Catherine Weiss, Director, ACLU Reproductive Freedom Project), available at http://energycommerce.house.gov/107/hearings/07112002Hearing632/Weiss1088print.htm.

[70] Religious Refusals and Reproductive Rights (2002), available at http://www.aclu.org/ReproductiveRights/ReproductiveRights.cfm?ID=10946&c=224.

[71] Id.

[72] See, e.g., *Smith v. Fair Employment and Housing Commission*, 913 P. 2d 909 (Cal. 1996), cert. denied, 521 U. S. 1129 (1997); *Swanner v. Anchorage Equal Rights Commission*, 874 P. 2d 274 (Alaska), cert. denied, 513 U. S. 979 (1994).

to the protection afforded to "core" religious activity.[73] The cases candidly state that if these landlords do not want to follow the prevailing secular wisdom then they can just get out of the business of being a landlord.[74] The same logic seems to be at work in the health care area – as the California contraceptive coverage mandate and the *Catholic Charities* litigation reveal. These religious institutions are being forced to abandon their distinctive missions – either "secularize" their operations or get out of the health care field altogether.

It seems clear that there is no solid basis for claiming that the United States Constitution, as currently interpreted, provides significant protection for those with a religious objection to being forced to comply with legislative mandates. There are, however, still some religious freedom arguments that can be made. In some situations, with respect to federal laws, there are certain statutory protections for religious freedom. In 1993, Congress passed The Religious Freedom Restoration Act as an effort to "overrule" the *Smith* decision.[75] In 1997, the Supreme Court invalidated RFRA as applied to state and local laws,[76] but RFRA still most likely provides a basis to argue for a religious exemption when faced with a federal mandate,[77] although such claims still may not succeed in a court of law.[78] And, with respect to state and local laws, there may be other possible bases to argue for a religious exemption. State constitutions sometimes provide broader protection for religious freedom than the federal Constitution,[79] and some

---

[73] The Swanner case is illustrative. There, the Supreme Court of Alaska stated: "Swanner has made no showing of a religious belief which requires that he engage in the property-rental business. Additionally, the economic burden, or 'Hobson's choice,' of which he complains, is caused by his choice to enter into a commercial activity that is regulated by anti-discrimination laws. Swanner is voluntarily engaging in property management. The law and ordinance regulate unlawful practices in the rental of real property and provide that those who engage in those activities shall not discriminate on the basis of marital status. Voluntary commercial activity does not receive the same status accorded to directly religious activity." Swanner, 874 P. 2d at 283 (citation omitted).

[74] Smith, 913 P. 2d at 925, 928–929.

[75] *City of Boerne v. Flores*, 521 U. S. 507, 512–516 (1997) (describing the Religious Freedom Restoration Act).

[76] *City of Boerne v. Flores*, 521 U. S. 507 (1997).

[77] See Lund, supra note 49, at 632 n. 26 (citing the cases that have so held and briefly discussing the controversy about this).

[78] See generally Ira C. Lupu, The Failure of RFRA, 20 U. Ark. Little Rock L. J. 575, 585–597 (1998). Professor Lupu's study concluded that "at least insofar as the litigation record demonstrates, RFRA resulted in surprisingly little protection for religion." Id. at 597.

[79] See Lund, supra note 49, at 632 n. 25.

states have passed state legislative counterparts to the Religious Freedom Restoration Act.[80]

The other protection for religious conscience arises on a case-by-case basis pursuant to other statutes. In certain contexts, Congress or individual states have provided protections for those with a conscientious objection to being forced to comply with legislative mandates. So, for example, in the United States there is fairly strong protection for doctors and nurses who do not wish to perform or participate in abortions.[81]

These case-by-case exemptions have very serious limitations.[82] They tend to only apply with respect to certain procedures, and the procedures covered may be interpreted narrowly (so that the morning-after pill may not be considered to cause an abortion if the pill acts prior to implantation). These exemptions only cover certain medical personnel. Sometimes the exemptions are limited to institutions and do not even potentially extend to individuals (a Catholic doctor who employs 5 or 6 people, for example). And these exemptions rarely deal with the serious issues involved in funding of health care, which, as the California situation demonstrates, is more and more becoming the focal point of the debate. With the exception of the states of Illinois and Mississippi, which have comprehensive statutes protecting the right of conscience in health care,[83] there is no comprehensive protection in the United States.

In sum, the US law on conscientious objection is not at all satisfactory. There are some bright spots in narrow areas, but there is no comprehensive protection in this area as a whole.

There is a pressing need for a more comprehensive strategy. One solution would be for a federal law to provide legal protection for those with a conscientious objection to being forced to comply with a governmental

---

[80] See Lund, supra note 49, at 632 n. 24.

[81] See Protecting the Rights of Conscience of Health Care Providers and a Parent's Right to Know: Hearing on H. R. 4691 Before the House Committee on Energy and Commerce, 107th Cong. (2002) (statement of Lynn Wardle) [hereinafter Wardle Testimony], available at http://energycommerce.house.gov/107/hearings/07112002Hearings632/Wardle1089print.htm; Katherine A. White, Note, Crisis of Conscience: Reconciling Religious Health Care Providers' Beliefs and Patients' Rights, 51 Stan. L. Rev. 1703, 1705–1711 (1999).

[82] Wardle Testimony, supra note 81.

[83] Until recently, Illinois was the only state with such protection. See Lynn D. Wardle, Protecting the Rights of Conscience of Health Care Providers, 14 J. Legal Med. 177, 179 (1993) ("Only one jurisdiction, Illinois, has enacted a comprehensive scheme of protections for the rights of conscience of health care providers."). On May 6, 2004, Mississippi's Governor signed the Mississippi Health Care Right of Conscience Act. See http://www.governorbarbour.com/ProLifeAgenda.htm.

mandate. This has been a non-starter. Even narrower conscience protections are often resisted because they allegedly interfere with the provision of mainstream medical care. In Arizona, the Governor vetoed a law that would have broadened Arizona's narrow exemption to its contraceptive mandate, a veto that was celebrated by Planned Parenthood.[84] Broadening exemptions allegedly conflicts with the obligation to provide basic medical care.

These efforts to seek protection for those with a conscientious objection to these mandates are important. In the current legal environment, such efforts to preserve the religious vision of health care by invoking the democratic process to protect religious liberty are about all that is available, given the narrow scope of the constitutional law in this area. There are, perhaps paradoxically, some risks to invoking the religious vision, at least in the way this tends to be articulated.

The argument in favor of conscience is often made in terms of the need to promote a genuine pluralism in health care – a vision that would protect Catholic or Jewish or Mormon visions of health care. I have a lot of sympathy for this view, but I have concerns about it as well. In many legal or policy discussions on these issues, a "religious" reason for acting is seen as inappropriate.[85] Such a vision is considered to be nonrational[86] or "irrational superstitious nonsense,"[87] in the words of the one of the leading constitutional scholars in the US. Certainly such a view cannot be the fit subject of public action.

There are many Supreme Court opinions that refer disparagingly to religiously informed moral judgments. Justice Stevens, for example, has expressed the view that the preamble to the Missouri abortion statute – which stated that "the life of each human being begins at conception" and that "unborn children have protectable interests in life, health, and well-being" – violated the Establishment Clause.[88] That conclusion was based on the view "that the preamble, an unequivocal endorsement of a religious

---

[84] Planned Parenthood Welcomes Governor's Veto of "Contraceptive Discrimination Bill." Press Release available at http://www.ppsaz.org/newpage25.htm.

[85] See Richard S. Myers, The United States Supreme Court and the Privatization of Religion, 6 Cath. Soc. Sci. Rev. 223, 228–230 (2001). See also Robert P. George, The Clash of Orthodoxies: Law, Religion, and Morality in Crisis (2001).

[86] See Steven G. Gey, Why is Religion Special?: Reconsidering the Accommodation of Religion Under the Religion Clauses of the First Amendment, 52 U. Pitt. L. Rev. 75 (1990). In this article, Professor Gey stated: "religion is an alternative system of nonrational and unprovable beliefs. As such, religion is fundamentally incompatible with the critical rationality on which democracy depends." Id. at 176.

[87] Suzanna Sherry, Outlaw Blues, 87 Mich. L. Rev. 1418, 1427 (1989).

[88] *Webster v. Reproductive Health Services*, 492 U. S. 490, 566 (1989) (Stevens, J, concurring in part and dissenting in part).

tenet of some but by no means all Christian faiths, serves no identifiable secular purpose."[89]

His opinion in the *Boy Scouts* case is similar. Justice Stevens referred to the Boy Scouts' views about homosexuality as "atavistic opinions... [whose] roots have been nourished by sectarian doctrine."[90] According to this opinion, it was not appropriate for the Court to permit the Boy Scouts to rely on such "prejudices;" "the light of reason" required that these prejudices be eradicated.[91]

The recent *Lawrence* opinion is to the same effect. The Court, in a majority opinion by Justice Kennedy, again referred to moral disapproval of homosexual conduct as evidencing unreflective animosity.[92] Justice Kennedy noted that the condemnation of homosexual conduct had "been shaped by religious beliefs, conceptions of right and acceptable behavior, and respect for the traditional family." "These views" were swept aside in favour of the extreme individual autonomy view expressed in *Casey*: ' "Our obligation is to define the liberty of all, not to mandate our own moral code." '[93]

This way of thinking is increasingly common, and potentially threatening to invoking "religious pluralism" in the effort to seek an exemption for conscientious objectors to health care mandates. It is risky to have issues such as abortion or contraception viewed as if they were "religious" issues.

A couple of years ago, when the DC City Council considered a law that would have required employers to pay for contraceptives in the prescription drug plans that they made available to their employees the Council refused to provide any conscience clause at all. (The law was later pocket vetoed by the Mayor.) One council member explained that his "problem [was with] surrendering decisions on public health to the [Catholic] Church [He said] I've spent years fighting church dogma."[94] Why the issue in question

---

[89] Id. at 566–567 (footnote omitted) (Stevens, J., concurring in part and dissenting in part).
[90] *Boy Scouts of America v. Dale*, 530 U. S. 640, 698 (2000) (Stevens, J., dissenting).
[91] Id. at 700 (Stevens, J., dissenting). See Richard S. Myers, The Supreme Court and the Privatization of Religion, 41 Cath. U. L. Rev. 19, 60 n. 232 (1991) (noting that Justice Stevens seems to be hostile to religion). See also Robert F. Nagel, Justice Stevens' Religion Problem, First Things, June/July 2003, at 9.
[92] Lawrence, 123 S. Ct. at 2482, 2484. See also *Goodrich v. Department of Public Health*, 798 N. E. 2d 941 (Mass. 2003).
[93] Lawrence, 123 S. Ct. at 2480 (quoting *Planned Parenthood v. Casey*, 505 U. S. 833, 850 (1992)).
[94] Report on D. C. Health Insurance Coverage for Contraceptives Act, 30 Origins 164, 165 (August 17, 2000) (quoting remarks made in the D. C. Council chambers). See also Msgr. Dennis Schnurr, Mandating Employer Coverage of Contraceptives: Protecting Conscientious Objection, 30 Origins 161 (August 17, 2000); Richard S. Myers, On the Need for a Federal Conscience Clause, 1 Nat'l Cath. Bioethics Q. 23, 23 (2001).

involved a matter of religious "dogma" – which a popular dictionary revealingly defines as "a point of view or tenet put forth as authoritative without adequate grounds"[95] – was never explained.

The same idea influenced the *Catholic Charities* case. There, the California court did not think that the contraceptive mandate impermissibly inhibited religion. The California Supreme Court was not even sure that Catholic Charities' religious beliefs were implicated at all. Catholic Charities had explained that paying its workers a just wage included, as a matter of justice and charity, coverage for prescription drugs. The Court couldn't seem to comprehend how "justice and charity" could be considered "religious."[96] In any event, these beliefs were entitled to little weight because Catholic Charities had entered "the general labor market."[97] We see here a very disturbing approach on the part of the court – simultaneously concluding that Catholic Charities is not really engaged in something "religious" when it provides social services, while also claiming that Catholic Charities' "religious" views on contraception are entitled to little weight.

These views are quite commonplace, and that is why I am concerned when people who are sympathetic to the rights of conscience describe issues such as abortion, euthanasia, human cloning, and stem cell research as "profoundly religious issues."[98] I understand why the religious vision of health care is invoked, but there are real risks because such views may be considered idiosyncratic, nonrational, irrational, not publicly accessible or what have you. (I want to make it clear that I don't accept any of these characterizations.[99]) On the disputed issues in play, we are not talking about "theological" issues at all, such as the nature of the Trinity or the Eucharist. We are talking about moral questions, and for many Catholics and others that means drawing on a rich tradition of natural law. But to the extent religious people persist in describing their moral vision of health care as "religious" they risk having this vision privatized and marginalized. It will only be protected when it doesn't matter very much. The moral vision won't be permitted to influence public business. Religion may be protected if practised in one's home or in a house of worship, but that will be it.

While the appeal to religious pluralism taps into the attractiveness many find in the "republic of choice," it risks being marginalized in the face of

---

[95] See Merriam-Webster Online Dictionary. See http://www.m-w.com.

[96] Catholic Charities of Sacramento, 32 Cal. 4th at 563.

[97] Id. at 565.

[98] Edmund D. Pellegrino, The Physician's Conscience, Conscience Clauses, and Religious Belief: A Catholic Perspective, 30 Fordham Urb. L. J. 221, 224 (2002).

[99] See, e.g., Myers, supra note 85; Myers, supra note 15.

the onslaught of the secular vision of health care, which is becoming increasingly aggressive in mandating its vision of the world. As a matter of first principle, then, an appeal to choice and in particular to religious choice has grave risks. The most desirable strategy is to promote a vision of health care that furthers a public morality with the substantive vision that promotes the truth about the dignity of the human person. On matters about which we are confident (that it is wrong to sexually abuse minors, for example), we are perfectly willing to limit choice. We should also be willing to do so on life and death issues in health care, where neutrality is really not possible. On these matters, it is imperative that we work to restore norms such as that it is wrong to intentionally take the life of an innocent human person. This is necessary, I believe, even though many hold this "moral" position because of the influence of deep theological commitments. Such moral positions, though, are fit subjects of public action, and in some areas – the prohibition against taking the life of an innocent human person – should be backed by law.

An appeal to religious choice has serious risks. The task ought to be to build up a public morality on these issues, so as to eliminate the clash between legislative mandates and the moral teachings of the Catholic Church; unfortunately, claiming a "religious" basis for acting may jeopardize this broader cultural effort. Building up the culture on these issues will also make the claim for conscientious objection, when that proves necessary to pursue, more likely to succeed, because we see in this area that claims for conscience are more likely to succeed the more support for the underlying moral position there is in the broader society. So, conscience claims in the area of abortion are more successful than those in the area of contraception, where the Catholic Church's position on the issue is held by so few and is not even comprehensible to most people.

But we are not just considering this from a position of first principle. We also ought to take account of current cultural realities. The moral vision of health care that would have been held in common by most religions in the United States a hundred years ago doesn't exist on a widespread basis any longer. We need to work to advance our moral vision, and it is altogether fitting and proper that we do so.[100] But in the interim, we also need to pursue a second-best approach. The individuals and groups who dissent from the public orthodoxy in areas such as abortion need to have the ability to preserve their distinctive witness. This requires protection for conscience –

---

[100] Cf. Abraham Lincoln, Address Delivered at the Dedication of the Cemetery at Gettysburg, reprinted in 7 Collected Works of Abraham Lincoln 23 (Roy P. Basler ed. 1953).

not as the best or most desirable strategy but because in face of the increasing demands of the secular vision of health care that is all that we are going to be permitted in the foreseeable future.

The choice is to pursue this second-best strategy of conscience – or go out of the vocation of health care altogether. The choice is really that stark.

Contributors

Bishop Donal Murray is Bishop of Limerick and Chairman of the Irish Bishops' Committee for Bioethics

Bishop Anthony Fisher is Auxiliary Bishop of Sydney and Episcopal Vicar for Life and Health

Jane Adolphe is Associate Professor of Law, Ave Maria School of Law

Mike Delany is a General Practitioner

John Finnis is Professor of Law and Legal Philosophy, University of Oxford, Biolchini Professor of Law, University of Notre Dame, and Vice-Chairman of the Linacre Centre

Luke Gormally is Senior Research Fellow and former Director of the Linacre Centre, and Research Professor, Ave Maria School of Law

Colin Harte is a doctoral student at Exeter University, and General Secretary of the charity Enable (Working in India)

Cathleen Kaveny is John P. Murphy Foundation Professor of Law and Professor of Theology, University of Notre Dame

Richard Myers is Professor of Law, Ave Maria School of Law

Charlie O'Donnell is a Consultant in Emergency and Intensive Care Medicine

Alexander Pruss is Assistant Professor in the Department of Philosophy, Georgetown University

Neil Scolding is Burden Professor of Clinical Neurosciences at the Institute of Clinical Neurosciences, Bristol, and Chairman of the Linacre Centre

Helen Watt is Director of the Linacre Centre

Index of names